I0072188

Advanced Dermatology for Clinicians

Advanced Dermatology for Clinicians

Edited by Heidi Mueller

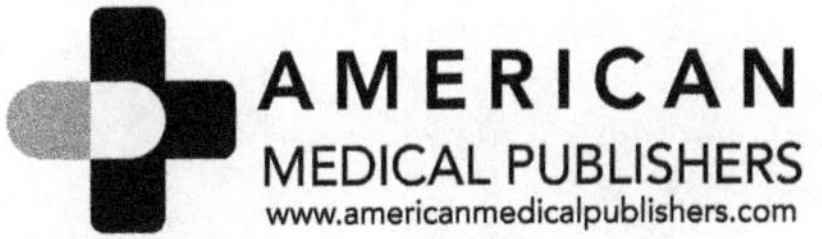

American Medical Publishers,
41 Flatbush Avenue,
1st Floor, New York,
NY 11217, USA

Visit us on the World Wide Web at:
www.americanmedicalpublishers.com

ISBN: 978-1-63927-063-7

Cataloging-in-Publication Data

Advanced dermatology for clinicians / edited by Heidi Mueller.
p. cm.
Includes bibliographical references and index.
ISBN 978-1-63927-063-7
1. Dermatology. 2. Skin--Diseases. 3. Skin--Diseases--Diagnosis. 4. Skin--Diseases--Treatment.
5. Dermatologists--Guidebooks. I. Mueller, Heidi.

RL72 .D473 2022
616.5--dc23

Table of Contents

Preface

The purpose of the book is to provide a glimpse into the dynamics and to present opinions and studies of some of the scientists engaged in the development of new ideas in the field from very different standpoints. This book will prove useful to students and researchers owing to its high content quality.

A branch of medicine which deals with the diseases of nails, hair and skin is known as dermatology. It involves the use of medications as well as surgeries. A few of the major fields of dermatology are dermatopathology, trichology and pediatric dermatology. Dermatopathology is primarily concerned with the pathology of the skin. Trichology focuses on the diseases of the hair such as hair abnormalities, scalp changes, hypertrichosis, etc. Pediatric dermatology includes the complicated diseases of infants such as hereditary skin diseases and various other problems of the neonates. Dermatology also includes various therapies such as excision and treatment of skin cancer, radiation therapy, phototherapy and laser therapy and allergy testing. This book contains some path-breaking studies in the field of dermatology. It traces the progress of this field and highlights some of its key concepts and applications. The book will provide comprehensive knowledge to the readers.

At the end, I would like to appreciate all the efforts made by the authors in completing their chapters professionally. I express my deepest gratitude to all of them for contributing to this book by sharing their valuable works. A special thanks to my family and friends for their constant support in this journey.

Editor

1

Specific Sensitization Age Dynamic in Patients with Atopic Dermatitis

N.G. Ilina[*,1], Yu M. Krinitsyna[1,2], M. Yu. Denisov[1] and I.G. Sergeeva [1,3]

[1]*Novosibirsk State University (NSU) 630090 Pirogova Street 2, Novosibirsk, Russia*

[2]*Institute of Regional Pathology and Pathomorphology 630117 Ak.Timakova street 2, Novosibirsk, Russia*

[3]*Institute International Tomography Center of the Russian Academy of Sciences, laboratory of translational brain research 630090 Institutskaia Street 3, Novosibirsk, Russia*

Abstract: *Background*: Specific sensitization characterizes increased serum level of IgE to different groups of allergens (food, dust, domestic and contact). Characteristic of specific sensitization changes with age of patient. Spectrum of specific sensitization determined environmental factors, conditions of habitation.

Objective: objective was to research characteristic of specific sensitization in patients with atopic dermatitis.

Methods: There were 108 patients with atopic dermatitis, 1st group – 31 patient (17 boys and 14 girls) 0-3y.o., 2nd group – 30 (13 boys and 17 girls) 4-13 y.o., 3rd group – 47 (16 men and 31 women) 16-63 y.o. In control group, there were 25 patients (4 men, 21 women) 16-64 y.o. with another dermatological diseases such as psoriasis, acne, rosacea and etc., without atopic dermatitis. In patients of all 4 groups evaluated personal, family allergic anamnesis, drug and food allergy, sensitization by measuring common and specific levels of immunoglobulin E.

Results: 10%, 32%, 27% patients of 1st, 2nd, 3rd groups had food allergy. The main allergens were citruses (37% cases), chocolate (27%) and milk (17%).

Conclusion: 44-52% patients with atopic dermatitis and 4% patients without atopy had non-specific sensitization, that characterized five-fold increased serum level of IgE and more.

50-60% patients with atopic dermatitis had specific sensitization. 60% infants at the age under 3 y.o. with atopic dermatitis had sensitization for epithelium of homepets, 50% - for milk, 30% - white-egg. Among adults with atopic dermatitis sensitization was the same, as in control group. 35% patients with dermatoses without atopy had specific sensitization.

Keywords: Atopic dermatitis, food allergy, immunoglobulin E, sensitization.

INTRODUCTION

There are currently two major pathogenetic forms of atopic dermatitis: truly allergic or allergic and atopiform or non-allergic. The allergic (extrinsic) form is associated with hypersensitivity to food and/or other allergens as well as increased levels of IgE in patients and is observed in 70–80% of patients. The non-allergic (intrinsic) form is characterised by normal levels of IgE and is observed in 20–30% of patients [1,2].

Specific hypersensitivity is characterised by increased levels of immunoglobulin E to various allergen groups (food, dust, household, and contact) [3]. Changes in the nature of food, dust, and household hypersensitivity are observed with age. The range of specific hypersensitivity is associated with environmental factors, living conditions, and everyday life. Thus, it has been shown that visiting a swimming pool with chlorinated water before the age of 3 increases the risk of specific hypersensitivity to house dust mites [4].

With the introduction of laboratory methods such as the measurement of the level of total immunoglobulin E and levels of specific immunoglobulin E in practice, the progression of the disease may be assessed, and case management tactics may be determined [5-7].

The purpose of the study was to determine the nature of specific hypersensitivity in patients with atopic dermatitis in relation to ageing.

MATERIALS AND METHODS

We observed 108 patients with atopic dermatitis aged 0 to 63 years. Depending on the age, the patients were divided into the following groups: Group 1 - 31 persons (17 boys, 14 girls) aged 0 to 3, Group 2 – 30 patients (13 boys and 17 girls) aged 4 to 13, and Group 3 – 47 patients (16 men and 31 women) aged 16 to 63. In all cases, the diagnosis of atopic dermatitis was made by a dermatologist; at the time of referral, all patients had clinical manifestations that met atopic dermatitis criteria. All patients were treated on an outpatient basis, depending on the nature and severity of the disease. To form a control group by the random sampling method, 25 patients with other skin diseases (acne, rosacea,

*Address correspondence to this author at the Novosibirsk State University (NSU) 630090 Pirogova Street 2, Novosibirsk, Russia;
E-mail: dr.natalia.ilina@gmail.com

psoriasis, contact dermatitis, allergic contact dermatitis), without having been diagnosed with atopic dermatitis at the time of examination or in the medical history, (4 men and 21 women) aged 16 to 64 were selected.

All patients were assessed for personal and family allergic history and for clinical manifestations of allergy to different groups of allergens (food, drugs, dust, and contact).

The prevalence of hypersensitivity was evaluated by the level of total immunoglobulin IgE according to age-based normal ranges.

To determine the nature of specific hypersensitivity, the standardised kit was used for immunoblot RIDA® Allergy Screen A2442 Panel No. 4 (paediatric), comprising 20 major allergens: food – cow's milk allergens (α-lactalbumin, β-lactalbumin, casein, and bovine serum albumin), and allergens of egg whites and yolks, soy, carrots, potatoes, wheat flour, hazelnuts, and peanuts; house dust mites – Dermatophagoides pteronyssinus and Dermatophagoides farinae; household allergens – cat and dog hair; fungal allergens – Alternaria alternata; and pollen allergens – birch and various grasses. Increased specific immunoglobulin IgE at a level above the threshold – i.e. over 0.35 IU/ml – was considered a criterion of positive specific hypersensitivity.

Statistical data were processed using the Student's t-test for qualitative parameters.

All patients gave signed informed consent for data examination and processing.

RESULTS

Based on the personal allergic history of patients with atopic dermatitis, an increasing incidence of bronchial asthma with age from 3.3% in infants to 10.6% in older patients and of allergic rhinitis from 3.2% in children to 14.9% in adults was observed (Table **1**). There were no cases of bronchial asthma or allergic rhinitis in the control group patients.

The family history of allergenic diseases was considered burdened if the patient stated cases of bronchial asthma, allergic rhinitis, Quincke's oedema, urticaria, or allergic reactions to foods and drugs in relatives of first and second lines of kinship. The family history of allergenic diseases was burdened in 43.3%, 38.7%, 36.2%, and 20.0% (p<0.05) of cases of patients from Groups 1, 2, 3, and 4 (Table **1**).

Among all cases of food allergies, the most common causes were citrus in 36.7% of cases, chocolate in 26.7%, and milk in 16.7%. According to parents, the group 1 patients were allergic to milk formula, vegetable solid foods, citrus fruits, and carrots; and group 2 patients to milk formula and in a few cases to tomatoes, kiwi, and fish. In individual cases, group 3 patients mentioned reactions to milk, grapes, strawberries, sea buckthorn, peaches, kiwi, cherries, watermelon, tomatoes, food additives, and honey. The control group patients had allergic reactions to Coca-Cola and chicken eggs.

Group 3 patients often indicated drug hypersensitivity compared with patients from groups 1 and 2 (p<0.005) (Table **1**). Among all allergic reactions to drugs, 20% of patients reported hypersensitivity to penicillin drugs. Moreover, group 1 patients had reactions when using drugs containing nifuroxazide, bacteriophage, and ibuprofen; and group 3 patients when using drugs containing azithromycin, fluoroquinolones, hexetidine, glycine, nicotinic acid, and phytopreparations. The control group patients had allergies to gentamicin and diphenhydramine.

The allergic history data obtained for patients are subjective, as reported by the patients or their parents. For an objective assessment of the allergic status of a patient, the levels of total and specific immunoglobulin E were utilised.

Increased total immunoglobulin in patients with atopic dermatitis was observed in 55.5%, 64.3%, and 52.4% of cases in groups 1, 2, and 3 significantly more often than in the control group of patients – 17.3% (p<0.01).

Total immunoglobulin IgE in patients with atopic dermatitis was consistent with normal age ranges in about half of the cases in patients of group 1 and about a third of the cases in patients of the groups 2 and 3. In the control group, 82.7% of patients had total immunoglobulin consistent with normal ranges (Table **2**). In half of the cases in patients with atopic dermatitis, 5 times or higher IgE

Table 1. Clinical parameters of the allergic status in observed patients %.

	Group 1 n=31	**Group 2 n=30**	**Group 3 n=47**	**Group 4 n=25**
Personal history of allergies				
Bronchial asthma	3.3	6.5	10.6	-
Allergic rhinitis	-	3.2	14.9	-
Quincke's oedema	-	3.2	6.4	4.0
Urticaria	-	-	4.3	8.0
Food allergy	10.0	32.3	27.7	16.0
Drug hypersensitivity	6.6	3.2	25.5	20.0
Family history of allergies				
Atopic dermatitis in family members	26.7	19.4	14.9	-
Other allergenic diseases in family members	36.7	22.6	25.5	20.0

levels were observed in 44.4%, 50.0%, and 52.4%, which was significantly higher than in the control group – 4.3% ($p<0.01$). A moderate increase in total immunoglobulin up to 5 times was observed in isolated cases – 11.1%, 14.3%, 9.5%, and 13.0% of patients of Groups 1, 2, 3, and 4.

Increased levels of IgE antibodies were observed in 60.0%, 57.1%, 50.0%, and 35.3% of patients of Groups 1, 2, and 3 as well as the control group. Only 4.5% of the patients with atopic dermatitis, who had a significant increase in total immunoglobulin (429 IU/ml), demonstrated no increase in specific immunoglobulins.

In patients of group 1, most significant were an increase

Table 2. Nature of the increase of total immunoglobulin IgE in observed patients,%

Group	Normal Range	Increase up to 5 Times	Increase up to 5 Times and Higher
Group 1 n=31	44.4	11.1	44.4
Group 2 n=30	35.7	14.3	50.0
Group 3 n=47	38.1	9.5	52.4
Group 4 n=25	82.7*	13.0	4.3*

Table 3. Detection rate of specific hypersensitivity in observed patients,%

Allergen	Group 1 n=31	Group 2 n=30	Group 3 n=47	Group 4 n=25
Aeroallergens				
House dust mites	-	7.1	16.6	23.6
Birch – pollen	10.0	7.1	5.6	5.9
Various grasses – pollen	-	-	11.1	11.8
Fungus Alternaria alternata	-	7.1	11.1	11.8
Household allergens				
Epithelium and animal hair (cat, dog)	60.0	14.2	27.8	5.9
Food allergens				
Milk and dairy products				
Milk	50.0	35.7	11.1	11.8
A-lactoglobulin	10.0	35.7	11.1	5.9
B-lactoglobulin	30.0	7.1	-	-
Casein	30.0	28.6	16.7	11.8
Egg white	30.0	-	5.6	11.8
Egg yolk	-	-	-	5.9
Bovine serum albumin	10.0	-	-	-
Vegetables				
Carrots	20.0	-	-	5.9
Potatoes	10.0	-	-	5.9
Soybeans	-	-	-	-
Nuts and cereals				
Wheat flour	20.0	7.1	5.6	11.8
Hazelnuts	20.0	-	-	11.8
Peanuts	10.0	-	-	-

of levels to epithelium and animal hair – 60.0%, to milk – 50.0%, and to lactoglobulin, casein, and egg whites – 30.0%. In patients of group 2, 37.5% had elevated levels of E-class antibodies, specific for alpha-lactoglobulin and milk, and 28.6% of the cases for casein. In the patients of group 3, 27.8% of the cases manifested higher frequency of detected immunoglobulin E to hair and dog epithelium, and 16.7% of the cases to casein. In patients in Group 3, 11.1% of the cases showed specific hypersensitivity to milk, which is consistent with this parameter in the control group. Hypersensitivity to the remaining dust and food allergens in older patients was observed in isolated cases. In patients of the control group, elevated specific immunoglobulins were observed in a few cases; no predominant allergens were identified (Table **3**).

In group 3, the frequency of specific hypersensitivity to foods did not differ from those obtained in the control group.

DISCUSSION

The prevalence of food allergies in patients with atopic dermatitis is from 35% to 90% according to the data of various authors, in patients with a children's form – 8.3% [8-10]. According to our data, 10.0%, 32.3%, and 27.7% of infants, children, and older patients had a food allergy.

It is important to bear in mind that, in all patients with atopic dermatitis with symptoms of food allergy, only 30-40% have specific hypersensitivity verified by enzyme immunoassay or food provocation in a double-blind, placebo-controlled study [11]. Food allergens indicated by patients are subjective. In most cases, the enzyme immunoassay revealed no specific hypersensitivity to the allergens indicated by the patients. Moreover, the allergens identified by the laboratory method point to existing hidden hypersensitivity.

The most common cause of food allergies in patients with atopic dermatitis is milk and dairy products. Cow's milk is the most allergenic food. Higher milk fat and increased protein content enhance its allergenic properties.

According to various sources, the frequency of hypersensitivity is from 8.4% to 41.2% [12,13]. In infants and children with atopic dermatitis, hypersensitivity to milk was observed in 50.0% and 35.7% of the cases. Unchanged hypersensitivity to milk in adults was observed in 11.1%, but these results were comparable in frequency with the control group patients – 11.8%. Based on the results of other studies, hypersensitivity to cow's milk proteins and casein in infants with severe atopic dermatitis is up to 92.3% [10].

However, protein fractions have the most allergenic properties. Cow's milk contains from 2.8 to 4.1 g of protein per 100 ml. Beta-lactoglobulin of cow's milk is considered the most allergenic, especially for children, as it is absent in human milk [14]. The incidence of allergic reactions to beta-lactoglobulin is 60–70%. Based on our data, hypersensitivity to beta-lactoglobulin was observed in 30.0% of infants, less frequently than in children – 7.1%. In paediatric patients, hypersensitivity to alpha-lactoglobulin was observed more frequently – 35.7%.

Based on the results of our study, 60.0% of infants with atopic dermatitis had hypersensitivity to epithelium and cat and dog hair. The need for maintenance of hypoallergenic living conditions has been discussed. Thus, the impact of prenatal exposure of the mother to farm animals significantly reduces the risk of atopic dermatitis in children by half [15]. According to EU guidelines, the exposure to aeroallergens should be minimal [16]. Hypersensitivity to epithelium and animal hair in the control group was lower (5.9%) compared with older patients with atopic dermatitis (27.8%) ($p<0.01$).

Hypersensitivity to egg and aeroallergens detected at an early age in children with atopic dermatitis is a compelling risk factor for bronchial asthma. In case of an allergy to egg protein, both intolerance to chicken meat and increased sensitivity to pillow feathers are sometimes identified. According to studies, the frequency of hypersensitivity to eggs is 32% [13]. Vetellin protein contained in egg yolk is characterised by less pronounced allergenic properties. Sometimes there is selective protein or egg yolk intolerance. According to our data, 30.0% of infants had hypersensitivity to chicken protein. Hypersensitivity to egg yolks was not identified in any cases in patients with atopic dermatitis, and only in 5.9% of control group patients.

Hypersensitivity to aeroallergens is more typical for patients with adolescent and adult forms of atopic dermatitis 16. According to the literature, the most common aeroallergen in patients with atopic dermatitis aged 3 to 6 is house the dust mite *Derm. farinae* [17]. According to the obtained data, hypersensitivity to house dust mites was observed more frequently in patients with children's and adult forms - 7.10% and 16.6%, respectively; hypersensitivity to birch pollen was observed in 10.0%, 7.1%, and 5.6% of cases in patients of all three groups.

Among foods, the significant allergens were carrots, potatoes, wheat, and certain products introduced as supplementary food for infants.

30.0% of infants with atopic dermatitis demonstrated hypersensitivity to nuts – hazelnuts and peanuts. Nuts are not a staple product among children or an introduced supplementary product; however, nuts may be added to foods as flavourings or additives.

The distribution of allergic and non-allergic forms of atopic dermatitis by total immunoglobulin was consistent with the data obtained in other studies 1. In 44.4%, 35.73%, and 38.1% of the cases, total immunoglobulin was within the normal age-based range, which was consistent with the non-allergic form of atopic dermatitis. A pronounced increase in the level of total immunoglobulin (5 times or higher) was observed in 44.4%, 50.0%, and 52.4% of patients with atopic dermatitis, significantly less than in control group patients.

Thus, specific hypersensitivity in atopic dermatitis varies with age and in patients older than 16 did not differ from hypersensitivity in patients with non-allergic dermatoses.

CONFLICT OF INTEREST

The authors confirm that this article content has no conflict of interest.

ACKNOWLEDGEMENTS

This work was financially supported by the Russian Science Foundation (project # 14-35-00020).

REFERENCES

[1] Suárez-Fariñas M, Dhingra N, Gittler J, *et al.* Intrinsic atopic dermatitis shows similar TH2 and higher TH17 immune activation compared with extrinsic atopic dermatitis. J Allergy Clin Immunol 2013; 132(2): 361-70.

[2] Liu FT, Goodarzi H, Chen HY. IgE, mast cells, and eosinophils in atopic dermatitis. Clin Rev Allergy Immunol 2011; 41(3): 298-310.

[3] Zheng T, Yu J, Oh MH, Zhu Z. The atopic march: progression from atopic dermatitis to allergic rhinitis and asthma (review). Allergy Asthma Immunol Res 2011; 3(2): 67-73.

[4] Voisin C, Sardella A, Bernard A. Risks of new-onset allergic sensitization and airway inflammation after early age swimming in chlorinated pools. Int J Hyg Environ Health 2014; 217(1): 38-45.

[5] Manam S, Tsakok T, Till S, Flohr C. The association between atopic dermatitis and food allergy in adults. Curr Opin Allergy Clin Immunol 2014; 14(5): 423-9.

[6] Gray CL, Levin ME, Zar HJ, *et al.* Food allergy in South African children with atopic dermatitis. Pediatr Allergy Immunol 2015 [Epub ahead of print].

[7] Just J, Deslandes-Boutmy E, Amat F, *et al.* Natural history of allergic sensitization in infants with early-onset atopic dermatitis: results from ORCA Study. Pediatr Allergy Immunol (E-pub at 2014 Oct 6).

[8] Lee CH, Kim HO, Cho SI, *et al.* Food Hy-persensitivity in patients with childhood atopic dermatitis in Korea. Ann Dermatol 2013; 25(2): 196-202.

[9] Kwon J, Kim J, Cho S, Noh G, Lee SS. Characterization of food allergies in patients with atopic dermatitis. Nutr Res Pract 2013; 7(2): 115-21.

[10] Sicherer SH, Sampson HA. Food allergy: epidemiology, pathogenesis, diag-nosis, and treatment. J Allergy Clin Immunol 2014; 133(2): 291-307.

[11] Campbell DE. Role of food allergy in childhood atopic dermatitis. J Paediatr Child Health 2012; 48: 1058-64.

[12] Bergmann MM, Caubet JC, Boguniewicz M, Eigenmann PA. Evaluation of food allergy in patients with atopic dermatitis. J Allergy Clin Immunol Pract 2013; 1(1): 22-28.

[13] Forsey RG. Prevalence of childhood eczema and food sensitization in the First Nations reserve of Natuashish, Labrador, Canada. BMC Pediatr 2014; 14: 76.

[14] Duan CC, Li AL, Yang LJ, Zhao R, Fan WG, Huo GC. Comparison of immunomodulating properties of Beta-lactoglobulin and its hydrolysates. Iran J Allergy Asthma Immunol 2014; 13(1): 26-32.

[15] Roduit C, Wohlgensinger J, Frei R. Prenatal animal contact and gene expres-sion of innate immunity receptors at birth are associated with atopic dermatitis. J Allergy Clin Immunol 2011; 127(1): 179-85.

[16] Schneider L, Tilles S. Atopic dermatitis: a practice parameter update 2012. J Allergy Clin Immunol 2013: 295-9.

[17] Kim EJ, Kwon JW, Lim YM, *et al.* As-sessment of total/specific IgE levels against 7 inhalant allergens in children aged 3 to 6 years in Seoul, Korea. Allergy Asthma Immunol Res 2013; 5(3): 162-9.

2

Evaluation of Arteriosclerosis Using the Brachial-Ankle Pulse Wave Velocity in Patients with Visceral Lesion-Free Systemic Lupus Erythematosus Characterized by Skin Lesions

Kimiko Maruyama, Takaharu Ikeda, Katsunori Tanaka and Fukumi Furukawa*

Department of Dermatology, Faculty of Medicine, Wakayama Medical University, Japan

Abstract: Recently, the cardio-/cerebrovascular lesion-related mortality rate has been high in patients with systemic lupus erythematosus (SLE). In these patients, the risk of cardio-/cerebrovascular lesions is also higher than in the general population. Cardio-/cerebrovascular lesions may occur during long-term follow-up. In this study, we evaluated arteriosclerosis using the brachial-ankle pulse wave velocity (baPWV) in visceral lesion-free SLE patients with skin lesions. In these patients, baPWV was higher than in healthy adults even at a young age. This suggests that baPWV is a possible tool to evaluate the patient's vascular function, which was difficult to evaluate using a conventional sera arteriosclerosis index. Even when conditions are characterized by skin lesions, it may be important to consider the influence on the cardio-/cerebrovascular systems, as indicated for patients with systemic symptoms.

Keywords: Arteriosclerosis, brachial-ankle pulse wave velocity, cutaneous lupus erythematosus, systemic lupus erythematosus.

INTRODUCTION

Previously, the frequent causes of death in patients with systemic lupus erythematosus (SLE) included nephropathy, central nervous system (CNS) lupus, and infectious diseases [1-3]. However, advances in clinical examination methods have facilitated the early diagnosis of SLE, and early treatments with corticosteroids or immunosuppressive drugs were established. Based on the background, there have recently been marked changes in the causes of death. According to the report of Bernatsky *et al.*, angiopathy accounts for approximately 25% of the mortality [4]. It results from arteriosclerosis in many cases. Manzi *et al.* reported that atherosclerosis progressed from a young age in patients with SLE, and that atherosclerotic plaques were detected in 40% of patients. They indicated that the relative risk of atherosclerosis was 5 times higher in SLE patients, and that it was 50 times higher in those aged under 45 years [5]. Therefore, the assessment and treatment of arteriosclerosis are particularly important in SLE patients involving a high proportion of young patients.

To evaluate arteriosclerosis, a blood test is basically performed. As indices of arteriosclerosis, the (total cholesterol (T-Cho)-HDL)/HDL and LDL/HDL ratios are used. The blood test is simple. However, a study indicated that there was no correlation between the incidence of myocardial infarction in SLE patients and risk factors previously reported; evaluation based on the results of a blood test alone is incomplete [6]. In addition, there are some patients primarily complaining of skin lesions among those with SLE, as a systemic disease. It should be examined whether or not arteriosclerosis is present in these patients.

Other evaluation methods include imaging procedures, represented by carotid ultrasonography [6] and electron-beam computed tomography (CT) [7], and measurement of the pulse wave velocity (PWV) [8]). Imaging procedures depend on examiners' skills and require a specific time. The results are influenced by the presence or absence of instruments. We used the brachial-ankle pulse wave velocity (baPWV) as a noninvasive examination procedure for a large number of patients in order to make an early diagnosis in clinical practice.

SUBJECTS AND METHODS

The subjects were 138 patients who had been treated in our department and from whom informed consent was verbally obtained. As a routine screening test, baPWV was measured once a year. They consisted of 29 patients with SLE meeting the new Systemic Lupus International Collaborating Clinics (SLICC) classification criteria 2012 (mean age: 47.8±12.0 years, 3 males, 26 females), 27 with systemic sclerosis (SSc) (mean age: 67.64±12.8 years, 3 males, 24 females), and 85 with other dermal diseases (eczema and dermatitis) (19 males, 66 females). Initially, a cuff for the limbs, an electrocardiographic clip for the wrist, and a heart sound sensor were attached to subjects. Subject information (age, sex, and body weight) necessary for measurement were input. After 5 minutes rest, baPWV is determined by simultaneously measuring the blood pressure and pulse wave in the limbs. In the subjects, excluding one case, facial erythema, discoid-shaped erythema, and photosensitivity were primarily observed at the time of

*Address correspondence to this author at the Department of Dermatology, Wakayama Medical University, Postal Code: 641-0012, 811-1, Kimiidera, Wakayama City, Wakayama Prefecture, Japan;
E-mail: dajs@wakayama-med.ac.jp

diagnosis. Although articular symptoms were noted in 50% of the subjects, no patient showed any cardiovascular/central nervous symptoms or kidney dysfunction, which was same in 85 with other dermal diseases (eczema and dermatitis). Follow-up periods ranged from 1 to 7 years.

The baPWV was measured using a blood pressure-/pulse wave-testing device (OMRON COLIN Co., Ltd, Japan). This parameter increases with age. The values obtained by the single regression analysis were compared with the mean baPWV in each age group, and dissociation was evaluated based on the standard deviation; individual baPWV values, which differed among age/sex groups, were corrected with the rate of change, facilitating assessment from the same perspective [9].

To measure conventional indices of arteriosclerosis, the (T-Cho - HDL)/HDL and LDL/HDL ratios, a blood test was simultaneously conducted at the baPWV measurement point in 13 subjects. Verbal informed consent was obtained. These parameters were calculated. Statistical analysis was performed by unpaired t-test.

Concerning the correlation with corticosteroid therapy, the steroid dose over a 5-year period was reviewed. The initial dose during this period was added to the last dose, multiplied by 5 (years), and divided by 2. The value was regarded as a coefficient (example: initial maintenance dose, 10 mg; after 5 years, 5 mg; and after 10 years, 3 mg: (10+5) 5/2 + (5+3) 5/2 = 57.5). When the initial dosing involved steroid pulse therapy, initial maintenance therapy was selected as the initial value.

After preliminary presentation of this study to our Ethics Committee, it was decided that ethical approval was not required because the method employed was standard. This study was performed in compliance with the ethical principles of the Declaration of Helsinki based on 2000 version.

RESULTS

The baPWV values in 29 patients with SLE characterized by skin lesions and those predicted by regression analysis are presented in Fig. (**1**). A comparison of the estimated baPWV values in SSc patients, which were calculated by regression analysis, with the mean in each age group is shown in Fig. (**2**). In the SLE patients, baPWV was high even at a young age. Among 29 patients, the standard deviation (SD) exceeded 2 in 13 patients and it exceeded one in 4 patients, respectively. In young SSc patients (30 to 39 years), there was no marked difference in comparison with the mean of healthy adults. However, the difference increased with age, and the standard deviation exceeded 2SD in more than 50% of the patients aged over 60 years.

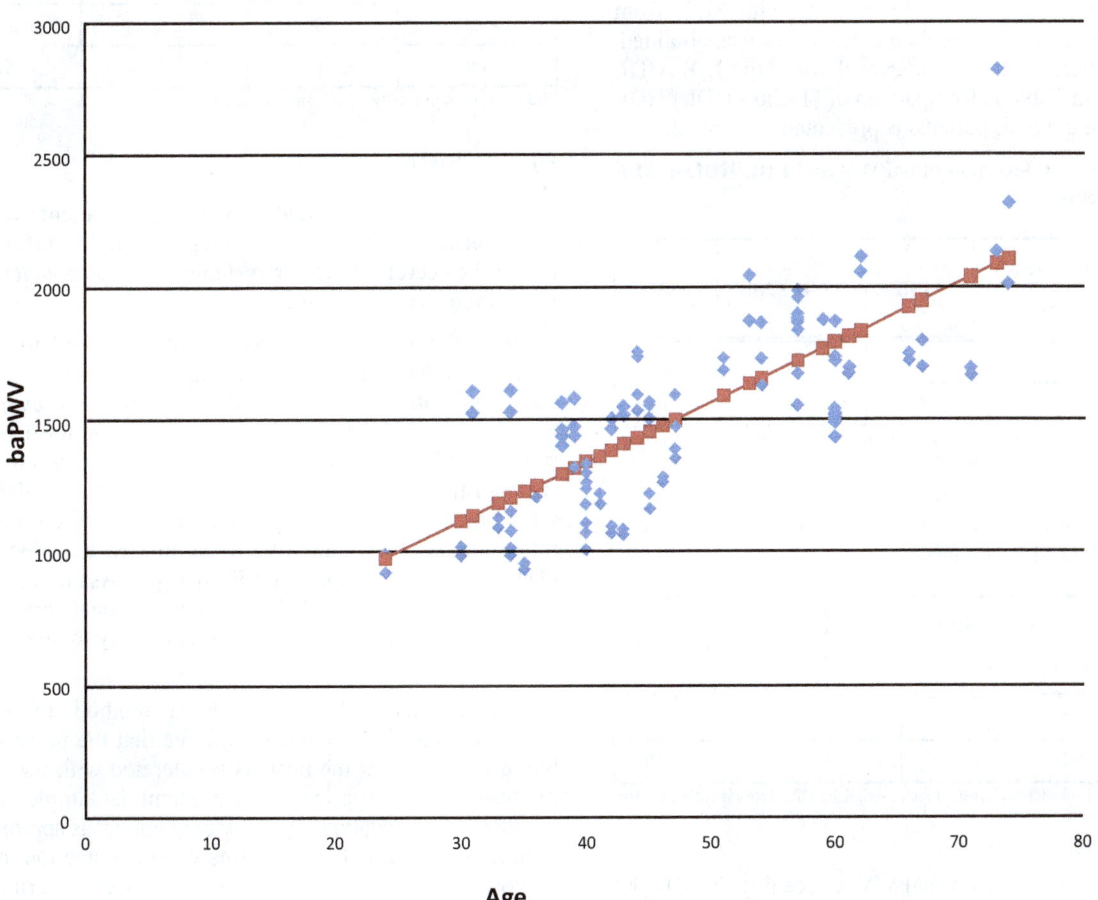

Fig. (1). Patient age and changes in baPWV. The predicted values, obtained by plotting the baPWV values in SLE patients and age on measurement and conducting regression analysis, are presented.

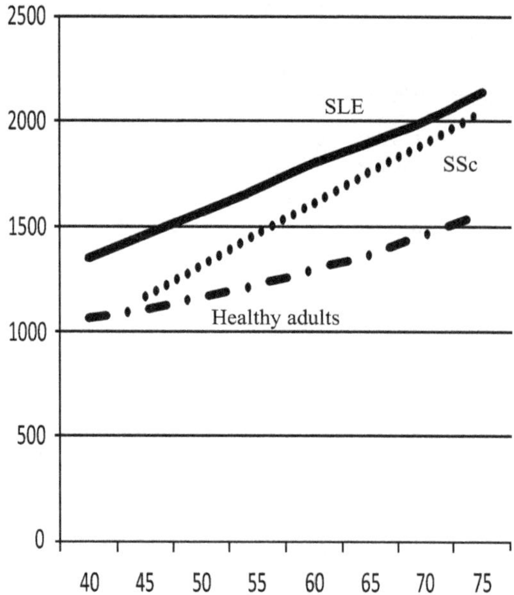

Fig. (2). The predicted values of baPWV in SLE, SSc patients and healthy adults with respect to age. The predicted values obtained through regression analysis in SLE and SSc patients were compared with the mean of 12517 healthy adults. The predicted values of baPWV in SLE and SSc (over 40 years old) and the mean of baPWV in the control (over 40 years old).

Comparison of baPWV in 13 patients with SLE, from whom informed consent regarding a blood test was obtained, with a conventional index of arteriosclerosis, the LDL/HDL ratio, is shown in Table **1**. Comparison of (T-cho - HDL)/HDL with baPWV in the SLE patients is presented in Table **2**.

Table 1. Standard deviation of baPWV and LDL/HDL in SLE patients.

SD of baPWV / LDL/HDL	<1SD	≥1SD, <2SD	≥2SD
≤2	3	1	2
>2	0	4	3

The standard deviation of baPWV in SLE patients was classified by 1 and 2SD, and the LDL/HDL value was classified by 2 (a normal value).

Table 2. Standard deviation of baPWV and (T-cho - HDL)/HDL in SLE patients.

SD of baPWV / (T-CHO-HDL)/HDL	<1SD	≥1SD, <2SD	≥2SD
≤4	3	4	3
>4	0	1	2

A conventional index of arteriosclerosis, (T-cho - HDL)/HDL, were classified by 4 (a normal value).

Among 5 patients with baPWV exceeding 2 SD, the LDL/HDL ratio was normal in 2 and high in 3 (normal range ≤2). Among 5 patients with baPWV from1SD to 2SD (≥1SD, <2SD), the LDL/HDL ratio was normal in 1 and high in 4. Among 3 patients with normal baPWV (<1SD), the LDL/HDL ratio was normal in 3. Among the patients with baPWV more than 1SD, the LDL/HDL ratio was relatively high but there were no statistical differences (by unpaired t test).

Among 5 patients with baPWV exceeding 2SD, the (T-cho - HDL)/HDL ratio was normal in 3 and high in 2 (normal range ≦ 4). Among 5 patients with baPWV from1SD to 2SD (≥1SD, <2SD), the (T-cho - HDL)/HDL ratio was normal in 4 and high in 1. Among 3 patients with normal baPWV, (T-cho - HDL)/HDL was normal in 3. When compared with the association of baPWV and LDL/HDL ratio, the inverse correlations were observed among groups of ≥1SD, <2SD and ≥2SD ($p<0.01$, unpaired t test)

As shown in Table **3**, there was no correlation between the coefficient of corticosteroid therapy and baPWV.

Table 3. Dose of corticosteroid (coefficient) and baPWV (as SD) in patients with SLE.

Coefficient	<1SD	≥1SD, <2SD	≥2SD
0-50	4	0	5
51-100	2	2	2
101-150	2	3	2
151-200	0	0	2
201-250	0	0	0
> 251	0	1	2
Total	8	6	13

There was no statistically significant correlation.

DISCUSSION

The results of this study involving 29 patients with SLE characterized by skin lesions suggest that the influence on the cardio-/cerebrovascular systems must be considered even when there are no systemic symptoms.

In this study, baPWV exceeded the mean +1 to +2SD of healthy adults in many subjects aged 40 years or older. In some patients with SLE, baPWV was high even when conventional risk factors for arteriosclerosis, the LDL/HDL ratio and (T-cho - HDL)/HDL, were normal. When baPWV was normal, the LDL/HDL ratio and (T-cho - HDL)/HDL were normal (2 and 4, respectively). Interestingly these two ratios varied from baPWV value in our examined group (Tables **2** and **3**). Reports by Roman [6], Asanuma *et al.* [7] and our study suggested that conventional management based on blood collection data alone is risky to determine the degrees of vascular damage.

Measurement of baPWV is a method to diagnose arteriosclerosis in which the principle that the pulse wave of blood ejected from the heart is accelerated with the stiffness of arteries was applied. Measurement is simple, and the duration of examination involving preparations is approximately 5 minutes. The baPWV facilitates the detection of early angiopathy. It reflects wall thickening of the arterial media. A study reported that baPWV was useful as an index of the grade of atherosclerosis or coronary risks, or as a parameter for predicting cardiovascular disease [10]. It is also possible to evaluate aortic sclerosis [11].

Thus, measurement of baPWV is a noninvasive method to manage/diagnose arteriosclerotic lesions in patients with SLE, and it may be useful in outpatient clinics. In addition, baPWV also tends to increase at an advanced age in patients with SSc. Therefore, this parameter should be considered for regular screening.

In SLE patients in whom baPWV was within the normal range at the first visit, we should continue the follow-up examination every year because as shown in Figs. (**1**, **2**) SLE patients have high risk of the increasing in baPWV. Another reason is that baPWV reached the mean plus 1SD of healthy adults during at least 5 years follow up which is based on the preliminary analysis of the present studies.

This suggests that baPWV is a possible tool to evaluate the patient's vascular function, which was difficult to evaluate using a conventional sera arteriosclerosis index. Even when conditions are characterized by skin lesions, it may be important to consider the influence on the cardio-/cerebrovascular systems, as indicated for patients with systemic symptoms.

CONFLICT OF INTEREST

The authors confirm that this article content has no conflict of interest.

ACKNOWLEDGEMENTS

Declared none.

REFERENCES

[1] Merrell M, Shulman LE. Determination of prognosis in chronic disease, illustrated by systemic lupus erythematosus. J Chronic Dis 1955; 1: 12-32.

[2] Dubois EL, Wierzchowiecki M, Cox MB, Weiner JM. Duration and death in systemic lupus erythematosus. An analysis of 249 cases. JAMA 1974; 227: 1399-402.

[3] Ofuji S, Miyawaki S. Epidemiological studies of systemic lupus erythematosus in Japan. Ryumachi 1975; 15: 310-25.

[4] Bernatsky S, Boivin JF, Joseph L, *et al.* Mortality in systemic lupus erythematosus. Arthritis Rheum 2006; 54: 2550-7.

[5] Manzi S1, Meilahn EN, Rairie JE, *et al.* Age-specific incidence rates of myocardial infarction and angina in women with systemic lupus erythematosus: comparison with the Framingham Study. Am J Epidemiol 1997; 145: 408-15.

[6] Roman MJ1, Shanker BA, Davis A, *et al.* Prevalence and correlates of accelerated atherosclerosis in systemic lupus erythematosus. N Engl J Med 2003; 349: 2399-406.

[7] Asanuma Y1, Oeser A, Shintani AK, *et al.* Premature coronary-artery atherosclerosis in systemic lupus erythematosus. N Engl J Med 2003; 349: 2407-15.

[8] Selzer F, Sutton-Tyrrell K, Fitzgerald S, Tracy R, Kuller L, Manzi S. Vascular stiffness in women with systemic lupus erythematosus. Hypertension 2001; 37: 1075-82.

[9] Tomiyama H, Yamashina A, Arai T, *et al.* Influences of age and gender on results of noninvasive brachial-ankle pulse wave velocity measurement-a survey of 12517 subjects. Atherosclerosis 2003; 166: 303-9.

[10] Lehmann ED, Riley WA, Clarkson P, Gosling RG. Non-invasive assessment of cardiovascular disease in diabetes mellitus. Lancet 1997; 350(Suppl 1): 14-9.

[11] Lehmann ED. Clinical value of aortic pulse wave velocity measurement. Lancet 1999; 354: 528-9.

3

Childhood Herpes Zoster-Triggered Guttate Psoriasis

V. Failla, N. Nikkels-Tassoudji, M. Sabatiello, V. de Schaetzen and A.F. Nikkels*

Department of Dermatology, University Hospital of Liège, Liège, Belgium

Abstract: Psoriasis is commonly triggered or exacerbated by various stress factors, certain drugs, or streptococcal throat infections. Viral infections such as HIV, CMV, chikungunya, or herpes simplex virus are very uncommon triggers for psoriasis. Cases of varicella-triggered psoriasis are exceptional. A 7-year-old boy with a previous history of guttate psoriasis presented with generalized acute guttate psoriasis shortly after an extensive herpes zoster infection affecting the first and second left lumbar dermatomes. INF-alpha and granulocyte monocyte colony stimulating factor influence peripheral monocytes to transform into INF-dendritic cells (DC's), similar to those involved in psoriasis. These INF-DC's express toll-like receptors 7 and 8, which are responsive to viral single stranded RNA. Hence, viral infections and interferon (INF)-alpha may play a role in triggering psoriasis.

A PubMed search revealed no previous reports of herpes zoster triggered acute guttate psoriasis in children.

Keywords: Herpes zoster, varicella zoster virus, psoriasis, child.

INTRODUCTION

Psoriasis, especially acute guttate psoriasis and plaque psoriasis, may be induced or exacerbated by a variety of trigger factors which may also impair the treatment response. The most common trigger is stress [1], probably mediated by a hypothalamic-pituitary-adrenal relationship with immunologic events. Medications such as lithium, beta blocking agents, or acetylsalicylic acid may also be involved [2-4]. However, the degree to which a drug may be responsible is not always easy to determine [2-5]. Smoking and alcohol abuse may also promote the development of psoriasis [6]. Furthermore, various infectious agents can trigger or aggravate psoriasis. The most common are beta-hemolytic streptococcal throat infections that can provoke acute guttate psoriasis or exacerbate preexisting plaque psoriasis [7,8]. Induction/exacerbation of psoriasis following viral infections is less common. Chikungunya infection [9], HIV/AIDS [10], persistent CMV infection [11] and herpes simplex virus (HSV)-related erythema multiforme [12] have all been reported as causal and/or aggravating factors. Acute guttate psoriasis in young children may also be seen after upper respiratory tract viral infections in connection with measles or influenza. Three publications have reported acute guttate psoriasis following varicella zoster virus (VZV) infections [13-15].

A PubMed search did not identify any previous reports of acute generalized guttate psoriasis following herpes zoster (HZ) in a child.

CASE REPORT

A 7-year-old boy without any significant medical history presented with an unilateral inguinal vesicular eruption (Fig. **1**). The boy was not taking any medication and had no atopic background. There was no family history of psoriasis. Vaccination status was assessed in accordance with local health regulations. The child had not been vaccinated against varicella. At the age of 1 he had presented with moderate varicella. Two years prior to the present consultation he had presented with acute generalized guttate psoriasis following a beta-hemolytic streptococcal throat infection. The lesions were clustered and scattered in a dermatomal distribution (L1, L2) and were almost perfectly semicircular in shape (Fig. **2**). All elements were vesicular. One week before the lesions appeared, the child had been complaining of burning and stinging pains in the inguinal area, prompting his mother to administer paracetamol. The child was not feverish and no lymph nodes were identified on physical examination. The typical unilateral distribution of the skin lesions and the presence of prodromal pains suggested the diagnosis of inguinal childhood HZ. A Tzanck smear was performed on one of the vesicular lesions and stained with PMS

Fig. (1). Herpes zoster in the left anterior L1 and L2 dermatomes, vesicular stage.

*Address correspondence to this author at the Department of Dermatology, CHU of Sart Tilman, University of Liège, B-4000 Liège, Belgium; E-mail: af.nikkels@chu.ulg.ac.be

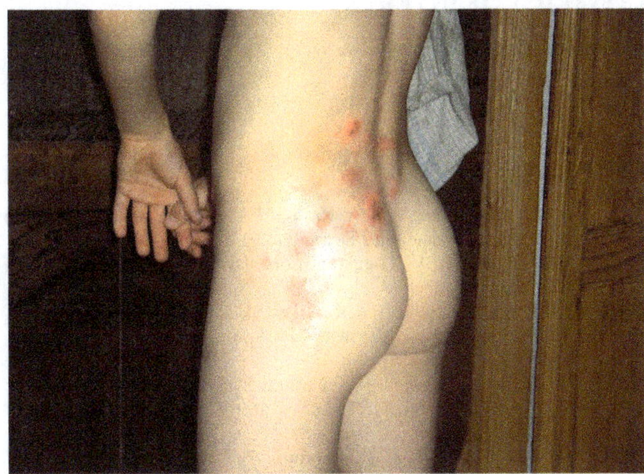

Fig. (2). Herpes zoster in the left posterior L1 and L2 dermatomes, vesicular stage.

(Polychrome Multiple Stain); this revealed syncitial giant cells, suggestive of an alpha-herpesvirus infection. Immunohistochemistry revealed the presence of the VZV-specific surface glycoprotein gE, whereas no HSV glycoproteins were detected [16]. As antiviral treatment is not recommended for HZ in children [17], the boy received only paracetamol 250 mg twice daily as supportive treatment. The pain was gradually alleviated and progressively disappeared over two weeks, with a simultaneous resolution of the skin lesions. One week later, the child represented to the dermatologist as he had rapidly developed an eruption of small erythematous and squamous well-circumscribed lesions over the entire body, suggestive of generalized acute guttate psoriasis (Fig. **3**). The child did not show any signs of a throat infection and had no fever, and no locoregional lymphadenopathies were palpated. The tonsils were neither swollen nor erythematous. A blood sample showed no evidence of any significant changes.

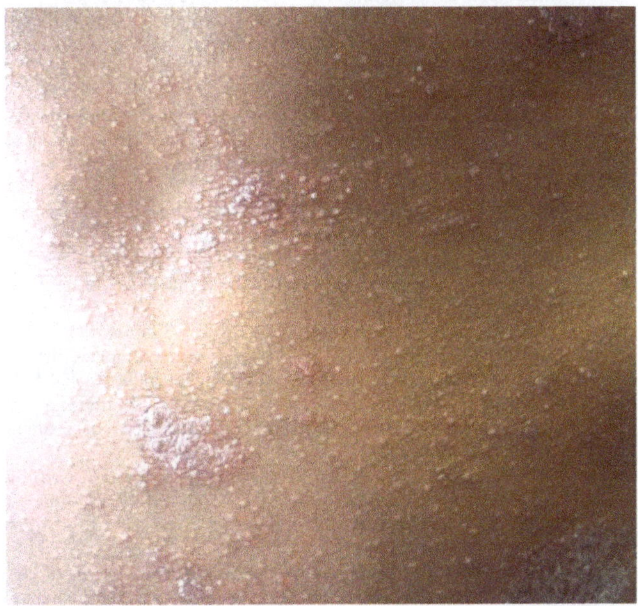

Fig. (3). Acute generalized guttate psoriasis.

Hepatic and renal function were both normal. The Antistreptolysin-O (ASLO) titer was negative, as was a throat culture. Topical application of potent corticosteroids (betamethasone dipropionate 0, 05% cream, 1x/d, 15 days) was commenced. The psoriasis lesions progressively resolved over approximately 3 weeks. The child showed no signs of any persisting post-zoster neuralgia, nor of any residual scarring from the cutaneous lesions.

DISCUSSION

Acute guttate psoriasis is a distinctive acute form of psoriasis that typically occurs in children and young adults. It is commonly associated with antecedent streptococcal throat infection or tonsillitis [7,8]. A study performed polymerase chain reaction (PCR) assays to detect universal 16S ribosomal DNA primers and specific primers for Streptococcus *pyogenes* in peripheral blood samples from 7 patients with guttate psoriasis, 6 patients with chronic plaque psoriasis, 7 chronic plaque psoriasis patients with associated guttate psoriasis, and 16 controls. Ribosomal bacterial DNA was found in all the psoriasis patients but not in the control group. Streptococci were found in 6 of 7 guttate psoriasis patients, whereas Staphylococci were identified in 9 of 13 patients with chronic plaque psoriasis. These findings suggest that distinct taxonomic bacterial groups are present in guttate and chronic plaque psoriasis [18]. Evidence of T cells recognizing common determinants to streptococcal M-protein and keratin have been found in psoriasis patients. CD8+ T cells in psoriatic epidermis respond mainly to such determinants, whereas CD4+ T cells in the dermis preferentially recognize determinants of the streptococcal peptidoglycan that might act as adjuvants [19]. A comparative one-year observational study showed that psoriasis patients reported having a sore throat significantly more often than controls (61/208 *vs* 3/116, $P < 0.0001$), and beta-hemolytic Streptococci of Lancefield groups A, C and G (M protein-positive Streptococci) were significantly more frequently cultured from the patients than the controls (19 of 208 *vs* one of 116, $P = 0.003$) (8). Despite the clear relationship between the streptococcal infection and recurrent acute guttate psoriasis or chronic plaque psoriasis, there is currently no evidence that antibiotics and/or tonsillectomy are beneficial for these patients [7]. Psoriasis has also been described after throat infections by Candida albicans [20].

Viral infections leading to acute guttate psoriasis are rarely reported and the pathomechanisms have not been elucidated (Table **1**). Some of the reported infections, including measles, influenza and HSV-related erythema multiforme [12] are localized in the throat, similar to Streptococcal infections. In contrast, Chikungunya infection [9], human immunodeficiency virus (HIV) infection [10], and persistent CMV infection [11] are systemic viral infections. Other authors have not been able to establish a link between CMV or human herpes viruses (HHV) 6 and 7 infections and a subsequent development of psoriasis [21]. HPV subtypes 5 and 36 are also pathogenic candidates, although their precise contribution remains to be clarified [22]. Three publications reported guttate psoriasis following varicella [13-15]. After the initial exposure to VZV, there is a phase of viral replication in the oropharyngeal area. These data suggest that bacterial, fungal or viral infections of the throat may play an important role in triggering psoriasis.

Table 1. Potential Infectious Agents Contributing to the Induction or Exacerbation of Psoriasis, or to Treatment Resistance

Risk Factors	Agents	References
Bacterial	Streptococcus Staphylococcus	[7,8]
Viral	HSV-related erythema multiforme	[12]
	VZV	[13-15, this report]
	CMV	[11]
	HIV	[10]
	HPV	[22]
	Influenza	[28]
	Measles	[28]
	Chikungunya	[9]
Fungal	Candidosis	[20]

HZ in children is uncommon but is probably underrecognized [17]. This child presented with chickenpox at the age of 1, which is a typical risk factor for childhood HZ. As far as we know, this is the first report of a child presenting with HZ followed by acute guttate psoriasis. Negative ASLO and the absence of drug intake ruled out any other potential triggers of acute guttate psoriasis. The extension and severity of the skin lesions suggest that an associated VZV-viremia was present, which may have played a role in the triggering of the psoriasis. Viral infections and interferon (IFN)-alpha play a role in triggering dendritic cell populations in psoriasis [23]. In fact, under the influence of INF-alpha and granulocyte monocyte colony stimulating factor (GM-CSF), peripheral monocytes transform into INF-dendritic cells (DC's) similar to those involved in psoriasis pathogenesis. The INF-DC's express a large range of toll-like receptors (TLR's) including TLR 7 and 8, responsive to (viral) single stranded RNA (ssRNA). In culture conditions, incubation with ssRNA increased the IFN-DCs mRNAs for interleukin (Il) IL-12p35, IL-12p40, IL-23p19, IL-27p28 and IL-27EBI [23]. Hence, viral infections may potentially trigger psoriasis [23]. Whether a similar molecular resemblance exists between some VZV constituents and epidermal keratins to that observed for streptococci, remains to be determined.

This phenomenon has to be distinguished from psoriasis lesions induced by a Koebner phenomenon after varicella skin lesions, which are defined as psoriasis lesions limited and restricted to the sites of previous varicella lesions [24-28].

In conclusion, HZ should be added to the list of potential triggers of generalized acute guttate psoriasis.

ACKNOWLEDGEMENT

Declared none.

CONFLICT OF INTEREST

Declared none.

REFERENCES

[1] Basavaraj KH, Navya MA, Rashmi R. Stress and quality of life in psoriasis: an update. Int J Dermatol 2011; 50: 783-92.

[2] Wolf R, Ruocco V. Triggered psoriasis. Adv Exp Med Biol 1999; 455: 221-5.

[3] Tsankov N, Angelova I, Kazandjieva J. Drug-induced psoriasis. Recognition and management. Am J Clin Dermatol 2000; 1: 159-65.

[4] Basavaraj KH, Ashok NM, Rashmi R, Praveen TK. The role of drugs in the induction and/or exacerbation of psoriasis. Int J Dermatol 2010; 49: 1351-61.

[5] Herman SM, Shin MH, Holbrook A, Rosenthal D. The role of antimalarials in the exacerbation of psoriasis: a systematic review. Am J Clin Dermatol 2006; 7: 249-57.

[6] Armstrong AW, Armstrong EJ, Fuller EN, Sockolov ME, Voyles SV. Smoking and Pathogenesis of Psoriasis: A Review of Oxidative, Inflammatory, and Genetic Mechanisms. Br J Dermatol 2011; 165(6): 1162-8.

[7] Owen CM, Chalmers RJ, O'Sullivan T, Griffiths CE. Antistreptococcal interventions for guttate and chronic plaque psoriasis. Cochrane Database Syst Rev 2000;(2):CD001976.

[8] Gudjonsson JE, Thorarinsson AM, Sigurgeirsson B, Kristinsson KG, Valdimarsson H. Streptococcal throat infections and exacerbation of chronic plaque psoriasis: a prospective study. Br J Dermatol 2003; 149: 530-4.

[9] Seetharam KA, Sridevi K. Chikungunya infection: A new trigger for psoriasis. J Dermatol 2011; 38: 1033-4.

[10] Blanco González OA, Larrondo Muguercia RJ, Blanco González BL, Rodríguez Barreras ME. Psoriasis and AIDS: a report of 2 cases. Rev Cubana Med Trop 2000; 52: 148-9.

[11] Weitz M, Kiessling C, Friedrich M, *et al.* Persistent CMV infection correlates with disease activity and dominates the phenotype of peripheral CD8+ T cells in psoriasis. Exp Dermatol 2011; 20: 561-7.

[12] Wiemers S, Krutmann J, Kapp A, Schöpf E. Postherpetic erythema exsudativum multiforme with concomitant exacerbation of psoriasis vulgaris. Hautarzt 1990; 41: 506-8.

[13] Ito T, Furukawa F. Psoriasis guttate acuta triggered by varicella zoster virus infection. Eur J Dermatol 2000; 10: 226-7.

[14] Veraldi S, Lunardon L, Dassoni F. Guttate psoriasis triggered by chickenpox. G Ital Dermatol Venereol 2009; 144: 501-2.

[15] Hellgren L. A statistical, clinical and laboratory investigation of 255 psoriatics and matched healthy controls. Acta Derma Venereol (Stockh) 1964; 44: 191-207.

[16] Nikkels AF, Debrus S, Sadzot-Delvaux C, Piette J, Rentier B, Piérard GE. Immunohistochemical identification of varicella-zoster virus gene 63-encoded protein (IE63) and late (gE) protein on smears and cutaneous biopsies: implications for diagnostic use. J Med Virol 1995; 47: 342-7.

[17] Nikkels AF, Nikkels-Tassoudji N, Piérard GE. Revisiting childhood herpes zoster. Pediatr Dermatol 2004; 21: 18-23.

[18] Munz OH, Sela S, Baker BS, Griffiths CE, Powles AV, Fry L. Evidence for the presence of bacteria in the blood of psoriasis patients. Arch Dermatol Res 2010; 302: 495-8.

[19] Valdimarsson H, Thorleifsdottir RH, Sigurdardottir SL, Gudjonsson JE, Johnston A. Psoriasis as an autoimmune disease caused by molecular mimicry. Trends Immunol 2009; 30: 494-501.

[20] Waldman A, Gilhar A, Duek L, Berdicevsky I. Incidence of Candida in psoriasis--a study on the fungal flora of psoriatic patients. Mycoses 2001; 44: 77-81.

[21] Kirby B, Al-Jiffri O, Cooper RJ, Corbitt G, Klapper PE, Griffiths CE. Investigation of cytomegalovirus and human herpes viruses 6 and 7 as possible causative antigens in psoriasis. Acta Derm Venereol 2000; 80: 404-6.

[22] Cronin JG, Mesher D, Purdie K, *et al.* Beta-papillomaviruses and psoriasis: an intra-patient comparison of human papillomavirus carriage in skin and hair. Br J Dermatol 2008; 159: 113-9.

[23] Farkas A, Tonel G, Nestle FO. Interferon-alpha and viral triggers promote functional maturation of human monocyte-derived dendritic cells. Br J Dermatol 2008; 158: 921-9.

[24] Skory L, Shearn MA. Psoriatic arthritis induced by varicella. West J Med 1979; 131: 440-1.

[25] Abraham A, Farber EM. The Köbner response to varicella in psoriasis. Int J Dermatol 1993; 32: 919-20.

[26] Varaldi S, Rizzitelli G. Varicella, Köbner phenomenon, and psoriasis. Int J Dermatol 1994; 33: 673-4.

[27] Kokolakis GP, Ioannidou D, Cholongitas E, Krüger-Krasagakis S. Guttate psoriasis occurring on varicella lesions. J Dermatol 2010; 37: 857-9.

[28] Müller H, Fäh J, Dummer R. Unusual Koebner phenomenon in psoriasis caused by varicella and UVB. Hautarzt 1997; 48: 130-2.

4

Alteration of the Structure of Human Stratum Corneum Facilitates Transdermal Delivery

Anne Mundstock, Rawad Abdayem, Fabrice Pirot and Marek Haftek*

Université Lyon 1, EA4169 "Fundamental, clinical and therapeutic aspects of the skin barrier function"; 8 avenue Rockefeller, 69373 Lyon, France

Abstract: Transdermal transport of pharmacologically active components into the skin depends on the ability of galenic formulations to overcome the *stratum corneum* (SC) barrier. Microemulsions (ME) are thermodynamically stable liquid systems composed of water, oil and surfactants which may be used for skin permeation and enhance penetration of hydrophobic as well as hydrophilic compounds. We investigated using transmission electron microscopy the effect of ME on human epidermis *ex vivo*, in order to establish relationship between the type of ME, i.e.: oil-in-water, water-in-oil, gel-like, thickened or not with colloidal silica, and the ultrastructural changes in SC barrier resulting from their topical application. ME induced various degrees of dissociation of the SC. The intercellular lipid matrix in the SC became disorganized, which contributed to the separation of corneocytes. This effect was intensified with the increasing oil content in the ME and also when ME were applied under occlusion. The observed morphological changes were in agreement with the increased permeability of ME-treated skin to both lipophilic and hydrophilic compounds reported in the literature. Severe deterioration of the SC barrier induced with the selected ME makes them suitable for selected indications only.

Keywords: Epidermal structure, microemulsion, skin barrier, transmission electron microscopy.

INTRODUCTION

Skin is a very effective barrier which protects the human body from environmental influences such as ultraviolet radiation, chemicals and pathogenic microorganisms. But it also forms a barrier against the loss of water and electrolytes [1]. It is the epidermis that elaborates the cornified layer (*stratum corneum*, SC) responsible for the skin barrier function [2]. Two parts of the normal SC can be distinguished. The lower part is the SC *compactum* which is composed of the first 4 to 6 cell layers of the SC [3]. It is this part of the horny layer that provides the effective barrier against water loss. The upper part is called the SC *disjunctum* and is composed of approximately 8-15 cell layers, more loosely structured, with only lateral cell-cell junctions persisting. The whole SC in human ventral skin consists of around 15-20 cell layers, but these numbers do vary according to the anatomical localization. They are significantly lower on the eyelids and markedly higher on the palms and soles. SC keratinocytes, called corneocytes, are flattened polyedric cells which are filled with keratin and amino acids issued from processing of profilaggrin. Corneocytes possess cornified envelope of cross-linked protein covered with a monolayer of ceramides forming a lipid envelope. The extracellular spaces are filled with lamellar sheets of lipids, primarily cholesterol, free fatty acids and ceramides in roughly equimolar proportions [1]. These lipid molecules organized in bi-layers provide the relative impermeability of the SC.

The aim of many pharmaceutical formulations is to overcome the epidermal barrier, in order to enable the transport of components into the skin. A former study showed that microemulsions (ME) may have a positive effect on the simultaneous permeation of the antioxidants, like vitamin C and vitamin E, into the skin [4]. A ME is a system of water, oil and surfactants, which is a transparent, optically isotropic and thermodynamically stable liquid solution. It forms easily, shows low viscosity with Newtonian behavior, displays a high specific surface area and has a very small size distribution. It is possible to dissolve in ME hydrophobic as well as hydrophilic substances. Several potential mechanisms have been described how such formulations can enhance drug permeation through the skin: i) swelling or increased hydration of intracellular keratin caused by denaturation or modification or its conformation; ii) action on desmosomes; iii) alteration of lipid bilayers that may lead to a decreased resistance to permeation; iv) modification of solvent properties of the SC, which changes drug partitioning; v) extraction of lipids from the horny layer with use of particular solvents [5, 6]. That is why detection of possible ultrastructural changes could be important for the explanation of the functional observations including an increased permeation of the SC. Electron microscopy is a technique which allows observation of such fine structural modifications. In the present study different ME, previously used for transcutaneous delivery of antioxidant vitamins [4], were prepared without any active ingredient. Transmission electron microscopy (TEM) observations of osmium and

*Address correspondence to this author at the Research Director with CNRS, Laboratory for Dermatological Research, EA4169 UCBL1, 8, Av. Rockefeller, 69373 Lyon, France;
E-mail: marek.haftek@univ-lyon1.fr

ruthenium tetroxide -stained biopsies were performed in order to explain with ultrastuctural clues the permeabilizing properties of different ME.

MATERIALS AND METHODS

Preparation of Microemulsions (ME)

Oil-in-water (o/W) ME, water-in-oil (w/O) ME, gel-like ME and Aerosil®-thickened ME were all prepared in the same manner using the same set of components (Table **1**). These ME previously showed their efficacy for simultaneous transdermal delivery of both hydrophobic and hydrophilic molecules, vitamins E and C [4,7,8]. Isopropyl myristate (IPM; Merck, Fleury les Aubrais, France) was used as the lipophilic phase and purified water as the hydrophilic one. The 1:1 mixture of surfactants Tween 40 (polyoxyethylene (20) sorbitan monopalmitate; Fluka Chemie, Buch, Switzerland) and Imwitor 308 (glyceryl caprylate; Condea, Hamburg, Germany) was kindly provided by the Faculty of Pharmacy, University of Ljubljana, Slovenia. The water phases and the oily phases were weighted into the same receptacle. Afterwards the mixture of surfactants was added and the formulations were stirred five minutes with a magnetic stirrer at 400 rpm. Gel-like ME was obtained by an increase of the water content at the expense of the lipophilic phase [7]. A thickening agent, colloidal silica (Aerosil® 200; Degussa, Dusseldorf, Germany) was added to o/w ME to obtain the formulation showing viscosity similar to that of the gel-like ME [8].

Ex Vivo Exposure of Human Skin to ME

Normal human skin of three female premenopausal donors was obtained from plastic surgery, following the agreement of the local ethics committee at the Civil Hospices of Lyon. The post-operatory fragments of ventral skin were recovered from the operating room, transported in a sterile container at 4°C, and immediately used for skin permeation experiments, typically within 1h after excision.

Each skin fragment was placed on wet tissue impregnated with Dulbecco's modified Eagle medium (DMEM; Gibco, Paris, France) enriched with 5% fetal calf serum (Gibco), on a heating plate maintained at 32°C. The permeation experiments were performed in duplicate. Glass chambers were affixed on the skin surface with Super Glue-3 (Loctite). One mL of each formulation was put into test chambers, two chambers per formulation. Two chambers remained empty, as controls. For each pair of formulations one chamber was left open to simulate non-occlusive conditions while the other chamber was closed with a plug to create occlusion. The control chambers were treated equally. After six hour incubation, the chambers with the applied formulations were carefully removed. Four millimeter punch biopsies were taken from the center of each incubated area and processed for routine histopathology and transmission electron microscopy (TEM).

Transmission Electron Microscopy

Small skin fragments were fixed with either 2% glutaraldehyde in sodium cacodylate buffer or 3% paraformaldehyde in PBS overnight. After washes in appropriate buffer solutions, they were post-fixed with 1% osmium tetroxide or 0.25% ruthenium tetroxide, respectively, as previously described [9]. Samples were than dehydrated in graded alcohol and embedded in epoxy resins. Semi-thin and ultra-thin sections were cut perpendicular to

Table 1. Composition of microemulsions used in the present study.

	Gel-like ME*	o/W ME	Thickened* o/W ME	w/O ME	Aerosil ® dispersion
Water	60%	45%	45%	10%	100%
Isopropyl myristate	10%	25%	25%	60%	-
Tween 40 (polyoxyethylene(20)sorbitan monopalmitate)	15%	15%	15%	15%	-
Imwitor 308 (glyceryl caprylate)	15%	15%	15%	15%	-
Aerosil ® (thickener)	-	-	10% in ME	-	10% in water

o/W = oil in water
w/O = water in oil

* similar viscosities

*) Thickening agents increase the viscosity of the system without affecting its stability and spontaneous formation.

the skin surface and counterstained, respectively, with toluidine blue and with uranyl acetate followed by lead citrate. For the samples post-fixed with osmium tetroxide, the magnifications ×28,000 and ×75,000 were used for ultrastructural examination, while the samples post-fixed with ruthenium tetroxide were observed at magnifications of ×125,000 and ×260,000.

RESULTS

Light Microscopy

Normal epidermal structure was observed in all the samples. No difference was noticed between the controls with and without occlusion. The Aerosil®-dispersion did not induce any notable changes either. The SC was often separated and partially lost in many samples during the preparatory procedures. However, treatment with the w/O ME consistently resulted in the nearly complete elimination of the horny cells, especially under occlusion, and the o/W ME induced a notable relaxation of the SC (Fig. **1**).

TEM of ME-Treated Human Skin Explants

Standard post-fixation with osmium tetroxide allowed observation of the tissue morphology, except of the fine structure of intercellular lipid lamellae in the SC [10,11]. When compared to the untreated control (Fig. **2a**), there was no major change in the SC morphology after application of the Aerosil®-dispersion alone, without lipophilic phase or surfactants (Fig. **2b**), (mean number of layers in the SC *compactum* +/-SD = 5.67 +/-0.52). Also the gel-like ME, with a relatively low contents of isopropyl myristate, induced only minor ultrastructural defects in the SC, such as discrete swelling of the intercellular spaces and the beginning of detachment in the SC *disjunctum* (mean number of layers in the SC *compactum* +/-SD = 5.33 +/-0.82; Fig. **3**). In contrast, the treatment with the o/W ME resulted in an extensive dissociation of the SC *disjunctum* and a correlated reduction of the SC *compactum* (mean number of layers in the SC *compactum* +/-SD = 3.67 +/-0.52; Fig. **4**). Additionally, amorphous and composite intercorneocyte inclusions were observed in the upper part of the cohesive SC (Fig. **4b**). The strongest effect was exerted by the w/O ME, application of which led to the pronounced dissociation between the SC cells. Typically, there were only a couple of corneocytes remaining at the surface of the living epidermis (mean number of layers in the SC *compactum* +/-SD = 1.83 +/-0.75; Fig. **5**). Occlusion, in general, amplified the degree of the observed ultrastructural changes whereas addition of the thickener had a somewhat attenuating effect (Fig. **6**). Ultrastructural changes were, thus, induced by all tested ME formulations and, with the constant proportion of surfactants, the extent of these modifications paralleled the increasing proportion of the lipophilic phase.

After ruthenium tetroxide staining, the controls showed intercellular spaces filled with the lipid lamellae in the SC *compactum* (Fig. **7a**). In the gel-like ME -treated samples, the deeper layers of the SC remained attached to the living epidermis and the intercorneocyte spaces were filled with the well-structured lipid lamellae (Fig. **3b**). A nearly complete

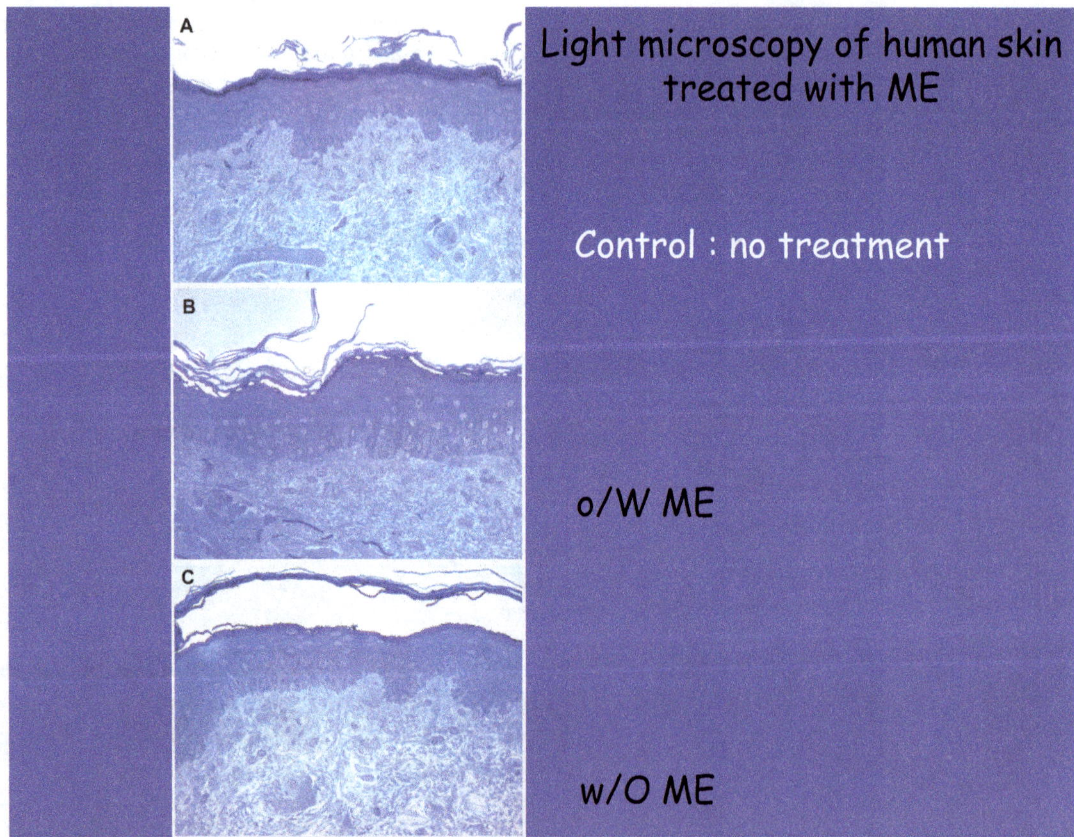

Fig. (1). Semi-thin sections observed at the light microscopy level do not show remarkable histological changes imputable to ME application, as compared to the non-treated controls (**A**), except of the SC relaxation (**B**: oil in water ME) and frequent loss of the upper SC layers in samples treated with the water in oil ME (**C**). Toluidine blue staining. Magnification: x400.

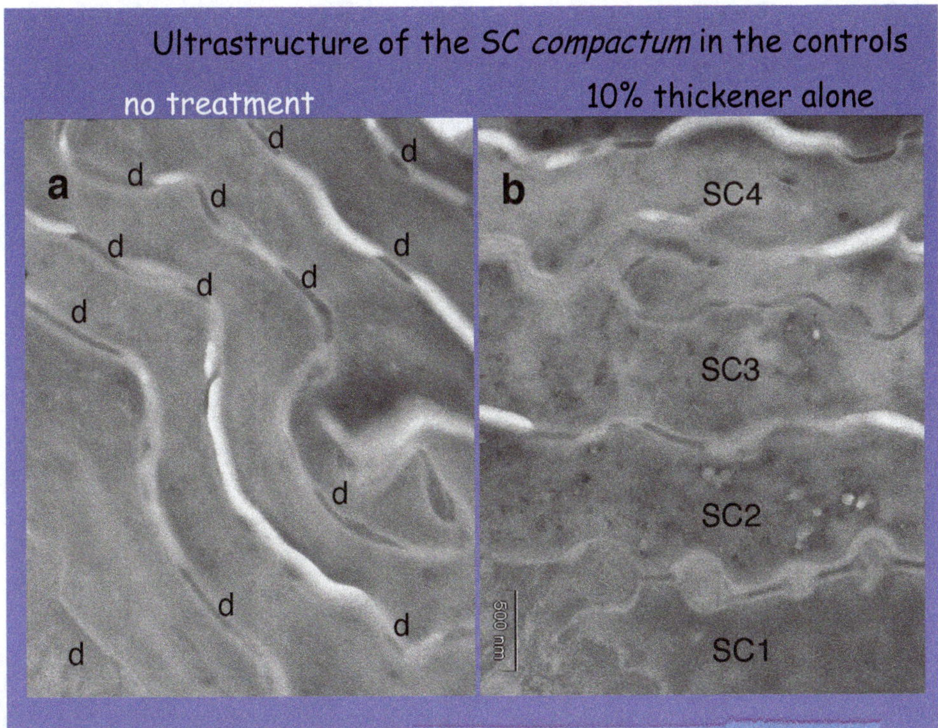

Fig. (2). TEM of the control SC. **a**) no treatment, normal SC *compactum*; **b**) no major influence due to the application of the thickener (Aerosil®). d, corneodesmosomes in (a); SC 1-4, the first four SC layers.

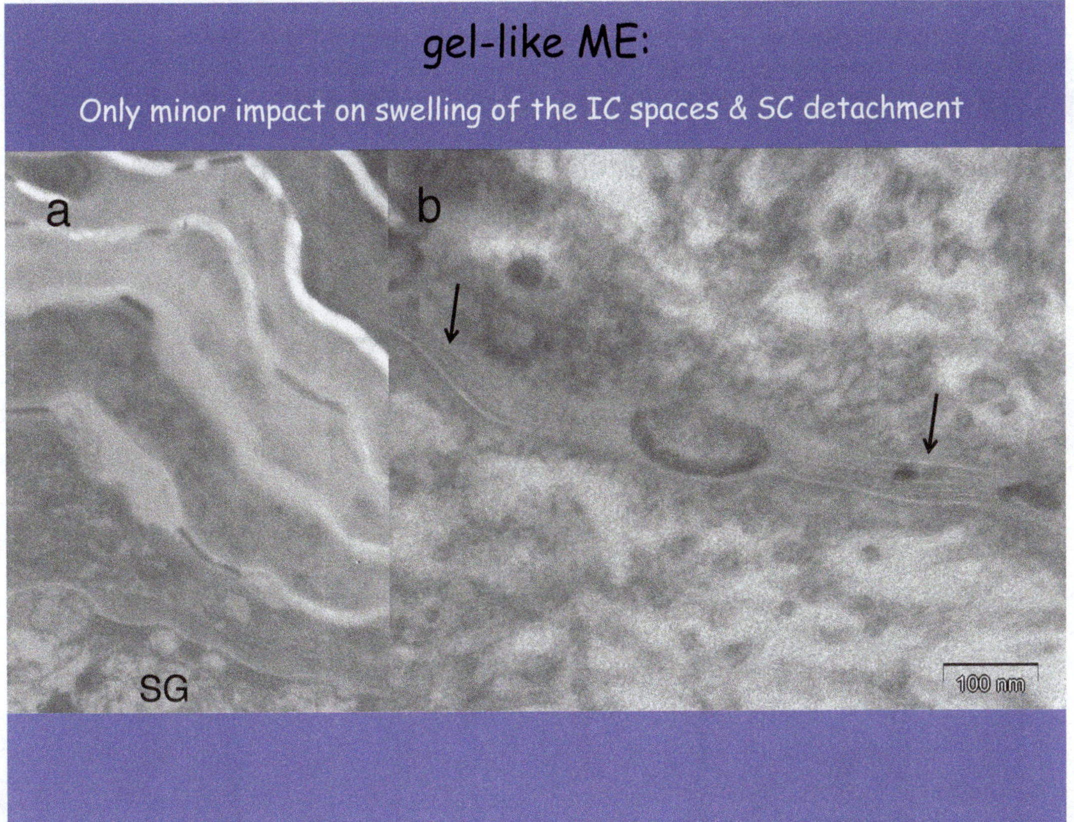

Fig. (3). TEM of the SC after application of the gel-like ME. **a**) Only minor impact on swelling of the intercellular spaces and SC detachment can be noticed. SG = *stratum granulosum*. Arrows in (**b**) indicate intact intercellular lipid lamellae in the SC visualized with RuO_4.

separation of the SC could be confirmed after incubation with w/O ME. Only the lipid envelopes stayed attached at the surface of the corneocytes, whereas loose intercellular lipid lamellae could be sometimes distinguished within the otherwise unstructured or altogether empty intercorneocyte spaces (Fig. **7b**).

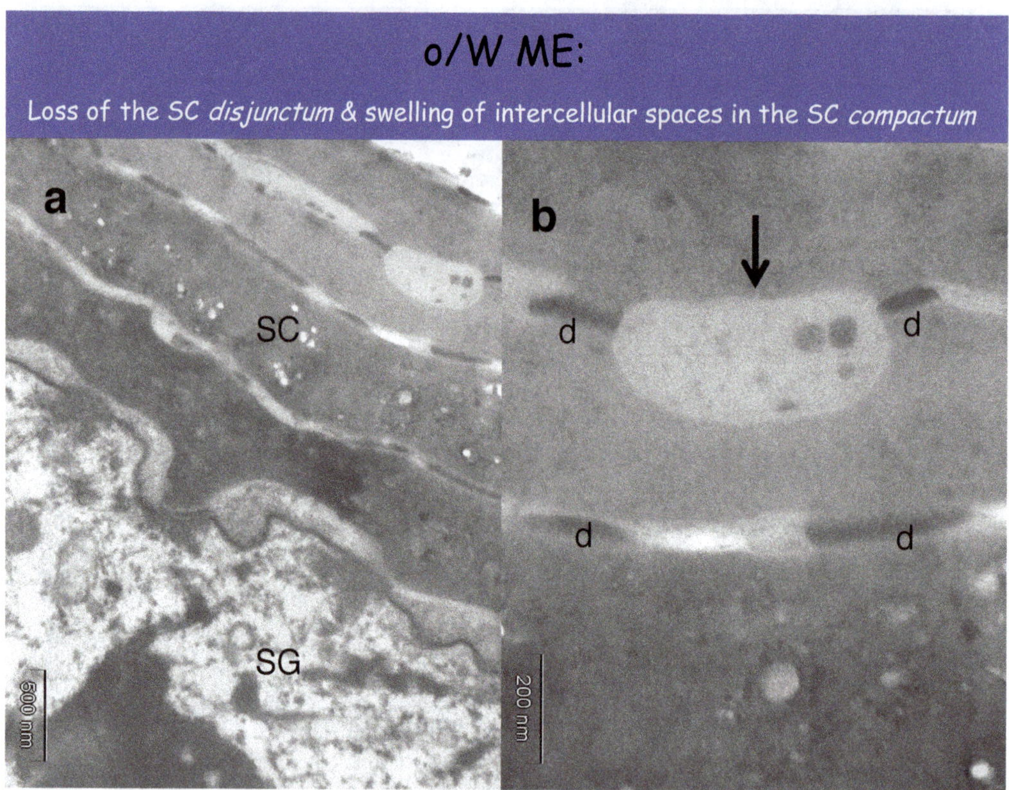

Fig. (4). Treatment of the SC with the oil in water ME provokes a partial loss of the SC *disjunctum* and swelling of intercellular spaces in the SC *compactum.* Here, only 4 corneocytes are left (**a**) and intercellular amorphous and composite inclusions are visible (arrow in **b**). d, corneodesmosomes. SG = *stratum granulosum*; SC = *stratum corneum*.

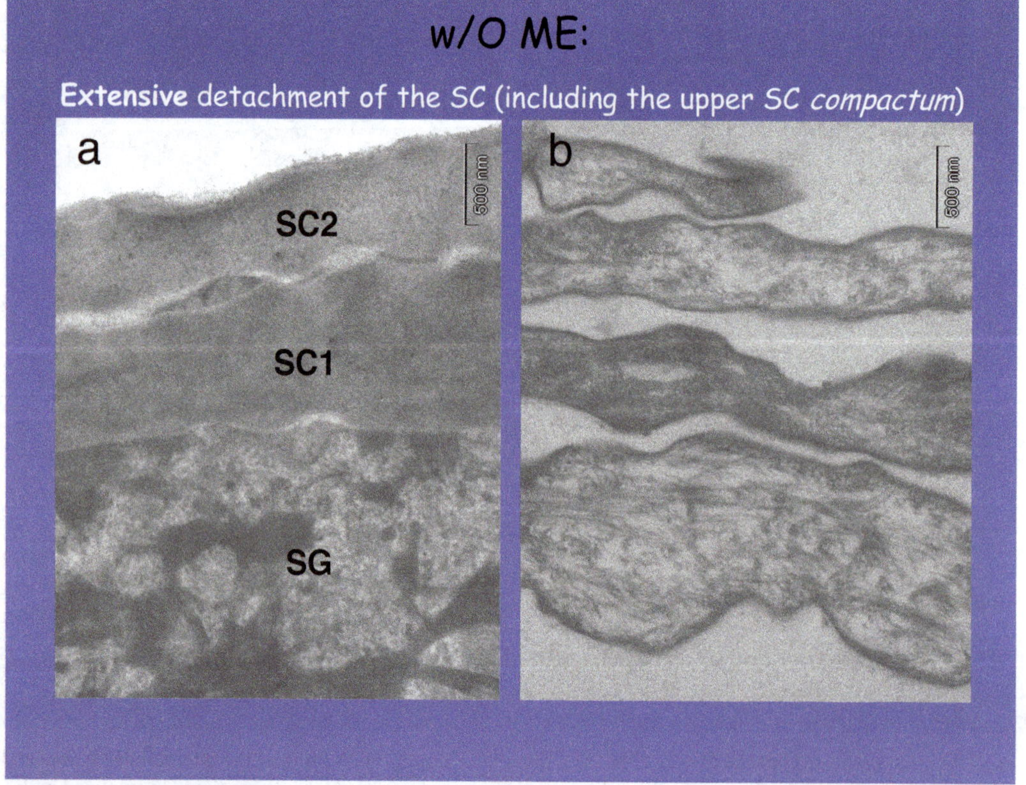

Fig. (5). Extensive detachment of the SC is observed after application of the water in oil ME. **a**) two corneocytes of SC *compactum* are left over the SG keratinocyte; **b**) loose corneocytes detaching from the sample in the upper part of the SC entirely separated from the remaining tissue; no corneodesmosomes.

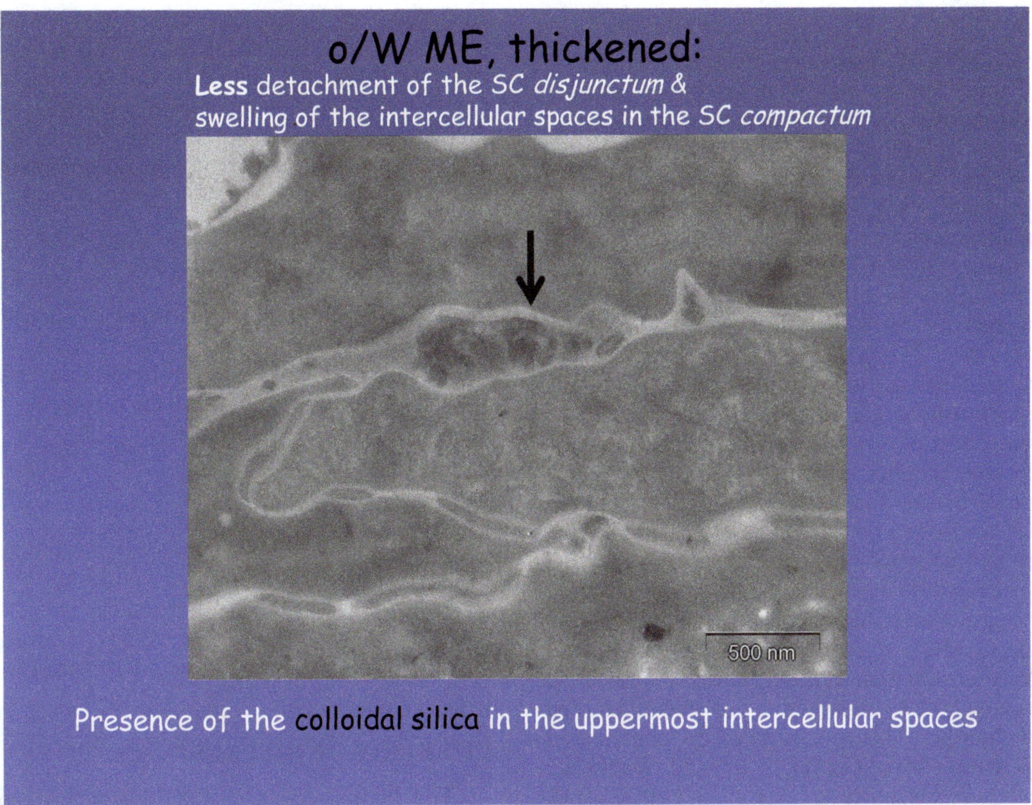

Fig. (6). Addition of thickener to the oil in water ME results in less detachment of the SC *disjunctum*. Intercellular deposits of the thickener are visualized in the upper SC (arrow).

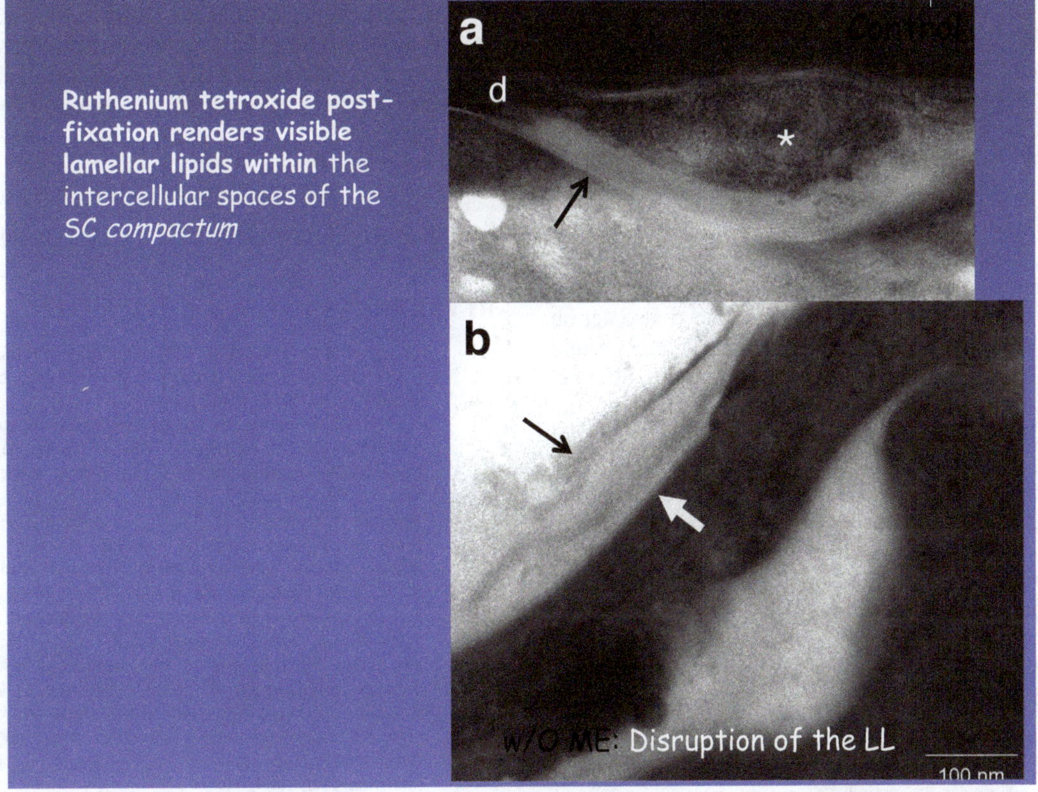

Fig. (7). Ruthenium tetroxide staining of the SC. a) intact lamellar lipids (LL) in the SC *compactum* of a control sample (arrow). b) Water/oil ME causes total disruption of the intercellular lipids. Residual lamellae are indicated with the black arrow. Thick white arrow points to the corneocyte lipid envelope. Corneodesmosome = d; Intercellular hydrophilic lacuna = asterisk.

DISCUSSION

It could be clearly demonstrated that the changes in morphology of the SC were dependent on the proportions between ingredients used for ME formulation. Specifically, the growing impact of ME on the SC overall structure and lamellar lipid disruption correlated with the increasing oil content: gel-like < o/W < w/O. Indeed, it has been previously observed using attenuated total reflectance Fourier transform infrared spectroscopy (ATR-FTIR) on pig ear substrates that ME –induced changes to the SC appear to be proportional to the level of uptake of individual ME components [12]. Consequently, isopropyl myristate and surfactant – co-surfactant mix used in our study, which segregate to the lipophilic compartment, could be predicted to disturb the intercellular lamellar lipids in a dose-dependent manner. Ruthenium tetroxide staining, which enabled us to observe the organization of the lipid lamellae in the spaces between the corneocytes, confirmed that the most profound changes in this compartment occurred after incubation with the w/O ME. Because intercellular lamellar lipids are considered essential for the skin barrier function [1,13], their disruption after application of ME with high lipophilic content should induce an increase in skin permeability. Indeed, it was found that ME of the same type as described in this study disturbed skin barrier function [4]. This was revealed by an increased transepidermal water loss (TEWL), a well-established method to determine integrity of the skin barrier [14]. However, in that earlier study [4], it was the gel-like formulation that showed the most pronounced « irritation potential » *ex vivo* (TEWL measurements on pig ear skin) and toxicity *in vitro* (MTT on reconstructed human epidermis). This indicates that despite of being a potentially interesting tool for prediction of skin penetration and tolerance, the ultrastructural examination of *ex vivo* treated human skin may yield results varying from the other tests, most probably depending on the different experimental settings.

In addition to the oil content, another possible reason for the observed dissociation of the SC could be the influence of surfactants used in the ME formulations. Apart from their impact on the extracellular lipids, surfactants can also act on proteins and possibly facilitate degradation of the protein structures [3], such as cell-cell junctions in the SC, i.e. corneodesmosomes. Nevertheless, in the present study, the proportions of surfactants in different ME were kept constant, so it is unlikely that this latter mechanism of action was primarily responsible for the observed differences in the degree of SC dissociation in the treated samples. The observed relaxation of the SC structure after application of ME and the resulting partial loss of the permeability barrier could contribute to the explanation of the fact that ME, even those with a low oil content, were able to increase simultaneously penetration of both hydrophilic and hydrophobic drugs [4,6,15].

Under our experimental conditions, no significant morphological alteration of the living epidermal layers was observed after 6 hour application of ME. This remains in agreement with the previous reports dealing with the same kinds of formulations tested *in vitro* on reconstructed human epidermis [4]. Nevertheless, based on this morphological study, our prediction is that with the constant proportion of surfactants, the permeation efficacy of ME should increase along with the proportion of the lipophilic fraction. The ransom of this effect could be the potential adverse effects. One has to keep in mind that a reduced barrier function facilitates penetration of various chemicals through the slightly damaged skin [16] and this represents a potential risk and limitation to the use of most "aggressive" formulations.

AUTHORS' CONTRIBUTIONS

All authors provided substantial contributions to the conception and design, acquisition of data, or analysis and interpretation of data, to the drafting of the article or revising it critically for important intellectual content.

ABBREVIATIONS

ME = Microemulsion

o/W = Oil in water

SC = *Stratum corneum*

SG = *Stratum granulosum*

TEM= Transmission electron microscopy

w/O = Water in oil

CONFLICT OF INTEREST

The authors confirm that this article content has no conflict of interest.

ACKNOWLEDGMENTS

The authors would like to thank Prof. Dr. Alfred Fahr and Prof. Françoise Falson for making possible student (AM) exchange between Friedrich-Schiller-Universität Jena, Germany and the Université Claude Bernard Lyon 1, France. The ultrastructural observations were performed at the Centre Technique des Microstructures (CTμ) belonging to the Lyon Bio Image platform of University Lyon 1.

The study was supported by COST action SKINBAD (BM0903).

REFERENCES

[1] Feingold KR, Elias PM. Role of lipids in the formation and maintenance of the cutaneous permeability barrier. Biochim Biophys Acta 2014; 1841: 280-94.

[2] Haftek M. 'Memory' of the stratum corneum: exploration of the epidermis' past. Br J Dermatol 2014; 171(Suppl 3): 6-9.

[3] Fartasch M. Ultrastructure of the epidermal barrier after irritation. Microsc Res Tech 1997; 37: 193-9.

[4] Rozman B, Gasperlin M, Tinois-Tessoneaud E, Pirot F, Falson F. Simultaneous absorption of vitamins C and E from topical microemulsions using reconstructed human epidermis as a skin model. Eur J Pharm Biopharm 2009; 72: 69-75.

[5] Kogan A, Garti N. Microemulsions as transdermal drug delivery vehicles. Adv Colloid Interface Sci 2006; 123-126: 369-85.

[6] Kreilgaard M. Influence of microemulsions on cutaneous drug delivery. Adv Drug Deliv Rev 2002; 54(Suppl 1): 77-98.

[7] Rozman B, Zvonar A, Falson F, Gasperlin M. Temperature-sensitive microemulsion gel: an effective topical delivery system for simultaneous delivery of vitamins C and E. AAPS PharmSciTech 2009; 10: 54-61.

[8] Rozman B, Gosenca M, Gasperlin M, Padois K, Falson F. Dual influence of colloidal silica on skin deposition of vitamins C and E simultaneously incorporated in topical microemulsions. Drug Dev Ind Pharm 2010; 36: 852-60.

[9] Haftek M, Teillon MH, Schmitt D. Stratum corneum, corneodesmosomes and ex vivo percutaneous penetration. Microsc Res Techn 1998; 43: 224-49.

[10] Schwartzendruber DC, Burnett IH, Wertz PW, Madison KC, Squier CA. Osmium tetroxide and ruthenium tetroxide are complementary reagents for the preparation of epidermal samples for transmission electron microscopy. J Invest Dermatol 1995; 104: 417-20.

[11] Fartasch M, Bassukas ID, Diepgen TL. Structural relationship between epidermal lipid lamellae, lamellar bodies and desmosomes in human epidermis: an ultrastructural study. Br J Dermatol 1993; 128: 1-9.

[12] Hathout RM, Mansour S, Mortada ND, Geneidi AS, Guy RH. Uptake of microemulsion components into the stratum corneum and their molecular effects on skin barrier function. Mol Pharm 2010; 7: 1266-73.

[13] Boddé HE, Kruithof MAM, Brussee J, Koerten HK. Visualisation of normal and enhanced $HgCl_2$ transport through human skin *in vitro*. Int J Pharm 1989; 53: 13–24.

[14] Netzlaff F, Kostka KH, Lehr CM, Schaefer UF. TEWL measurement as a routine method for evaluation the integrity of epidermis sheets in static Franz type diffusion cells *in vitro*. Limitations shown by transport data testing, Europ J Pharm Biopharm 2006; 63: 44-50.

[15] Lopes LB. Overcoming the cutaneous barrier with microemulsions. Pharmaceutics 2014; 6: 52–77.

[16] Nielsen JB, Nielsen F, Sorensen JA. Defence against dermal exposure is only skin deep: significantly increased penetration through slightly damaged skin. Arch Dermatol Res 2007; 299: 423-31.

5

Current Trends in Photoprotection - A New Generation of Oral Photoprotectors

Salvador Gonzalez[*,1,2], Yolanda Gilaberte[3], Neena Philips[4] and Angeles Juarranz[5]

[1]*Dermatology Service, Memorial Sloan-Kettering Cancer Center, New York, USA*

[2]*Dermatology Service, Ramon y Cajal Hospital, Madrid, Spain*

[3]*Dermatology Service, Hospital San Jorge, Huesca, Spain*

[4]*School of Natural Sciences, University College, Fairleigh Dickinson University, Teaneck, NJ, USA*

[5]*Biology Department, Sciences School, Universidad Autónoma de Madrid, Madrid, Spain*

Abstract: This review provides an overview of important concepts and trends in photoprotection. From the use of protective clothing to latest-generation oral photoprotectives, this article covers these topics from two points of view: 1) the physical blockade (absorption and/or reflection) of UV photons by topical sunscreens; 2) topical compounds with antioxidant properties that thereby protect of the consequences of UV-mediated photooxidation. The last section is devoted to the development of strong antioxidant oral compounds and discusses their possibilities as adjuvants in skin protection and repair and regeneration.

Keywords: Photoprotection, sunscreens, oral antioxidants, dietary photoprotectants.

INTRODUCTION

UV filters ("sunscreens") are designed to protect the skin from the harmful effects of solar radiation, particularly the UV band. UV radiation can be roughly divided into two segments according to wavelength: UVB (~290-320 nm) and UVA (~320-400 nm). UVB is erythematogenic, carcinogenic, induces photoaging and mutagenic damage to nucleic acids, e.g. RNA and DNA. UVA, on the other hand, is also mildly erythematogenic, but promotes ROS (Reactive Oxygen Species) accumulation. ROS also induce direct cell damage, carcinogenesis and contribute to photoaging.

The basic idea underlying photoprotection is to establish a physical barrier between the sun and the skin; hence most of these compounds exert their protective effect when used topically. However, a new trend is emerging, consisting of increasing the basal antioxidant threshold of the body to improve the response to oxidative damage, including that due to exposure to the sun. Thus, new substances that include potent antioxidant capability are starting to be used systemically, for example orally.

UV-based skin damage can be divided into two major categories: 1) acute, including necrosis, erythema and inflammation, and 2) chronic, termed photoaging, and characterized by the appearance of wrinkles, changes in skin color and skin cancer. The acute effects of UV exposure are mainly caused by high energy-containing photons, which are relatively easy to stop using molecules or molecular complexes that absorb, reflect, or scatter high-energy UV photons. Consequently, the major components of most topical sunscreens include barrier components as described above. However, most sunscreens cannot stop the lower-energy UV photons that cause photoaging. These photons do not cause erythema, but they can induce immunosupression as well as mutations in the DNA of the most exposed cells of the epidermis and superficial dermis. These effects are amplified by the increased oxidative damage that results from the energy transfer of these photons to destroy naturally-occurring photoprotective molecules in the skin as well as to produce reactive oxygen species (ROS). The consequences of increased oxidation include extracellular matrix (e.g. collagen) deterioration, cellular apoptosis, plasma membrane destruction, direct DNA damage and increased mutagenesis [1-5].

Visible light can also harm the skin if there is a previous skin condition, e.g. chronic actinic dermatosis, or erythropoietic porphiria. Current UV filters do not protect against visible light; opaque filters are required, including clothing or "old school" preparations of physical filters, such as ZnO or TiO_2 ([6] and see below).

From these facts, it can be inferred that proactive strategies to combat oxidative damage are highly desirable. This concept underlies the possibility of using oral antioxidants to combat the effects of photoaging. Some of the new substances used as oral photoprotectives contain one, or many, antioxidant active principles that can stop UV-induced skin damage, or even collaborate to repair previously induced damage. Future scenarios in the treatment and prevention of sun-induced skin pathologies contemplate synergic protection conferred by complementation of topical and oral sunscreens.

*Address correspondence to this author at the Dermatology Service, Memorial Sloan-Kettering Cancer Center, 160 East 53rd Street, New York, NY-10022 USA;
E-mail: gonzals6@mskcc.org

THOU SHALL NOT PASS! PREVENTING UV PHOTONS FROM REACHING THE SKIN

1. Clothing and Glasses

Appropriate clothing and sunglasses are basic tools to fight sun-induced damage from both the UV and visible parts of the spectrum. The American Society of Photobiology and the American Academy of Dermatology have highlighted the importance of the use of adequate cloths, hats and eyewear to protect from UV radiation. Clothing photoprotection directly depends on thickness (thicker is usually better), color (reflective colors, such as white), moisture and tightness. Highly efficient photoprotective textiles are available, e.g. nylon made from BASF fibers, which has TiO2 particles embedded in the fabric. Also, some laundry products can endow or enhance photoprotection. For example, Rit Sun Guard® contains Tinosorb® FD, which is a UVA/UVB filter. Hats protect the scalp, forehead and neck, whereas gloves can prevent the appearance of lentigo on the hands, which has important cosmetic implications [7].

Solar erythema in the eyes often appears as "pink eye" (inflammation of the conjunctiva). In more severe cases, it can cause solar keratitis and irreversible damage to the vision [8, 9]. Chronic damage includes cataracts and macular degeneration [3, 4]. Interestingly, use of appropriate goggles significantly decreases the risk of these events. There are well-defined, FDA-approved parameters for sunglasses: less than 0.001% of photons between 200-320 nm are accepted through the protective material, whereas the percentage is <0.01 % for less damaging wavelengths (320-400 nm) [10].

2. Topical Sunscreens

Topical sunscreens include substances: 1) that reflect or scatter UV photons, 2) that absorb them, preventing their incidence on the cells of the skin acceptors; 3) substances with antioxidant properties. The main goals are to protect against UVB radiation [11] and long-wavelength UVA radiation [12]; scavenge ROS; activate cellular repair systems, including DNA repair (Table **1**).

Their activity is established according to their SPF (Sun Protection Factor), which is a measurement of their capability to stop UV photons: higher SPF means higher efficiency. A sunscreen SPF is usually measured using solar-simulated radiation (SSR) and a defined sunscreen application density (2 mg·cm^{-2}), and calculated according to the following formula:

$$\text{SPF} = \frac{\text{Minimal Erythema Dose (MED) with sunscreen}}{\text{MED without sunscreen}}$$

Other parameters utilized are: 1) Ery-PF (Erythema protection factor), which only takes into account the erythematous response after 24 hours; 2) PFA (Protection Against UVA), which is mainly used in the European Union; 3) Immune protection factor, for which there is no standardized protocol. One of the most utilized is the suppression of contact hypersensitivity by UV [13]. Additionally, sunscreens should (and some are) be tested for their antimutagenic and antioxidant properties.

Table 1. Main Photoprotector Groups

1. **Topical Photoprotective Agents**
   a) Physical blockers
      i) Zinc oxide (ZnO)
      ii) Titanium dioxide (TiO_2]
   b) Chemical and biological filtres
      i) Cinnamates
      ii) Benzophenones
         - Oxybenzone
         - Avobenzone
      iii) Mexoryl SX
      iv) Mexoryl XL
      v) Tinosorb M
      vi) Tinosorb S
   c) Antioxidants
      i) Hydroxycinnamic acids
      ii) Polyphenolics
         - Flavonoids
         - Green tea Extract
         - Astaxantin
      iii) Anthocyanins and tannins
      iv) Pycnogenol® (*French Maritime pinus* extract)
      v) Fernblock® (*Polypodium leucotomos* extract)
      vi) Others
         - Diydroxyacetone
         - Caffeine and caffeine sodium benzoate
         - Polygonum multiflorum thumb
         - N-(4-pyridoxylmethylene)-l-serine
         - Creatine
         - Idebenone
         - COX-2 inhibitors
         - DNA repair systems
           - Photolyase
           - T4 endonuclease
         - DNA oligonucleotides
         - AC-11

2) **Oral Photoprotective Agents**
   a) Vitamin derivatives
   b) Dietary animal and botanic extracts
      i) Genistein
      ii) ω3 polyunsaturated fatty acids
      iii) Fernblock® (*Polypodium leucotomos* extract)
      iv) Green teat polyphenols

High SPF sunscreens always contain a physical filter and at least two organic filters; one with optimal screening for UVB wavelengths and the other for UVA photons.

Topical sunscreens are presented as ointments, lotions, creams or sprays. Due to their ease of use, they are the most common photoprotective measure in environments of high exposure, e.g. seaside, mountain and countries with with low incidence of rain, e.g. countries in Oceania. Population studies have been conducted in some of these countries. For example, a study in Australia showed that consistent use of sunscreens (SPF ≥15) significantly reduced the occurrence of some types of skin cancers [14]. A major caveat of most of these studies is that they fail to address the long-term effect of sunscreens in preventing photoaging. A few studies are emerging on the use of sunscreens to prevent photoaging. An early clinical trial in humans showed that use of a sunscreen (SPF=29) for two years reduced photoaging [15]; recently, sunscreens containing Mexoryl SX were found to reduce wrinkle depth in long-term studies [16]. However, these studies need to be standardized for future use as a general screening for topical sunscreens and to avoid false claims on efficacy.

Components of Topical Sunscreens

- **Physical blockers**: Blocking agents are made of big particles (diameter is ~0.1-1 μm) that scatter, reflect or absorb solar radiation in the UV, visible and even infrared wavelengths. By far, the two most common physical blockers are zinc oxide (***ZnO***) and titanium dioxide (***TiO_2***). Microfine zinc oxide is a better blocker than titanium dioxide [17]. However, both components are somewhat photosensitive and can react with light, inhibiting their efficiency or even causing tissue damage [18]. In addition, microfine ZnO or TiO2 do not protect against visible light. To prevent this, both compounds are usually caged. The most common caging substances are dimethicone or silica [19]. Additional stabilizers include carnauba wax, which contains cinnamates that synergize with TiO_2 resulting in stable solutions that can hold SPF up to 50 [20-22].
- Filters (chemical or biological): These include:
    a) ***UVB filters***: They are efficient (90%) UVB blockers [23]. Cinnamates are frequently used in combination with other substances, e.g. salicylates, which are very stable and insoluble in water, which allows them to retain their properties once applied on the skin [24, 25]. Salicylates can also be used to dissolve other sunscreen ingredients, such as benzophenones [26].
    b) ***UVA Filters***: Most sunscreens protect well from UVB; however, these do not necessarily protect from UVA as well. Specific filters exist to absorb UVA photons, including oxybenzone (Bp-3; Eusolex 4360) and avobenzone (Parsol 1789) [23]. A major caveat is that these are easily oxidized and degraded.
    c) ***Dual UVB/ UVA filters***: Newer filters have been developed that can absorb both UVA and UVB. Some examples include the Mexoryl series. Mexoryl SX is the commercial name of terephthalylidene dicamphor sulfonic acid. This compound is quite stable, and frequently used together with avobenzone in broad-spectrum sunscreens [1]. Several studies suggest a significant effect for Mexoryl SX-based formulations in preventing several aspects of photoaging [16, 27, 28]. Mexoryl XL is drometrizol trisiloxane and it absorbs UVB and UVA2 radiation. Mexoryl XL synergizes with Mexoryl SX for enhanced photoprotection [28]. Other dual filters include Tinosorb M (methylene-bis-benzotriazolyl tetramethylbutylphenol), which is made of microfine, water-soluble organic particles [25]; Tinosorb S (bis-ethylhexyloxyphenol methoxyphenyl triazine), which is another high-molecular mass broadband sunscreen filter (280-380 nm) that can absorb and also reflect UV photons. It also synergizes with other blocking substances, such as OMC (2-ethylhexyl-4-methoxycinnamate) and avobenzone [29]. Different biophysical techniques have been used to improve the efficacy and applicability of these filters, e.g. their encapsulation in sol-gel glass silica microcapsules of ~1 μm diameter [30]. These approaches decrease penetration beyond the epidermis and immunogenicity and improve photostability.
- **Antioxidants**: Antioxidants are commonly included in commercial sunscreens to reduce the photo-oxidative damage that results from UV-induced ROS production. These include several well-characterized vitamins including vitamins C, E and β-carotene [31]. Other common substances are:
    - **Hydroxicinnamic acids,** e.g. caffeic or ferulic acids. They prevent UVB-induced erythema *in vivo* and *in vitro* [24], and decrease UV-induced oxidative damage in skin cells and lymphocytes [32-34].
    - ***Polyphenolics,*** e.g. flavonoids and phenolic acids. Several of them have antioxidant, antiinflammatory and antitumoral activities [35]. Several of these are used in sunscreens, including:
        - Flavonoids: they are vegetal isoflavones endowed with antioxidant and antitumoral properties [36, 37]. Genistein is a specific inhibitor of protein tyrosine kinases and a phytoestrogen that effectively blocks UVB induced erythema [38, 39], as well as PUVA-induced photodamage and molecular alterations in hairless mouse skin [40, 41]. It also bears antiphotocarcinogenic and antiphotoaging properties [39]. Silymarin is a plant flavonoid isolated from the seeds of milk thistle (*Silybum marianum).* It is a combination of of silybin, silydianin and silychristin that prevents ultraviolet light-induced immune suppression and oxidative stress in a mouse model [42]. Equol can be purified from red clover (*Trifolium pretense)* in its precursor form, daidzein [43], and also from *Punica granatum* [44]. Equol protects from UV erythema and may prevent photocarcinogenesis [45, 46] and photoaging [47]. Quercetin is a very potent antioxidant used to successfully inhibit UVB-induced skin damage in rodent models [48, 49]. Apigenin decreases UV-induced skin tumorigenesis and inhibits tumor cell growth *in vitro* [50, 51]. Its mechanism includes inhibition of UV-induced upregulation of COX-2 [52].

- *Green tea polyphenols (GTPP)* is used to refer to several potent antioxidants that appear in green tea leaves. The most abundant is epigallocatechin-3-gallate (EGCG). EGCG reduces lipid peroxidation induced by UVB, and also decreases UVA-induced skin damage and immunosupression [53]. EGCG inhibits activation of pro-inflammatory transcription factors such as AP-1 and NF-κB, collagenase expression and collagen cross-linking [54, 55]. Due to its intrinsic instability on skin, it needs to be mixed with butylated hydroxytoluene [56].
- *Resveratrol* is a polyphenolic phytoalexin present in several fruits, particularly grapes. Its topical use on hairless mice before UVB irradiation decreased erythema, ROS production and inflammation [57, 58]. Its effect on delaying UV-induced tumorigenesis has also been reported [59].
- *Astaxanthin* is a natural xantophilic pigment that sequesters ROS and thus inhibits accumulation of free polyamines induced by UVA [60]. It also attenuates the UVA-induced up-regulation of matrix metalloproteinases and elastase in human dermal fibroblasts [61].

- **Anthocyanins and tannins** are present in several fruits, e.g. grapes or pears, and are endowed with antioxidant and anti-inflammatory properties. Used topically, they protect against the adverse effects of UV radiation, inhibiting UVB-dependent activation of NF-κB, MAP kinase and COX-2 pathways downstream of the signaling kinases MKK4, MEK1, and Raf-1 [62, 63].
- **Pycnogenol®** is an extract of French maritime pine (*Pinus pinaster Ait*). It bears antioxidant, anti-inflammatory and anticarcinogenic properties. Pycnogenol prevents UV-induced erythema as well as longer-term effects, such as immunosuppression and tumor formation [64, 65]. It also possesses regenerative skin properties [66], and prevents UVB-induced photoaging [67].
- **Fernblock®** is an extract obtained from the fern *Polypodium leucotomos*. Topical application of *Polypodium leucotomos* extract (PL) inhibited UVB- and PUVA therapy-induced erythema *in vivo* [68]. PL is a potent antioxidant and has shown immunomodulating capability and inhibition of pro-inflammatory cytokines, such as TNF-α or IL-6 [69]. PL also inhibits the depletion of Langerhans cells induced by irradiation with UV light and PUVA therapy [68, 70, 71] and reduces chronic elastosis and matrix metalloprotease expression [72, 73].
- **Other photoprotective agents:** We include miscellanea of compounds that have been used in different skin formulations. Some are:

- **Dihydroxyacetone** is a photoprotective agent that provides SPF 3-4 and protects against UVA photons [74]. Its main drawback is that it tints the skin and rare cases of contact dermatitis have been reported [75].
- **Caffeine and caffeine sodium benzoate (SB)** inhibit UVB-induced apoptosis. Additional studies have shown that caffeine-SB strongly inhibited UVB-induced carcinogenesis [76].
- ***Polygonum multiflorum* thumb (PM)** is an extract that possesses antibacterial properties. PM decreases oxidative stress induced by UVB irradiation [77].
- **N-(4-pyridoxylmethylene)-L-serine (PYSer)** is an antioxidant that suppresses iron-catalyzed ROS generation, and has shown promise in the treatment of UVB-induced photoaging [78].
- **Creatine** is a metabolic reservoir of energy in the muscle. It has been suggested that boosting the energy metabolism in the skin may improve skin aging and photoaging [79]. Consistently, topical use of creatine has been shown to decrease UV-induced damage *in vitro* and *in vivo* [80], and postulates it use to fight photoaging [81].
- **Idebenone** is a synthetic analog of coenzyme Q10 [82, 83]. A clinical study using a compound based on idebenone has suggested its efficacy in preventing photoaging [84], but other studies have suggested otherwise [85, 86]. In addition, cases of contact dermatitis have been documented [87].
- **COX-2 inhibitors:** COX-2 (cyclooxygenase-2) is a metabolic enzyme linked to tumorigenesis and cancer progression. Consequently, COX-2 makes an excellent target for the development of antitumor drugs, which has turned out a bumpy road due to unforeseen side effects [88]. Regarding their topical use, celecoxib, a COX-2 inhibitor, has been shown to decrease UVB-mediated erythema, inflammation and prostaglandin E2 (PGE_2) production [89, 90]. It also inhibited UVB-induced papilloma formation [91] as well as the appearance of skin tumors after adoptive transfer of tumor cells [92].
- **DNA repair enzymes** constitute an emerging approach to enhance DNA repair after UV exposure. Some examples are:
- Photolyase is isolated from the cyanobacteria *Anacystis nidulans.* It promotes DNA repair and also decreases the number of UV-induced thymidine dimers [93, 94].
- T4 endonuclease has been assayed in patients with xeroderma pigmentosum [95, 96]. Treatment with a liposomal preparation of T4 endonuclease, T4N5, prevents sunburn and local

suppression of contact- and delayed-type hypersensitivy [95, 97].

- **DNA oligonucleotides** can enhance the cellular response to subsequent UV irradiation, regardless the existence of previous DNA damage [98]. The most commonly assayed are thymidine dinucleotides as well as homologues of the telomere 3-prime overhang sequence (T-oligos). The latter exhibited enhanced melanogenesis and increased DNA repair in response to UV irradiation [99].

- **AC-11 (C-Med-100)** is obtained from cat's claw (*Uncaria tomentosa*). It promotes DNA repair (8-hydroxyguanine and strand breaks) after UVB exposure. Possible mechanisms include enhanced base excision repair or an inherent antioxidant effect. A single-blind, right side-left side beach sun exposure pilot study described a significant decrease in erythema and blistering by application of 0.5% topical AC-11 with an SPF-15 sunscreen compared to application of SPF-15 sunscreen alone [100].

THE ROAD LESS TAKEN: ORAL PHOTOPROTECTIVE AGENTS

Oral photoprotection is a novel approach to skin care. Evidently, they cannot be used in lieu of topical sunscreens, as they do not prevent erythema but they complement their use by preventing photoaging and photocarcinogenesis. The amount of mechanistic information on their effects is still limited, but they are believed to increase the basal threshold of systemic antioxidant, actively collaborating in the refreshing of the skin natural antioxidant systems [101, 102]. Different active principles have been assayed for their oral photoprotective effect (Table **1**). These are:

- Vitamin derivatives: They include:

- **Carotenoids.** Lycopene is the major carotenoid present in tomatoes and a very efficient singlet oxygen quencher. Recent studies have suggested beneficial photoprotective effects [103]. Lutein and zeaxanthin are xanthophyllic carotenoids that exhibit a moderate photoprotective effect in combination with topical application [104].

- **Tocopherol** and **ascorbate** exhibit moderate oral photoprotective effect when used in combination [105]; interestingly, a combination of **lycopene, beta-carotene, alpha-tocopherol and selenium** yeast reduced UV-induced damage [106]. Other combinations include **Seresis®**, which contains carotenoids (β-carotene and lycopene), ascorbate, tocopherol, selenium yeast and proanthocyanidins. Oral use of Seresis® delays the onset of UVB-induced erythema and inhibits the expression of matrix metalloproteinases, postulating an effect on photoaging [107].

- **Dietary animal and botanical extracts:** Their composition is rather heterogenenous, but most contain dietary flavonoids and phenolics. Some examples include:

- **Genistein**, which can be used as a dietary complement as well as in topical formulations (see above). Oral genistein decreases UVB-induced skin photoaging and tumorigenesis in a rodent model [39], postulating its use as a natural cancer preventive [108].

- **ω-3 polyunsaturated fatty acids** are a popular dietary supplement obtained from fish oil. Regarding their use as oral skin photoprotectors, high doses have been shown to decrease UVB-induced erythema and inflammation [109].

- ***Polypodium leucotomos* extract (PL)** can also be administered orally with very low toxicity. In addition to its antioxidant properties, PL can exert immunomodulatory effects. Oral PL scavenges free radicals and reactive oxygen species such superoxide anion, singlet oxygen, hydroxyl radical and hydrogen peroxide, and prevents lipid peroxidation [110, 111]. Oral administration also induced photoprotection against UVB radiation and during PUVA therapy without significantly affecting the efficacy of the treatment [70, 71]. Supplementation with PL significantly decreased erythema and depletion of Langerhans cells [70, 71]. PL also prevents oxidative DNA damage (8-hydroxyguanine) and accelerates repair of thymine dimers [71, 112]. In addition, it also inhibited *trans*-urocanic acid photo-induced isomerization and inactivation [113]. Analysis of its *in vivo* and *in vitro* protective effects have revealed several molecular mechanisms of action [68, 114, 115], including abrogation of UV-induced TNF-α and nitric oxide (NO) production [116]; potentiation of the endogenous antioxidant response [117]; inhibition of photoimmunosupression [118]; and modulation of the inflammatory response [112]. A recent study notes that oral administration reduces UVA-induced cyclobutane pyrimidine dimer deletions and mitochondrial DNA damage [119].

- **Green tea polyphenols (GTPPs)**, e.g. epigallocatechin-3-gallate (EGCG). Oral use of EGCG prevents UV-induced skin tumorigenesis in mice. Several mechanisms underlie this effect, e.g. induction of interleukin 12, which prevents immunosupression and boosts DNA repair through excision repair mechanisms dependent; inhibition of angiogenic factors and stimulation of T cell-dependent cytotoxicity and tumor cell clearance [120]. Oral GTPPs can also decrease UV-induced expression of skin matrix metalloproteinases, postulating an effect in photoaging [121].

CONCLUDING REMARKS AND FUTURE PERSPECTIVES

This review offers a non-comprehensive account of several compounds with proven effect in photoprotection. Most of the topical compounds used topically are well proven tools to prevent erythema and the acute deleterious effects of UV exposure; However, the jury is still out regarding their efficacy in preventing chronic damage and photoaging. On the other hand, oral photoprotectives exert often modest effects. It is necessary to mention that they are not meant to be silver bullets in photoprotection, i.e. they cannot and are not intended to substitute sunscreens or to increase the threshold of what is considered healthy exposure to the sun. It is the general consensus that they are intended to fight the long term effects of UV exposure, particularly photoaging and skin tumorigenesis. Future studies will undoubtedly reveal the complementary effect of topical and oral photoprotection.

The mechanisms of photoprotection of most of these compounds are not fully defined yet; most of them are based on powerful antioxidant activities; others promote regeneration through yet-unknown mechanisms, making this an active and attractive field for basic and clinical research. Therefore, further clinical trials will be required to validate the preventive and therapeutic value of these products. In summary, oral sunscreens have a demonstrated therapeutic value in the prevention and treatment of sun damage, and are likely in their way to become a mainstream method of protection that complements traditional screening methods.

ACKNOWLEDGMENTS

Salvador Gonzalez is a consultant for Industrial Farmaceutica Cantabria (IFC), which supports some of the studies reviewed in this article. This work has been partially supported by a grant from the Carlos III Health Institute, Ministry of Science and Innovation, Spain (PS09/01099).

REFERENCES

[1] Seite S, Colige A, Piquemal-Vivenot P, *et al.* A full-UV spectrum absorbing daily use cream protects human skin against biological changes occurring in photoaging. Photodermatol Photoimmunol Photomed 2000; 16(4): 147-55.

[2] Moyal D. Immunosuppression induced by chronic ultraviolet irradiation in humans and its prevention by sunscreens. Eur J Dermatol 1998; 8(3): 209-11.

[3] van der Pols JC, Xu C, Boyle GM, Parsons PG, Whiteman DC, Green AC. Expression of p53 tumor suppressor protein in sun-exposed skin and associations with sunscreen use and time spent outdoors: a community-based study. Am J Epidemiol 2006; 163(11): 982-8.

[4] Al Mahroos M, Yaar M, Phillips TJ, Bhawan J, Gilchrest BA. Effect of sunscreen application on UV-induced thymine dimers. Arch Dermatol 2002; 138(11): 1480-5.

[5] Bernerd F, Vioux C, Asselineau D. Evaluation of the protective effect of sunscreens on *in vitro* reconstructed human skin exposed to UVB or UVA irradiation. Photochem Photobiol 2000; 71(3): 314-20.

[6] Kaye ET, Levin JA, Blank IH, Arndt KA, Anderson RR. Efficiency of opaque photoprotective agents in the visible light range. Arch Dermatol 1991; 127(3): 351-5.

[7] Menter JM, Hatch KL. Clothing as solar radiation protection. Curr Probl Dermatol 2003; 31: 50-63.

[8] Cullen AP. Photokeratitis and other phototoxic effects on the cornea and conjunctiva. Int J Toxicol 2002; 21(6): 455-64.

[9] Young RW. The family of sunlight-related eye diseases. Optom Vis Sci 1994; 71(2): 125-44.

[10] Dain SJ. Sunglasses and sunglass standards. Clin Exp Optom 2003; 86(2): 77-90.

[11] Sano T, Kume T, Fujimura T, Kawada H, Moriwaki S, Takema Y. The formation of wrinkles caused by transition of keratin intermediate filaments after repetitive UVB exposure. Arch Dermatol Res 2005; 296(8): 359-65.

[12] Krutmann J. Ultraviolet A radiation-induced biological effects in human skin: relevance for photoaging and photodermatosis. J Dermatol Sci 2000; 23 Suppl 1: S22-6.

[13] Young AR. Methods used to evaluate the immune protection factor of a sunscreen: advantages and disadvantages of different *in vivo* techniques. Cutis 2004; 74(5 Suppl): 19-23.

[14] Neale R, Williams G, Green A. Application patterns among participants randomized to daily sunscreen use in a skin cancer prevention trial. Arch Dermatol 2002; 138(10): 1319-25.

[15] Boyd AS, Naylor M, Cameron GS, Pearse AD, Gaskell SA, Neldner KH. The effects of chronic sunscreen use on the histologic changes of dermatoheliosis. J Am Acad Dermatol 1995; 33(6): 941-6.

[16] Fourtanier A, Moyal D, Seite S. Sunscreens containing the broad-spectrum UVA absorber, Mexoryl SX, prevent the cutaneous detrimental effects of UV exposure: a review of clinical study results. Photodermatol Photoimmunol Photomed 2008; 24(4): 164-74.

[17] Pinnell SR, Fairhurst D, Gillies R, Mitchnick MA, Kollias N. Microfine zinc oxide is a superior sunscreen ingredient to microfine titanium dioxide. Dermatol Surg 2000; 26(4): 309-14.

[18] Wamer WG, Yin JJ, Wei RR. Oxidative damage to nucleic acids photosensitized by titanium dioxide. Free Radic Biol Med 1997; 23(6): 851-8.

[19] Van Reeth I. Beyond skin feel: innovative methods for developing complex sensory profiles with silicones. J Cosmet Dermatol 2006; 5(1): 61-7.

[20] Villalobos-Hernandez JR, Muller-Goymann CC. Novel nanoparticulate carrier system based on carnauba wax and decyl oleate for the dispersion of inorganic sunscreens in aqueous media. Eur J Pharm Biopharm 2005; 60(1): 113-22.

[21] Villalobos-Hernandez JR, Muller-Goymann CC. Sun protection enhancement of titanium dioxide crystals by the use of carnauba wax nanoparticles: the synergistic interaction between organic and inorganic sunscreens at nanoscale. Int J Pharm 2006; 322(1-2): 161-70.

[22] Villalobos-Hernandez JR, Muller-Goymann CC. *In vitro* erythemal UV-A protection factors of inorganic sunscreens distributed in aqueous media using carnauba wax-decyl oleate nanoparticles. Eur J Pharm Biopharm 2007; 65(1): 122-5.

[23] Lowe NJ. An overview of ultraviolet radiation, sunscreens, and photo-induced dermatoses. Dermatol Clin 2006; 24(1): 9-17.

[24] Saija A, Tomaino A, Trombetta D, De Pasquale A, Uccella N, Barbuzzi T, *et al.* *In vitro* and *in vivo* evaluation of caffeic and ferulic acids as topical photoprotective agents. Int J Pharm 2000; 199(1): 39-47.

[25] Kullavanijaya P, Lim HW. Photoprotection. J Am Acad Dermatol 2005; 52(6): 937-58; quiz 959-62.

[26] Chatelain E, Gabard B, Surber C. Skin penetration and sun protection factor of five UV filters: effect of the vehicle. Skin Pharmacol Appl Skin Physiol 2003; 16(1): 28-35.

[27] Seite S, Moyal D, Richard S, de Rigal J, Leveque JL, Hourseau C, *et al.* Mexoryl SX: a broad absorption UVA filter protects human skin from the effects of repeated suberythemal doses of UVA. J Photochem Photobiol B 1998; 44(1): 69-76.

[28] Moyal D. Prevention of ultraviolet-induced skin pigmentation. Photodermatol Photoimmunol Photomed 2004; 20(5): 243-7.

[29] Chatelain E, Gabard B. Photostabilization of butyl methoxydibenzoylmethane (Avobenzone) and ethylhexyl methoxycinnamate by bis-ethylhexyloxyphenol methoxyphenyl triazine (Tinosorb S), a new UV broadband filter. Photochem Photobiol 2001; 74(3): 401-6.

[30] Lapidot N, Gans O, Biagini F, Sosonkin L, Rottman C. Advanced sunscreens: UV absorbers encapsulated in sol-gel glass microcapsules. J Sol-Gel Sci Technol 2003; 26: 67-72.

[31] Pinnell SR. Cutaneous photodamage, oxidative stress, and topical antioxidant protection. J Am Acad Dermatol 2003; 48(1): 1-19; quiz 20-2.

[32] Prasad NR, Jeyanthimala K, Ramachandran S. Caffeic acid modulates ultraviolet radiation-B induced oxidative damage in human blood lymphocytes. J Photochem Photobiol B 2009; 95(3): 196-203.

[33] Di Domenico F, Perluigi M, Foppoli C, Blarzino C, Coccia R, De Marco F, *et al.* Protective effect of ferulic acid ethyl ester against oxidative stress mediated by UVB irradiation in human epidermal melanocytes. Free Radic Res 2009; 43(4): 365-75.

[34] Kang NJ, Lee KW, Shin BJ, *et al.* Caffeic acid, a phenolic phytochemical in coffee, directly inhibits Fyn kinase activity and UVB-induced COX-2 expression. Carcinogenesis 2009; 30(2): 321-30.

[35] Lambert JD, Hong J, Yang GY, Liao J, Yang CS. Inhibition of carcinogenesis by polyphenols: evidence from laboratory investigations. Am J Clin Nutr 2005; 81(1 Suppl): 284S-291S.

[36] Cazarolli LH, Zanatta L, Alberton EH, Figueiredo MS, Folador P, Damazio RG, *et al.* Flavonoids: prospective drug candidates. Mini Rev Med Chem 2008; 8(13): 1429-40.

[37] Dinkova-Kostova AT. Phytochemicals as protectors against ultraviolet radiation: versatility of effects and mechanisms. Planta Med 2008; 74(13): 1548-59.

[38] Afaq F, Mukhtar H. Botanical antioxidants in the prevention of photocarcinogenesis and photoaging. Exp Dermatol 2006; 15(9): 678-684.

[39] Wei H, Saladi R, Lu Y, *et al.* Isoflavone genistein: photoprotection and clinical implications in dermatology. J Nutr 2003; 133(11 Suppl 1): 3811S-3819S.

[40] Liu Z, Lu Y, Lebwohl M, Wei H. PUVA (8-methoxy-psoralen plus ultraviolet A) induces the formation of 8-hydroxy-2'-deoxyguanosine and DNA fragmentation in calf thymus DNA and human epidermoid carcinoma cells. Free Radic Biol Med 1999; 27(1-2): 127-33.

[41] Shyong EQ, Lu Y, Lazinsky A, Saladi RN, Phelps RG, Austin LM, *et al.* Effects of the isoflavone 4',5,7-trihydroxyisoflavone (genistein) on psoralen plus ultraviolet A radiation (PUVA)-induced photodamage. Carcinogenesis 2002; 23(2): 317-21.

[42] Katiyar SK. Treatment of silymarin, a plant flavonoid, prevents ultraviolet light-induced immune suppression and oxidative stress in mouse skin. Int J Oncol 2002; 21(6): 1213-22.

[43] Widyarini S, Spinks N, Husband AJ, Reeve VE. Isoflavonoid compounds from red clover (Trifolium pratense) protect from inflammation and immune suppression induced by UV radiation. Photochem Photobiol 2001; 74(3): 465-70.

[44] Park HM, Moon E, Kim AJ, *et al.* Extract of Punica granatum inhibits skin photoaging induced by UVB irradiation. Int J Dermatol 2010; 49(3): 276-82.

[45] Lin JY, Tournas JA, Burch JA, Monteiro-Riviere NA, Zielinski J. Topical isoflavones provide effective photoprotection to skin. Photodermatol Photoimmunol Photomed 2008; 24(2): 61-6.

[46] Widyarini S, Husband AJ, Reeve VE. Protective effect of the isoflavonoid equol against hairless mouse skin carcinogenesis induced by UV radiation alone or with a chemical cocarcinogen. Photochem Photobiol 2005; 81(1): 32-7.

[47] Reeve VE, Widyarini S, Domanski D, Chew E, Barnes K. Protection against photoaging in the hairless mouse by the isoflavone equol. Photochem Photobiol 2005; 81(6): 1548-53.

[48] Casagrande R, Georgetti SR, Verri WA Jr, Dorta DJ, dos Santos AC, Fonseca MJ. Protective effect of topical formulations containing quercetin against UVB-induced oxidative stress in hairless mice. J Photochem Photobiol B 2006; 84(1): 21-7.

[49] Vicentini FT, Simi TR, Del Ciampo JO, *et al.* Quercetin in w/o microemulsion: *in vitro* and *in vivo* skin penetration and efficacy against UVB-induced skin damages evaluated *in vivo*. Eur J Pharm Biopharm 2008; 69(3): 948-57.

[50] Wei H, Tye L, Bresnick E, Birt DF. Inhibitory effect of apigenin, a plant flavonoid, on epidermal ornithine decarboxylase and skin tumor promotion in mice. Cancer Res 1990; 50(3): 499-502.

[51] Wang W, Heideman L, Chung CS, Pelling JC, Koehler KJ, Birt DF. Cell-cycle arrest at G2/M and growth inhibition by apigenin in human colon carcinoma cell lines. Mol Carcinog 2000; 28(2): 102-10.

[52] Tong X, Van Dross RT, Abu-Yousif A, Morrison AR, Pelling JC. Apigenin prevents UVB-induced cyclooxygenase 2 expression: coupled mRNA stabilization and translational inhibition. Mol Cell Biol 2007; 27(1): 283-96.

[53] Katiyar SK, Vaid M, van Steeg H, Meeran SM. Green Tea Polyphenols Prevent UV-Induced Immunosuppression by Rapid Repair of DNA Damage and Enhancement of Nucleotide Excision Repair Genes. Cancer Prev Res (Phila Pa) 2010.

[54] Rutter K, Sell DR, Fraser N, *et al.* Green tea extract suppresses the age-related increase in collagen crosslinking and fluorescent products in C57BL/6 mice. Int J Vitam Nutr Res 2003; 73(6): 453-60.

[55] Xia J, Song X, Bi Z, Chu W, Wan Y. UV-induced NF-kappaB activation and expression of IL-6 is attenuated by (-)-epigallocatechin-3-gallate in cultured human keratinocytes *in vitro*. Int J Mol Med 2005; 16(5): 943-50.

[56] Dvorakova K, Dorr RT, Valcic S, Timmermann B, Alberts DS. Pharmacokinetics of the green tea derivative, EGCG, by the topical route of administration in mouse and human skin. Cancer Chemother Pharmacol 1999; 43(4): 331-5.

[57] Afaq F, Adhami VM, Ahmad N. Prevention of short-term ultraviolet B radiation-mediated damages by resveratrol in SKH-1 hairless mice. Toxicol Appl Pharmacol 2003; 186(1): 28-37.

[58] Nichols JA, Katiyar SK. Skin photoprotection by natural polyphenols: anti-inflammatory, antioxidant and DNA repair mechanisms. Arch Dermatol Res 2010; 302(2): 71-83.

[59] Aziz MH, Reagan-Shaw S, Wu J, Longley BJ, Ahmad N. Chemoprevention of skin cancer by grape constituent resveratrol: relevance to human disease? Faseb J 2005; 19(9): 1193-5.

[60] Goto S, Kogure K, Abe K, Kimata Y, Kitahama K, Yamashita E, *et al.* Efficient radical trapping at the surface and inside the phospholipid membrane is responsible for highly potent antiperoxidative activity of the carotenoid astaxanthin. Biochim Biophys Acta 2001; 1512(2): 251-8.

[61] Suganuma K, Nakajima H, Ohtsuki M, Imokawa G. Astaxanthin attenuates the UVA-induced up-regulation of matrix-metalloproteinase-1 and skin fibroblast elastase in human dermal fibroblasts. J Dermatol Sci 2010; 58(2): 136-42.

[62] Kwon JY, Lee KW, Kim JE, *et al.* Delphinidin suppresses ultraviolet B-induced cyclooxygenases-2 expression through inhibition of MAPKK4 and PI-3 kinase. Carcinogenesis 2009; 30(11): 1932-40.

[63] Kim JE, Kwon JY, Seo SK, *et al.* Cyanidin suppresses ultraviolet B-induced COX-2 expression in epidermal cells by targeting MKK4, MEK1, and Raf-1. Biochem Pharmacol 2010; 79(10): 1473-82.

[64] Saliou C, Rimbach G, Moini H, *et al.* Solar ultraviolet-induced erythema in human skin and nuclear factor-kappa-B-dependent gene expression in keratinocytes are modulated by a French maritime pine bark extract. Free Radic Biol Med 2001; 30(2): 154-60.

[65] Bito T, Roy S, Sen CK, Packer L. Pine bark extract pycnogenol downregulates IFN-gamma-induced adhesion of T cells to human keratinocytes by inhibiting inducible ICAM-1 expression. Free Radic Biol Med 2000; 28(2): 219-27.

[66] Sime S, Reeve VE. Protection from inflammation, immunosuppression and carcinogenesis induced by UV radiation in mice by topical Pycnogenol. Photochem Photobiol 2004; 79(2): 193-8.

[67] Cho HS, Lee MH, Lee JW, *et al.* Anti-wrinkling effects of the mixture of vitamin C, vitamin E, pycnogenol and evening primrose oil, and molecular mechanisms on hairless mouse skin caused by chronic ultraviolet B irradiation. Photodermatol Photoimmunol Photomed 2007; 23(5): 155-62.

[68] Gonzalez S, Pathak MA, Cuevas J, Villarubia VG, Fitzpatrick TB. Topical or oral administration with an extract of *Polypodium leucotomos* prevents acute sunburn and psolaren-induced phototoxic reactions as well as depletion of Langerhans cells in human skin. Photodermatol. Photoimmunol Photomed 1997; 13: 50-60.

[69] Brieva A, Guerrero A, Pivel JP. Immunomodulatory properties of an hydrophilic extract of *Polypodium leucotomos*. Inflammopharmacol 2002; 9: 361-371.

[70] Middelkamp-Hup MA, Pathak MA, Parrado C, *et al.* Orally administered Polypodium leucotomos extract decreases psoralen-UVA-induced phototoxicity, pigmentation, and damage of human skin. J. Am. Acad. Dermatol. 2004; 50(1): 41-49.

[71] Middelkamp-Hup MA, Pathak MA, Parrado C, Goukassian D, Rius-Diaz F, Mihm MC, *et al.* Oral Polypodium leucotomos extract decreases ultraviolet-induced damage of human skin. J Am Acad Dermatol 2004; 51(6): 910-918.

[72] Alcaraz MV, Pathak MA, Rius F, Kollias N, González S. An extract of *Polypodium leucotomos* appears to minimize certain photoaging changes in a hairless albino mouse animal model. Photodermatol. Photoimmunol Photomed 1999; 15: 120-126.

[73] Philips N, Conte J, Chen YJ, Natrajan P, Taw M, Keller T, *et al.* Beneficial regulation of matrixmetalloproteinases and their inhibitors, fibrillar collagens and transforming growth factor-beta

by Polypodium leucotomos, directly or in dermal fibroblasts, ultraviolet radiated fibroblasts, and melanoma cells. Arch Dermatol Res 2009; 301(7): 487-495.

[74] Draelos ZD. Self-tanning lotions: are they a healthy way to achieve a tan? Am J Clin Dermatol 2002; 3(5): 317-8.

[75] Morren M, Dooms-Goossens A, Heidbuchel M, Sente F, Damas MC. Contact allergy to dihydroxyacetone. Contact Dermatitis 1991; 25(5): 326-7.

[76] Lu YP, Lou YR, Xie JG, *et al.* Caffeine and caffeine sodium benzoate have a sunscreen effect, enhance UVB-induced apoptosis, and inhibit UVB-induced skin carcinogenesis in SKH-1 mice. Carcinogenesis 2007; 28(1): 199-206.

[77] Hwang IK, Yoo KY, Kim DW, *et al.* An extract of Polygonum multiflorum protects against free radical damage induced by ultraviolet B irradiation of the skin. Braz J Med Biol Res 2006; 39(9): 1181-8.

[78] Kitazawa M, Ishitsuka Y, Kobayashi M, *et al.* Protective effects of an antioxidant derived from serine and vitamin B6 on skin photoaging in hairless mice. Photochem Photobiol 2005; 81(4): 970-4.

[79] Blatt T, Lenz H, Koop U, *et al.* Stimulation of skin's energy metabolism provides multiple benefits for mature human skin. Biofactors 2005; 25(1-4): 179-85.

[80] Lenz H, Schmidt M, Welge V, *et al.* The creatine kinase system in human skin: protective effects of creatine against oxidative and UV damage *in vitro* and *in vivo*. J Invest Dermatol 2005; 124(2): 443-52.

[81] Knott A, Koop U, Mielke H, *et al.* A novel treatment option for photoaged skin. J Cosmet Dermatol 2008; 7(1): 15-22.

[82] Farris P. Idebenone, green tea, and Coffeeberry extract: new and innovative antioxidants. Dermatol Ther 2007; 20(5): 322-9.

[83] Dong KK, Damaghi N, Kibitel J, Canning MT, Smiles KA, Yarosh DB. A comparison of the relative antioxidant potency of L-ergothioneine and idebenone. J Cosmet Dermatol 2007; 6(3): 183-8.

[84] McDaniel D, Neudecker B, Dinardo J, Lewis J, 2nd, Maibach H. Clinical efficacy assessment in photodamaged skin of 0.5% and 1.0% idebenone. J Cosmet Dermatol 2005; 4(3): 167-73.

[85] Tournas JA, Lin FH, Burch JA, *et al.* Ubiquinone, idebenone, and kinetin provide ineffective photoprotection to skin when compared to a topical antioxidant combination of vitamins C and E with ferulic acid. J Invest Dermatol 2006; 126(5): 1185-7.

[86] Bruce S. Cosmeceuticals for the attenuation of extrinsic and intrinsic dermal aging. J Drugs Dermatol 2008; 7(2 Suppl): s17-22.

[87] Mc Aleer MA, Collins P. Allergic contact dermatitis to hydroxydecyl ubiquinone (idebenone) following application of anti-ageing cosmetic cream. Contact Dermatitis 2008; 59(3): 178-9.

[88] Psaty BM, Furberg CD. COX-2 inhibitors--lessons in drug safety. N Engl J Med 2005; 352(11): 1133-5.

[89] Fischer SM, Lo HH, Gordon GB, Seibert K, Kelloff G, Lubet RA, *et al.* Chemopreventive activity of celecoxib, a specific cyclooxygenase-2 inhibitor, and indomethacin against ultraviolet light-induced skin carcinogenesis. Mol Carcinog 1999; 25(4): 231-240.

[90] Zhan H, Zheng H. The role of topical cyclo-oxygenase-2 inhibitors in skin cancer: treatment and prevention. Am J Clin Dermatol 2007; 8(4): 195-200.

[91] Wilgus TA, Koki AT, Zweifel BS, Kusewitt DF, Rubal PA, Oberyszyn TM. Inhibition of cutaneous ultraviolet light B-mediated inflammation and tumor formation with topical celecoxib treatment. Mol Carcinog 2003; 38(2): 49-58.

[92] Fegn L, Wang Z. Topical chemoprevention of skin cancer in mice, using combined inhibitors of 5-lipoxygenase and cyclo-oxygenase-2. J Laryngol Otol 2009; 123(8): 880-4.

[93] Stege H, Roza L, Vink AA, Grewe M, Ruzicka T, Grether-Beck S, *et al.* Enzyme plus light therapy to repair DNA damage in ultraviolet-B-irradiated human skin. Proc Natl Acad Sci USA 2000; 97(4): 1790-5.

[94] Essen LO, Klar T. Light-driven DNA repair by photolyases. Cell Mol Life Sci 2006; 63(11): 1266-77.

[95] Yarosh D, Klein J, O'Connor A, Hawk J, Rafal E, Wolf P. Effect of topically applied T4 endonuclease V in liposomes on skin cancer in xeroderma pigmentosum: a randomised study. Xeroderma Pigmentosum Study Group. Lancet 2001; 357(9260): 926-9.

[96] Zahid S, Brownell I. Repairing DNA damage in xeroderma pigmentosum: T4N5 lotion and gene therapy. J Drugs Dermatol 2008; 7(4): 405-8.

[97] Cafardi JA, Elmets CA. T4 endonuclease V: review and application to dermatology. Expert Opin Biol Ther 2008; 8(6): 829-38.

[98] Goukassian DA, Helms E, van Steeg H, van Oostrom C, Bhawan J, Gilchrest BA. Topical DNA oligonucleotide therapy reduces UV-induced mutations and photocarcinogenesis in hairless mice. Proc Natl Acad Sci USA 2004; 101(11): 3933-8.

[99] Arad S, Konnikov N, Goukassian DA, Gilchrest BA. T-oligos augment UV-induced protective responses in human skin. Faseb J 2006; 20(11): 1895-7.

[100] Emanuel P, Scheinfeld N. A review of DNA repair and possible DNA-repair adjuvants and selected natural anti-oxidants. Dermatol Online J 2007; 13(3): 10.

[101] Pattison DI, Davies MJ. Actions of ultraviolet light on cellular structures. Exs 2006(96): 131-57.

[102] DeBuys HV, Levy SB, Murray JC, Madey DL, Pinnell SR. Modern approaches to photoprotection. Dermatol Clin 2000; 18(4): 577-90.

[103] Stahl W, Heinrich U, Aust O, Tronnier H, Sies H. Lycopene-rich products and dietary photoprotection. Photochem Photobiol Sci 2006; 5(2): 238-42.

[104] Palombo P, Fabrizi G, Ruocco V, *et al.* Beneficial long-term effects of combined oral/topical antioxidant treatment with the carotenoids lutein and zeaxanthin on human skin: a double-blind, placebo-controlled study. Skin Pharmacol Physiol 2007; 20(4): 199-210.

[105] Eberlein-Konig B, Ring J. Relevance of vitamins C and E in cutaneous photoprotection. J Cosmet Dermatol 2005; 4(1): 4-9.

[106] Cesarini JP, Michel L, Maurette JM, Adhoute H, Bejot M. Immediate effects of UV radiation on the skin: modification by an antioxidant complex containing carotenoids. Photodermatol Photoimmunol Photomed 2003; 19(4): 182-9.

[107] Greul AK, Grundmann JU, Heinrich F, Pfitzner I, Bernhardt J, Ambach A, *et al.* Photoprotection of UV-irradiated human skin: an antioxidative combination of vitamins E and C, carotenoids, selenium and proanthocyanidins. Skin Pharmacol Appl Skin Physiol 2002; 15(5): 307-15.

[108] Gullett NP, Ruhul Amin AR, *et al.* Cancer prevention with natural compounds. Semin Oncol 2010; 37(3): 258-81.

[109] Rhodes LE, O'Farrell S, Jackson MJ, Friedmann PS. Dietary fish-oil supplementation in humans reduces UVB-erythemal sensitivity but increases epidermal lipid peroxidation. J Invest Dermatol 1994; 103(2): 151-4.

[110] Gonzalez S, Pathak MA. Inhibition of ultraviolet-induced formation of reactive oxygen species, lipid peroxidation, erythema and skin photosensitization by *Polypodium leucotomos*. Photodermatol Photoimmunol Photomed 1996; 12: 45-56.

[111] Gomes AJ, Lunardi CN, Gonzalez S, Tedesco AC. The antioxidant action of Polypodium leucotomos extract and kojic acid: reactions with reactive oxygen species. Braz J Med Biol Res 2001; 34(11): 1487-1494.

[112] Zattra E, Coleman C, Arad S, *et al.* Oral Polypodium leucotomos decreases UV-induced Cox-2 expression, inflammation, and enhances DNA repair in Xpc +/- mice. Am J Pathol 2009; 175: 1952-1961.

[113] Capote R, Alonso-Lebrero JL, Garcia F, Brieva A, Pivel JP, Gonzalez S. Polypodium leucotomos extract inhibits trans-urocanic acid photoisomerization and photodecomposition. J Photochem Photobiol B 2006; 82(3): 173-9.

[114] Gonzalez S, Joshi PC, Pathak MA. *Polypodium leucotomos* extract as an antioxidant agent in the therapy of skin disorders. J Invest Dermatol 1994; 102: 651-659.

[115] Alonso-Lebrero JL, Domínguez-Jiménez C, Tejedor R, Brieva A, Pivel JP. Photoprotective properties of a hydrophilic extract of the fern *Polypodium leucotomos* on human skin cells. J Photochem Photobiol B 2003; 70: 31-37.

[116] Janczyk A, Garcia-Lopez MA, Fernandez-Penas P, *et al.* A Polypodium leucotomos extract inhibits solar-simulated radiation-induced TNF-alpha and iNOS expression, transcriptional activation and apoptosis. Exp Dermatol 2007; 16(10): 823-829.

[117] Mulero M, Rodriguez-Yanes E, Nogues MR, *et al.* Polypodium leucotomos extract inhibits glutathione oxidation and prevents Langerhans cell depletion induced by UVB/UVA radiation in a hairless rat model. Exp Dermatol 2008; 17: 653-658.

[118] Siscovick JR, Zapolanski T, Magro C, *et al.* Polypodium leucotomos inhibits ultraviolet B radiation-induced immunosuppression. Photodermatol. Photoimm-unol. Photomed 2008; 24(3): 134-141.

[119] Villa A, Viera MH, Amini S, *et al.* Decrease of ultraviolet A light-induced "common deletion" in healthy volunteers after oral Polypodium leucotomos extract supplement in a randomized clinical trial. J Am Acad Dermatol 2010; 62(3): 511-3.

[120] Katiyar S, Elmets CA, Katiyar SK. Green tea and skin cancer: photoimmunology, angiogenesis and DNA repair. J Nutr Biochem 2007; 18(5): 287-96.

[121] Vayalil PK, Mittal A, Hara Y, Elmets CA, Katiyar SK. Green tea polyphenols prevent ultraviolet light-induced oxidative damage and matrix metalloproteinases expression in mouse skin. J Invest Dermatol 2004; 122(6): 1480-7.

6

Skin Care Habits of Dermatology Patients in Yaounde, Cameroon

Anne Cécile Zoung-Kanyi Bissek[1], Guillaume Chaby[2], Earnest N. Tabah[1], Emmanuel Kouotou[1], Julius Y. Fonsah[1], Catherine Lok[2], Alfred K. Njamnshi[*,1], Paul Koueke[1] and Walinjom F.T. Muna[1]

[1]*Department of Internal Medicine and Specialties (Dermatology & Neurology Units), Faculty of Medicine & Biomedical Sciences, University of Yaoundé I, Yaoundé, Cameroon*

[2]*Centre Hospitalier Universitaire, Amiens Sud, France*

Abstract: *Introduction*: Black and satinee skin has been a beauty quality in our environment. Then bleaching became very popular in our communities but not much is known about skin habits. The objective of this study was to identify skin care habits of patients in Yaoundé.

Patients and Methods: This study took place in the dermatology clinic of the Yaounde General Hospital, including all patients seen from October 2001 to September 2002. The skin care habits were compared with respect to sex and age. The level of statistical significance was $p < 5\%$.

Results: During the study period, 714 medical files (418 females and 296 males) were reviewed. In men as well as in women, *savon de Marseille* and antiseptic soap were respectively the first and second most used bathing soaps. However, women had a statistically significant preference for bleaching, super fat and exfoliative soaps (78.0% *vs* 22.0%, 69.0% *vs* 31.0%, 87.0% *vs* 13.0%) with respect to men. Users of antiseptic soaps had eczemas (35%). Only 16.0% of women did not apply daily body lotions as against 84% of men ($p = 0.0001$). The use of bleaching lotion (13% overall) was clearly more widespread in women than in men (87.0% *vs* 13.0%; $p = 0.0001$). The use of topical corticosteroids was associated with acne.

Conclusion: A relatively high proportion of our patients use bleaching products and antiseptic soaps. The use of antiseptic soaps and the additional of topical steroids in commercial preparations may become a serious health problem if left uncontrolled.

Keywords: Skin care, black, bleaching.

INTRODUCTION

Black, bright and satinee skin used to be a beauty criterion in our environment. Smith *et al.* declare in an article on hair and skin care in black children, that the skin and hair that were well appreciated before the time of slavery had lost their value after the contact with the whites [1]. Progressively, the desire for skin bleaching by African Americans in the USA and later in African populations became widespread throughout the black population, reaching prevalences of 80% in some African towns [1-3]. Skin bleaching then became a sign of well being for those who practiced it.

Bleaching has thus become a very popular practice in several communities, in spite of its many well known side effects. Besides skin bleaching, other habits which appear to be less dangerous should equally be of interest to health practitioners in our context in order to promote good cosmetologic practices. The objective of this work was to identify the different skin care habits of patients received at the dermatology outpatient clinic in the Yaoundé General Hospital.

*Address correspondence to this author at the Department of Internal Medicine (Dermatology & Neurology Units), Faculty of Medicine & Biomedical Sciences, University of Yaoundé I, Yaoundé, Cameroon; E-mail: aknjamnshi@yahoo.co.uk

PATIENTS AND METHODS

The survey was done at the Yaoundé General Hospital. We reviewed 714 files of all patients consecutively received at the dermatology outpatient consultation either on appointment or as an emergency, during the period from October 2001 to September 2002. The main inclusion criterion was any patient presenting with a skin problem at the dermatology outpatient clinic, irrespective of age or sex. The dermatology service of the Yaoundé General Hospital is one of the main departments of the teaching hospitals of Yaoundé, and has had a consultant dermatologist since 1999. All patients in this department were seen by the same dermatologist and data were systematically collected irrespective of the main complaint. The pathologic conditions observed were recorded according to the following groups: allergies, scars, systemic diseases, infections, sexually transmissible disease (STD) syndromes (genital ulceration, urethral discharge, vaginal discharge, scrotal swelling, lower abdominal pains), HIV infection, lichenification, disorders of epidermal appendages, disorders of epidermal differentiation, pigmentation disorders, tumours and others. The following variables were extracted from the case files for analysis: chief presenting complaint, sociodemographic data (age, sex), cosmotologic history (nature of body lotions and bathing soaps used on a daily basis). Any soap or body lotion prescribed during the medical consultation was considered as an integral part of the treatment and were thus not included as habitual use in the analysis.

The pharmacological composition of the soaps and body lotions was not taken into consideration for this study. Information collected from patients and vendors of cosmetic products facilitated the classification of products unknown to the dermatologist. The different soaps recorded were separated into seven types: *savon de Marseille*, antiseptic soaps, bleaching soaps, super fat soaps, ordinary soaps, exfoliative soaps and the unclassified. The term "ordinary soaps" groups all soaps with perfume, in solid or liquid form available in the market. The expression "*savon de Marseille*" referred to non perfumed neutral soaps. The nature of the soap was described as undetermined when no information concerning it could obtained.

The different products used to moisten or smoothen the skin were classified into 5 categories: pure glycerine, oils (palm kernel, palm, maize, olive, almond), dermo-cosmetic lotions, (specific non perfumed lotions, available only in the pharmacy), bleaching lotions (irrespective of the active ingredient), ordinary moisturing lotions (neither bleaching nor antiseptic, perfumed or not available in the open market). Any lotion was considered "indeterminate" if the patient did not know its nature. It was considered that there was "no lotion" when the patient was not applying any emollient or moisturizers after bathing and douching.

The extracted data were analysed using Epi Info version 6.0 for Windows (CDC Atlanta). Qualitative variables were expressed as frequencies or percentages. The cosmetologic habits of males were compared with those of females and also between different age groups and with reference to the chief presenting complaint using the Chi^2 test. The level of statistical significance was set at 5% (p<0,05).

RESULTS

Of 714 files studied (59.0% female and 41.0% male) with ages varying from 6 weeks to 89 years, the five most frequent reasons for consultation in decreasing order were: pruritus (46.0%), asymptomatic eruption (20%), acne (8.0%), pigmentary disorders (6.0%) and pain (5.0%). The five main diagnostic groupings recorded in decreasing order were: allergic reactions (34.0%); infections (20.0%); skin appendage disorders (15.0%) and pigmentation disorders (4.0%). The allergic conditions were dominated by eczema (66.00%). Fungal infections were the most frequent (32.0%) followed by parasitic infections (28.0%) among all infectious conditions. Acne was the most frequent skin appendage condition recorded (86.0%). Globally there was a statistically significant difference in the percentage of chief complaints in both sexes (see Table **1**). More women than men had as chief complaint acne, pruritus and pigment disorders (p = 0.000001, 0.008110, 0.003900 respectively) but more men than women consulted for scars and ulcerations (p = 0.028300 and 0.000591 respectively).

Six types of bathing soaps were currently used, in the following decreasing order: *savon de Marseille*, antiseptic soap, bleaching soap, super soap, ordinary soap, and exfoliative soap. *Savon de Marseille* and antiseptic soap were the first and second choices respectively for men as well as for women. However, women had a statistically significant preference for bleaching, super fat, and exfoliative soaps (78.0% *vs* 22.0%, p = 0.0435; 69.0% *vs* 31.0%, p = 0.0398; 87.0% *vs* 13.0%, p = 0.0008) with respect to men (Table **2**).

Among all the case files reviewed, 11.06% of patients did not know the nature of the soap they used. In the group of those who knew the nature of the soap (635/714), *savon de Marseille* was the most preferred (53.0%) and exfoliative soap the less preferred (1.0%). The use of antiseptic soap (123) was introduced within the age-group 0-10 years in 2.0% of the sample population with a knowledge of the nature of the soap (data not shown on table). Antiseptic soaps were most used by the 11-20 and 21-30 age groups (Table **3**) and this represented 11.0% of the sample population with a knowledge of the nature of the soap. Users

Table 1. Chief Complaint as a Function of Sex

Sex	Women		Men		Total		P
Chief Complaint	N	%	N	%	N	%	
Total	418	58.5	296	41.5	714	100	0.000002
Acne	50	12.0	5	1.7	55	7.7	**0.000001**
Skin appendage lesions	14	3.3	10	3.4	24	3.4	***0.052100***
Scars	13	3.1	20	6.8	33	4.6	***0.028300***
Pain	18	4.3	19	6.4	37	5.2	*0.378100*
Asymptomatic eruption	73	17.5	70	23.6	143	20	*0.093520*
Pruritus	200	47.8	128	43.2	328	45.9	***0.008110***
Pigmentation disorders	27	6.5	14	4.7	41	5.7	***0.003900***
Tumors / infiltration	3	0.7	5	1.7	8	1.1	*0.074300*
Ulcers	7	1.7	17	5.7	24	3.4	***0.000591***
Others	13	3.1	8	2.7	21	2.9	*0.076100*

of antiseptic soap were found to have the following skin disorders (data not shown): 43 presented with allergies, of which 33 were eczemas; 4 cheloid scars; 1 systemic disease; 31 infections (5 fungal infections, 9 parasitic infections, 12 viral infections, 1 bacterial infections, 4 dermatophytoses); 2 STDs; 3 lichenification; 17 disorders of epidermal appendages (acne); 3 disorders of epidermal differentiation, 2 pigmentation disorders, 4 tumours and 17 others.

Table 2. Soap Using Habits of Patients with Respect to Sex

Type of Soap	N	Female (%)	Male (%)	P Value
Total	714	59	41	
Antiseptic soap	123	60	40	0.1503
Exfoliative soap	8	87	13	**0.0008**
Savon de Marseille	334	56	44	0.0576
Bleaching soap	63	78	22	**0.0435**
Ordinary soap	52	58	42	0.0757
Super-fat soap	55	69	31	**0.0398**
Indeterminate soap	79	42	58	0.0569

Bleaching soap was also introduced early in life, within the age-group 0-10 years and mostly used by the age group 21 to 50 years. Super fat soap was mostly used for children less than 10 years (Table **3**).

In the case files, 87.00% practiced daily body care after a bath, with a significant difference between men and women: only 16.0% of women do not apply daily body lotion as against 94.0% for men ($p = 0.0001$). The analysis of skin care habits showed in the two sexes a preference for ordinary moisturizing body milk (65% in women *vs* 35.0% in men). The use of bleaching lotions was clearly more widespread in women than in men (87.0% *vs* 30.0%; $p = 0.0004$). Some patients (1.8%) could not determine the nature of products used (Table **4**).

The addition of some other substance into commercial moisturizers or emollient preparations was observed in 18.0% of cases (data not shown). Glycerin (13.0%) and topical corticosteroids (2.0%) were the substances most frequently added (data not shown). The other products added represented 3.0% (21/714) of the cases (data not shown).

Among the 714 case files, 13.0% of patients did not use any body lotion (92/714). Within the group that used body lotion after a bath, ($n = 622$), 12.0% did not know the nature of the lotion (Table **5**). Ordinary moisturising lotions were the most used (67.0%) while dermo cosmetic lotions were the least preferred (1.0%). Bleaching lotions were introduced within the age-group 0-10 years (4.0%) and mostly used by the age group 21 to 30 years (24.0%). The analysis of users of body moisturizers/emollients with respect to bathing soap type showed that 16.0% of those who habitually used antiseptic soaps did not apply any body lotion at all (Table **6**). An analysis of chief presenting complaints and cosmetologic habits revealed that amongst patients who presented with acne, the proportion that added other products in their body lotion was significantly higher than those who did not, $p = 0.025$ (Table **7**). Furthermore, it was observed that 63.0% added glycerin, 19.0% unspecified products and 13.0% topical corticosteroids (Table **8**).

DISCUSSION

This is the first study in Cameroon focusing on skin care habits. It shows the importance of skin care habits amongst patients consulting for various skin problems. Our results reveal that the habitual use of antiseptic soap comes second place after *savon de Marseille* in Yaoundé. Furthermore, our data shows that antiseptic soap is introduced very early in life. It is well known that these products indiscriminately destroy the flora of the skin thereby modifying one of the defense mechanisms of the body against microbes, namely the saprophyte flora [6]. It is also well established that the prolonged use of antiseptic soap alters the protective hydrolipid film of the skin [6]. The combination of these two consequences of antiseptic soap use certainly modifies the physiology of the skin in the long term, fragilising and rendering it susceptible to further external aggression. This situation is even more serious given the early introduction of antiseptic soaps, before age 10 years, to physiologically immature skin of subjects in our environment. To the best of our knowledge, no longitudinal study has been conducted in Cameroon (and in sub Saharan Africa) to determine the long term effect of these practices on the skin.

Fitoussi and Cabotin had already reported the practice of aggressive and irritating body washing attitudes of Africans living in France [4]. In fact, these people habitually use detergents and antiseptics for bathing, and scrub the skin with exfoliative commercial or traditional sponges, scrubbing stone [4, 5]. The observation of essentially

Table 3. Soap-Using Habits with Respect to Age (n = 635)

Age Group	N	*Savon de Marseille* (%)	Antiseptic Soap (%)	Exfoliative Soap (%)	Ordinary Soap (%)	Bleaching Soap (%)	Super Fat Soap (%)
Total	635	53	19	1	8	10	9
0-10	116	63	11	0	6	2	18
11-20	97	53	28	2	7	4	6
21-30	175	43	25	3	5	15	7
31-40	99	58	14	0	7	15	6
41-50	80	51	18	0	15	13	4
>51	68	53	16	0	15	7	9

inflammatory skin disorders in this group has led to the development of the new concept of "adaptation pathology" described by these authors in dermatological practice on black skin in the temperate regions.

Table 4. The Distribution of Daily Skin Care with Moisturiser/ Emollient by Sex

Moisturizer/ Emollient Use	N	Female (%)	Male (%)	P Value
Total	714	59	41	
Pure glycerine	19	53	47	0.0956
Pure oils	11	45	55	0.0726
Dermo-cosmetic body lotion	4	100	0	**0.0019**
Bleaching lotion	93	87	13	**0.0004**
Ordinary moisturizing body milk	418	65	35	0.0521
Indeterminate body lotion	77	40	60	0.0683
No body lotion	92	16	84	**0.0001**

We think that in the tropical environment, daily body rubbing probably attenuates this irritability of the skin, but the precarious equilibrium of skin physiology is rapidly broken once the climatic conditions are modified. In our current study, it was observed that 12.20% of those who habitually used antiseptic soaps did not apply any body lotion at all. Some African authors have described an increase in the prevalence of atopic dermatitis and contact eczema to the detriment of infectious dermatoses that were formerly the most encountered [7, 8]. Their explanation for this modification is based on an increased level of environmental allergens and nutritional factors. We however, suggest as a possible additional hypothesis to understand this phenomenon, namely, the habitual use of antiseptic products on the skin. Our finding of a high proportion of antiseptic soap users who presented with allergic skin disorders (35%) especially eczemas lends some support to this hypothesis.

The use of bleaching agents is not uncommon in Yaoundé, as 13% of subjects were involved in our series. It is very likely that this figure is an underestimation of the reality, given the retrospective nature of our study, and that 12.38% of those who admitted the use of body lotion did not reveal the nature of the lotion. This latter attitude could be an attempt to conceal the use of bleaching agents as the

Table 5. Daily Skin Care Habits with Respect to Age (n=622)

Age Group	N	Pure Glycerine (%)	Oils (%)	Dermo-Cosmetic Lotion (%)	Bleaching Lotion (%)	Ordinary Moisturizing Body Lotion (%)	Undetermined Body Lotion (%)
Total	622	3	2	1	15	67	12
0-10	114	1	4	0	4	89	3
11-20	97	2	0	1	15	72	9
21-30	184	3	2	2	24	54	15
31-40	100	4	0	0	15	60	21
41-50	69	6	1	0	16	61	16
>51	58	5	2	0	7	78	9

Table 6. The Use of Emollient/Moisturizing Body Lotions with Respect to Bathing Soap Type

	n	Antiseptic Soap (%)	Bleaching Soap (%)
Total	714	17	9
Pure Glycerine	19	26	11
Oils	11	18	18
Dermo-cosmetic lotion	4	0	0
Bleaching body lotion	93	18	28
Ordinary Moisturizing body lotion	418	20	7
Indeterminate body lotion	77	0	0
No body lotion	92	16	3

Table 7. Analysis of Main Complaints *vs* Additives to Body Lotion

Main Complaint	Total		Additives to Body Lotion				
			Yes		No		P Value
	N	%	N	%	N	%	
Total	714	100	126	100	588	100	
Lesions of skin appendages	24	3	7	6	17	3	0.098
Acne	55	8	16	13	39	7	**0.025**
Others	25	4	5	4	20	3	0.561
Skin eruptions	179	25	27	21	152	26	0.240
Pruritus	322	45	57	45	265	45	1.000
Ulceration/scars	51	7	5	4	46	8	0.117
Pigmentation disorders	41	6	7	6	34	6	1.000
Swelling/ inflammations	17	2	2	2	15	3	0.539

Table 8. Distribution of Types of Additives to Body Lotion with Respect to Main Complaint

	n	Aloevera (%)	Corticosteroids (%)	Fruits (%)	Glycerine (%)	Others (%)
Total	126	2	11	2	72	12
Skin appendages lesions	7	0	0	0	86	14
Acnea	16	6	13	0	63	19
Others	5	0	20	20	40	20
Skin eruptions	27	7	7	0	74	11
Pruritus	57	0	12	4	74	11
Ulceration/scars	5	0	0	0	100	0
Pigmentation disorders	7	0	29	0	57	14
Swellings/inflammations	2	0	0	0	100	0

sentiment of guilt in users of these products is well described in the literature [9-12]. Several authors have described higher rates of use of this type of agents in Africa: 25 to 67% in the general population and 27 to 92% in hospital populations. The practice of bleaching agents, whose complications have been proven, constitute a public health problem in many countries [2, 3, 8, 10-12].

The tendency of patients to add other substances to emollients and commercialized moisturizers (17.7%) is not specific to our context. This practice is not without risk as it may result in a product with a modified composition, not respecting quality norms. Many women in search of bleaching are familiar with this fact [2]. However, the proportion of those who added pure glycerin in our study sample was not negligible. This probably suggests an inadequacy between the products sold on the market and the cosmetic needs of black skin especially in terms of moisturizing characteristics. In spite of the efforts of producers to meet the needs of consumers with respect to products adapted to the black skin, the best cosmetics remain inaccessible [13], the majority of the population using products of lower quality making those who are unsatisfied to turn to artisanal preparations. Okeke had reported the insufficiencies related to the quality assurance of products available to consumers in Nigeria [13]. He emphasized on the high bacterial load of products from recognized cosmetic industries and the infectious risk they represent [13], especially with local compositions. Concerning the association of acne as a chief presenting complaint and the addition of topical corticosteroids in body lotions, a causal relationship is highly probable in our sample, given that this has been established in the literature. On the other hand, the observation that significantly more women than men had as chief complaint acne and pigmentation disorders, could constitute a justification for the use of inappropriate cosmetic products.

This preliminary study has some limitations for example: patients generally would not be able to give precise information such as duration of skin care habits. Another limitation is that the association of chief presenting complaints and cosmetologic habits may not have a causal relationship. Furthermore, as the study was conducted in a specialized department of a tertiary health institution, the results cannot be extrapolated to the general population. Nevertheless, the study provides the baseline for further work that will hopefully answer some of the many issues raised by the use of these skin modifying agents for habitual skin care.

CONCLUSION

A relatively high proportion of patients seen in the Dermatology outpatient clinic in Yaoundé use antiseptic soap and bleaching products, and this is done quite early in life. Furthermore, the addition of some harmful substances in commercial preparations by these patients may become a serious health problem if left uncontrolled. There is a need for more studies on these issues in our environment.

REFERENCES

[1] Smith W, Burns C. Managing the hair and skin of African American pediatric patients. J Pediatr Health Care 1999; 13(2): 72-8.

[2] Ly F. Complications dermatologiques de la dépigmentation artificielle en Afrique. Ann Dermatol Venereol 2006; 133: 899-906.

[3] Gathse A, Obengui P, Ibara JR. Motifs de consultation liés à l'usage des dépigmentants chez 104 utilisatrices à Brazzaville, Congo. Bull Soc Pathol Exot 2005; 98: 387-9.

[4] Fitoussi C. Pathologie d'adaptation de la peau noire en France métropolitaine. Ann Dermatol Venereol 2006; 133: 871-5.

[5] Cabotin PP. Cosmétologie de la peau noire. Encycl Med Chir (Editions Scientifiques et Médicales Elsevier SAS, Paris, Cosmétologie et Dermatologie Esthétique), 50-220-110, 2000; p. 4.

[6] Pons-Guiraud A. Les cosmétiques et la peau, Edition du Rocher 1997.

[7] Nnoruka EN. Skin diseases in south-east Nigeria: a current perspective. Int J Dermatol 2005; 44(1): 29-33.

[8] Ogunbiyi AO, Daramola OO, Alese OO. Prevalence of skin diseases in Ibadan, Nigeria. Int J Dermatol 2004; 44(1): 31-6.

[9] Mahe A, Blanc L, Halna JM, Keita S, Sanogo T, Bobin P. Enquête épidémiologique sur l'utilisation cosmétique de produits dépigmentants par le femmes de Bamako (Mali). Ann Dermatol Venereol 1993; 120: 870-3.

[10] Raynaud E, Cellier C, Perret JL. Depigmentation cutanée à visée cosmétique: Enquête de prévalence et effets indésirables, dans une population féminine sénégalaise. Ann Dermatol Venereol 2001; 128: 720-4.

[11] Petit A. Prise en charge des complications de la dépigmentation volontaire en France. Ann Dermatol Venereol 2006; 133: 907-16.

[12] Petit A, Cohen-Ludmann C, Clevenbergh P, Bergmann JF, Dubertret L. Skin lighteningand its complications among African people living in Paris. J Am Acad Dermatol 2006; 55: 873-8.

[13] Okeke IN, Lamikanra A; Bacteriological quality of skin – moisturizing creams and lotions distributed in a tropical developing country. J Appl Microbiol 2001; 91: 922-8.

A Hydroxypropyl Chitosan (HPCH) Based Medical Device Prevents Fungal Infections: Evidences from an *In Vitro* Human Nail Model

Anna Bulgheroni*, Linda Frisenda, Alessandro Subissi and Federico Mailland

Scientific Department, Polichem S.A., Lugano CH, Switzerland

Abstract: A long lasting, protective and film forming HPCH-based medical device was developed and tested in a novel *in vitro* human nail infection model. HPCH-treated and untreated human distal fingernail fragments were disposed on the culture surface of *Trychophyton rubrum, T. mentagrophytes, Scopulariopsis brevicaulis* or *Candida parapsilosis*. After incubation for one or three weeks, the fragments were collected and histological analysis was performed. Results obtained in untreated nails evidenced, as expected, that the fungal invasion was different depending on the species: it was completed with *Trichophyton* spp., partial with *Scopurlariopsis* sp. and limited to the surface with *Candida* sp.. On the other hand, HPCH-treated nails were not invaded by fungal elements, neither dermatophytes nor moulds or yeasts. Besides showing the barrier effect of HPCH this paper describes a novel *in vitro* model of nail infection that is simple, reproducible and closely represents the *in vivo* human situation.

Keywords: Dermatophytes, hydroxypropyl chitosan, *in vitro* human nail model, moulds, onychomycosis, prevention, yeasts.

INTRODUCTION

Onychomycosis is responsible for up to 40% of all nail disorders, most of which (90-95%) are caused by dermatophytes, especially *T. rubrum* and *T. mentagrophytes*. Yeasts (*Candida* spp.) and non-dermatophytic moulds (*Aspergillus* spp., *Acremonium* spp., *Fusarium* spp. and *Scopulariopsis brevicaulis*) account for the rest of nail infections [1]. Dermatophytes are soil saprophytes that evolved as parasites of animal keratinous tissues. They invade the nail structure directly and deeply [2]. Conversely, yeast and non-dermatophyte moulds, which are devoid of keratinolytic enzymes, infect firstly the soft tissues around the nails and they reach the nail secondarily, infecting only its surface [2].

The impaired integrity of nail structure plays an essential role in onychomycosis. Several risk factors promote fungal colonisation and infections: nail trauma, aging, damage in the nail structure such as enlarged porosity and intercellular spaces. The preventive measures commonly suggested to reduce the risk of infection are the implementation of hygienic measures, the use of comfortable and perspiring shoes and, in some cases, the treatment with antimycotic agents at a reduced dosage. However, no clear evidence of efficacy was ever proved with any of these measures. In addition, the use of low-dose antifungal agents is at high risk of inducing resistances [3]. In the light of these considerations, any non-pharmacological measure capable of protecting the nail of subjects at high risk of onychomycosis is of considerable value.

A new medical device (Myfungar®, Polichem S.A.), based on Hydroxypropyl Chitosan (HPCH), was developed by Polichem S.A. HPCH, a semisynthetic water-soluble derivative of chitosan, is a film forming water-soluble biopolymer endowed with several medically and cosmetically useful properties. Among them its capability to form a protective and long lasting barrier, when applied on the nail surface, is of utmost importance in the prevention of onychomycosis [4-6].

Procedures to test the efficacy of ready-to-use formulations have been set up but they are not devoid of limitations such as the absence of a nail substrate or of keratin [7].

In these regards, a fungal infection model based on human nails was set up. The experimental conditions, to monitor the fungal invasion of human nails in the presence or absence of the barrier formed by the HPCH-based medical device, were developed and tested with dermatophytes, yeasts and moulds responsible for onychomycosis.

MATERIALS AND METHODS

Test Item

Nail solution (Myfungar®, Polichem S.A.) containing 1% hydroxypropyl chitosan, and preservatives in a hydroalcoholic solution.

Fungal Strains

The species selected for these experiments represent the main causative agents of onychomycosis [5]: reference strains representative of dermatophytes, moulds and yeasts were obtained from the Deutsche Sammlung von Mikroorganismen und Zellkulturen GmbH (German Collection of Microorganisms and Cell Cultures: *T. rubrum* DSM 4167, *T. mentagrophytes* DSM 4870, *C. parapsilosis* DSM 11224 and

*Address correspondence to this author at the Scientific Department, Polichem S.A., *via* Senago 42D, 6912 Lugano Pazzallo, Switzerland;
E-mail: anna.bulgheroni@polichem.com

S. brevicaulis DSM 9122). Strains were grown on Sabouraud Dextrose Agar (SDA) at 35±1°C.

Preparation of Human Fingernail Fragments

Distal fingernail clippings (0.9 cm minimum) were obtained from four healthy adult volunteers. Inclusion criteria were: no use of nail varnish or polish and no signs of fingernail disease for at least six months. Subjects were required to cut and collect the distal free edge of their fingernails using scissors or standard nail clippers. Cut nail fragments were soaked and shaken for 1 h in 70% ethanol, removed, dried and finally stored in sterile vials until the time of the experiment.

Experimental Procedures

The aim of this experiment was to evaluate the protective effects of an HPCH on human nails against fungal infections. SDA plates were inoculated with fungi (*T. rubrum, T. mentagrophytes, S. brevicaulis* or *C. parapsilosis*) and incubated until a well defined fungal growth was visible all over the plate surface. The size of the fragments was approximately 0.9-1.5 cm in length and 350-500 µm thick. A volume of 20 µl of the test product (HPCH-based medical device) was applied as a thin layer on the nail fragments by means of a brush and let dry. Controls were left untreated. Treated and untreated fragments were subsequently placed on the surface of the plates inoculated with the fungi and incubated for 7 or 21 days. At day 7 and day 21, nails were

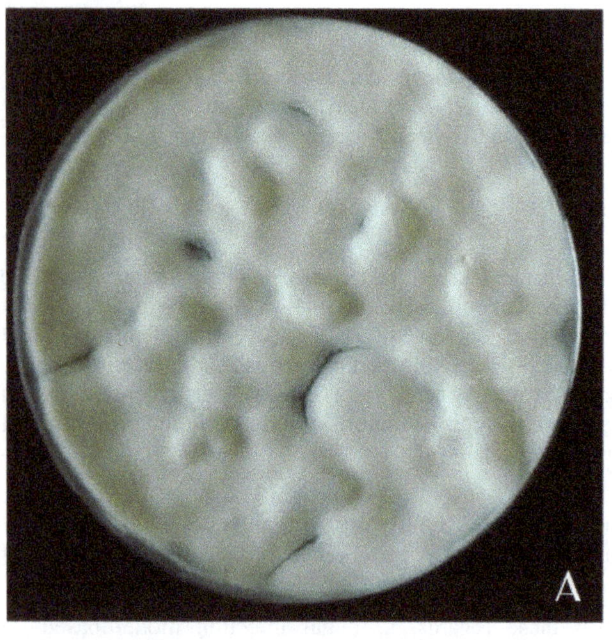

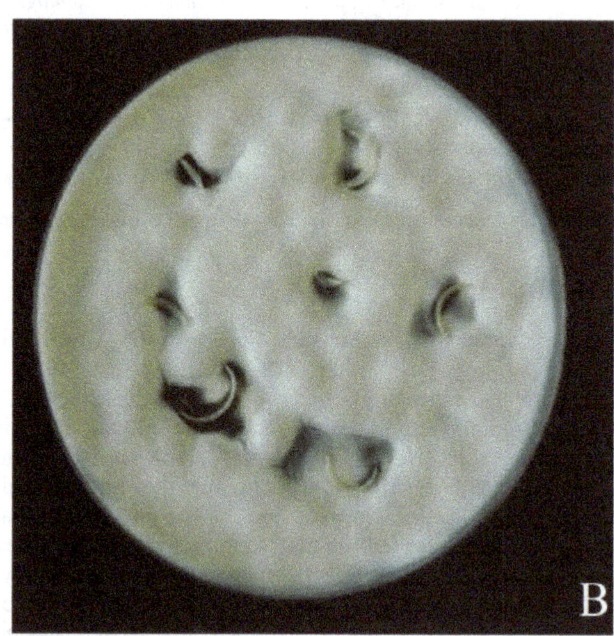

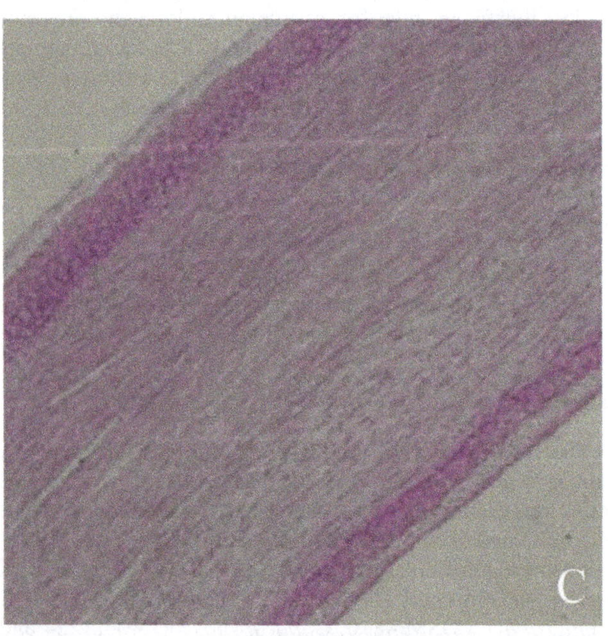

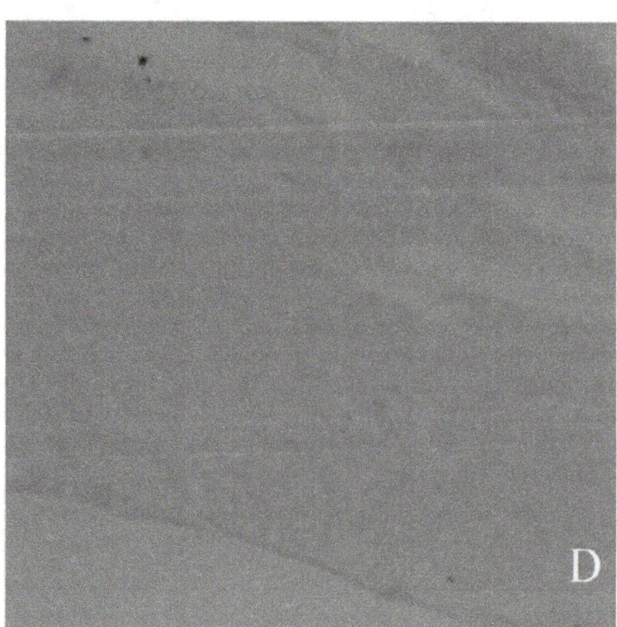

Fig. (1). *Trichophyton rubrum* following 7 days of incubation. Fungal growth on untreated (**A**) and treated nails (**B**). Fungal invasion of the nails of untreated (**C**) and treated (**D**) nails (100X; PAS stained).

removed from the culture and observed macroscopically and microscopically, following PAS (Periodic acid-Schiff) staining.

RESULTS

Results here reported are representative of 3 to 4 different experiments.

Dermatophytes - All untreated nails were completely surrounded by fungal mycelium when put in contact with *T. rubrum* and *T. mentagrophytes* (Fig. **1A**: *T. rubrum*; Fig. **2A**: *T. mentagrophytes*) already after 7 days of incubation; on the contrary, those treated with the HPCH solution remained free from fungal colonization (Fig. **1B**: *T. rubrum*; Fig. **2B**: *T. mentagrophytes*). At PAS stain, both dermatophytes were able to invade the whole thickness of untreated nails already after 7 days (Fig. **1C**: *T. rubrum*; Fig. **2C**: *T. mentagrophytes*). Conversely in the HPCH treated nails only few fungal elements were visible at the external margins that had been in contact with the fungal culture (Fig. **1D**: *T. rubrum*; Fig. **2D**: *T. mentagrophytes*).

Moulds and yeasts - No macroscopically visible growth was observed on either untreated or HPCH treated nails, following incubation with *S. brevicaulis* or *C. parapsilosis* (Fig. **3A**, **B**: *S. brevicaulis*; Fig. **4A**, **B**: *C. parapsilosis*). As far as *S. brevicaulis* is concerned, in the untreated nails, PAS stain results were suggestive of a mild invasion of the nail, limited to the external margins. Contrary to the other test

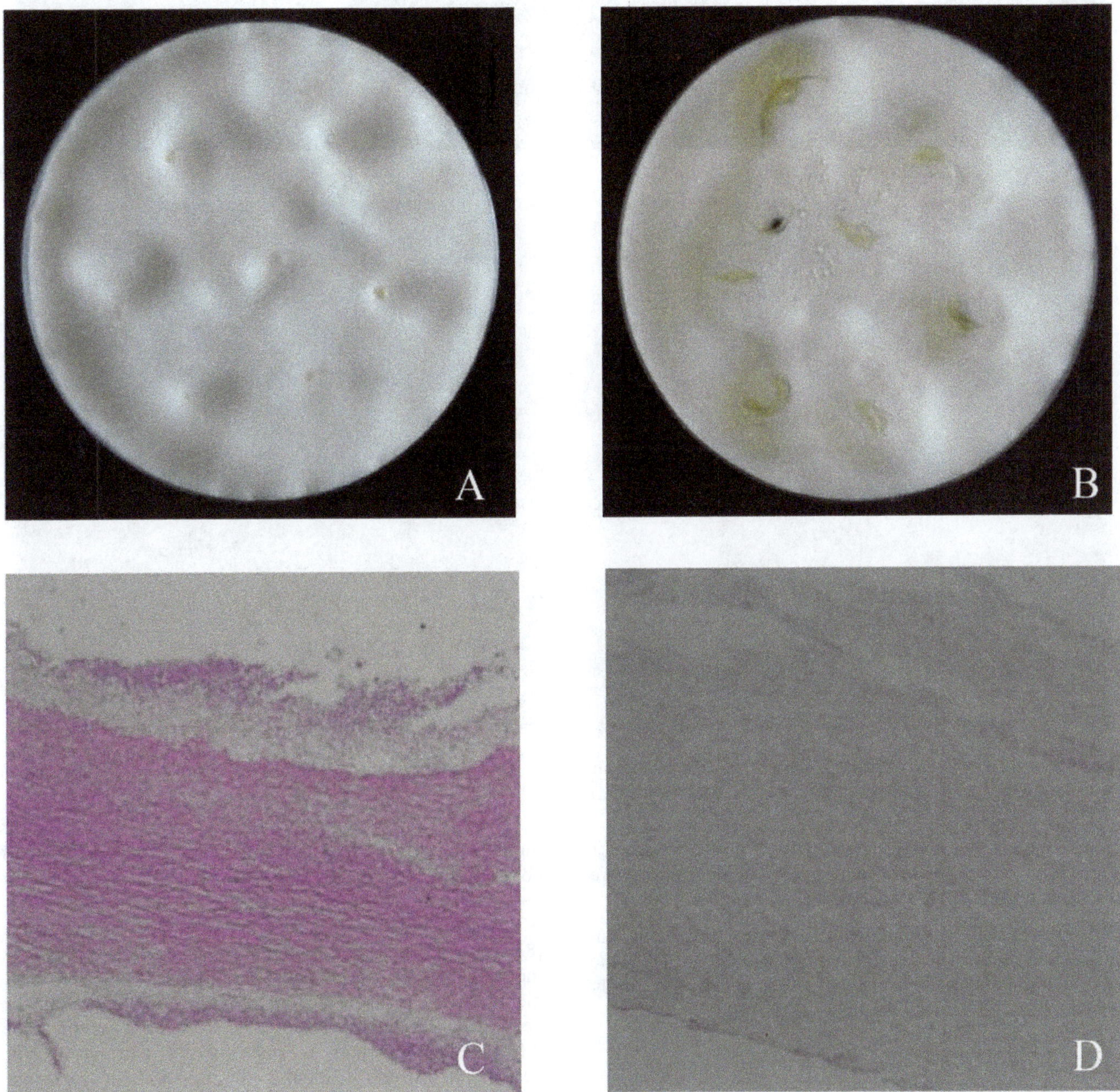

Fig. (2). *Trichophyton mentagrophytes* following 7 days of incubation. Fungal growth on untreated (**A**) and treated nails (**B**). Fungal invasion of the nails of untreated (**C**) and treated (**D**) nails (100X; PAS stained).

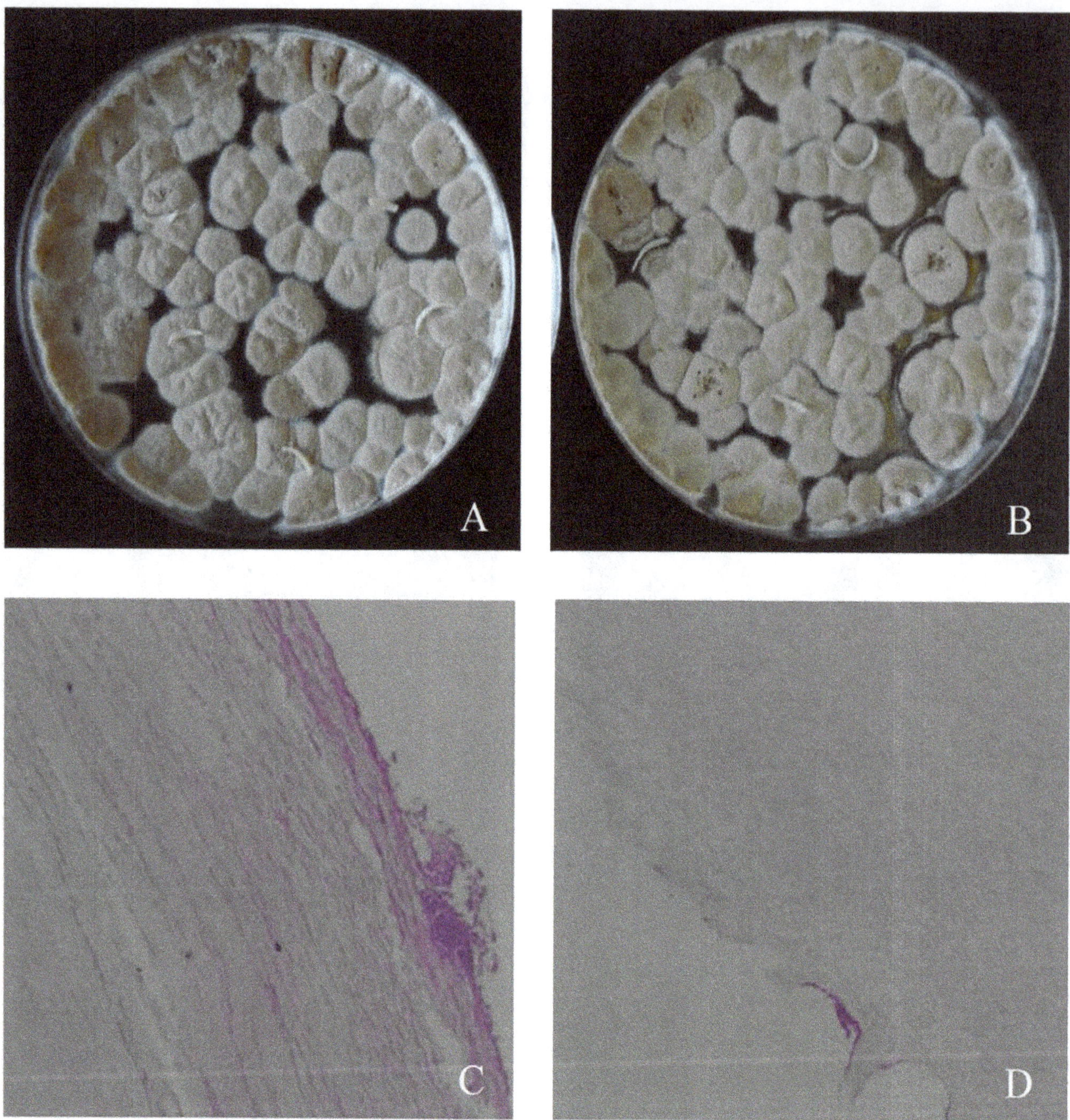

Fig. (3). *Scopulariopsis brevicaulis,* following 7 days of incubation. Fungal growth on untreated (**A**) and treated nails (**B**). Fungal invasion of the nails of untreated (**C**) and treated (**D**) nails (100X; PAS stained).

strains, fungal invasion progressed from day 7 to day 21 (Fig. **3C**). No signs of colonisation or invasion were observed in the HPCH-treated nails (Fig. **3D**).

Untreated nails incubated with *C. parapsilosis* showed an intense and uniform violet staining at PAS but limited to the surface of the preparation (Fig. **4C**). PAS staining was totally absent in the HPCH treated samples (Fig. **4D**).

DISCUSSION

It is increasingly being recognised that onychomycosis is a disorder that needs to be prevented and treated, providing impetus for the search of new models for the identification of novel antimycotic agents/formulations [2]. Procedures to test the efficacy of actives are available: the M27-A3 and M38-A2 assays from Clinical and Laboratory Standards Institute [8] use drug solutions brought into a medium previously inoculated with suspended fungi or spores. However, these methods do not consider other factors involved in the development of the disease, e.g. the presence of keratin at the infected site. Keratin is not only a nutrient to the dermatophytes but it is also the up-regulator for some putative virulence factors [5]. The importance of keratin for mimicking the *in vivo* situation was the object of various studies [9-11], where the medium was supplemented with

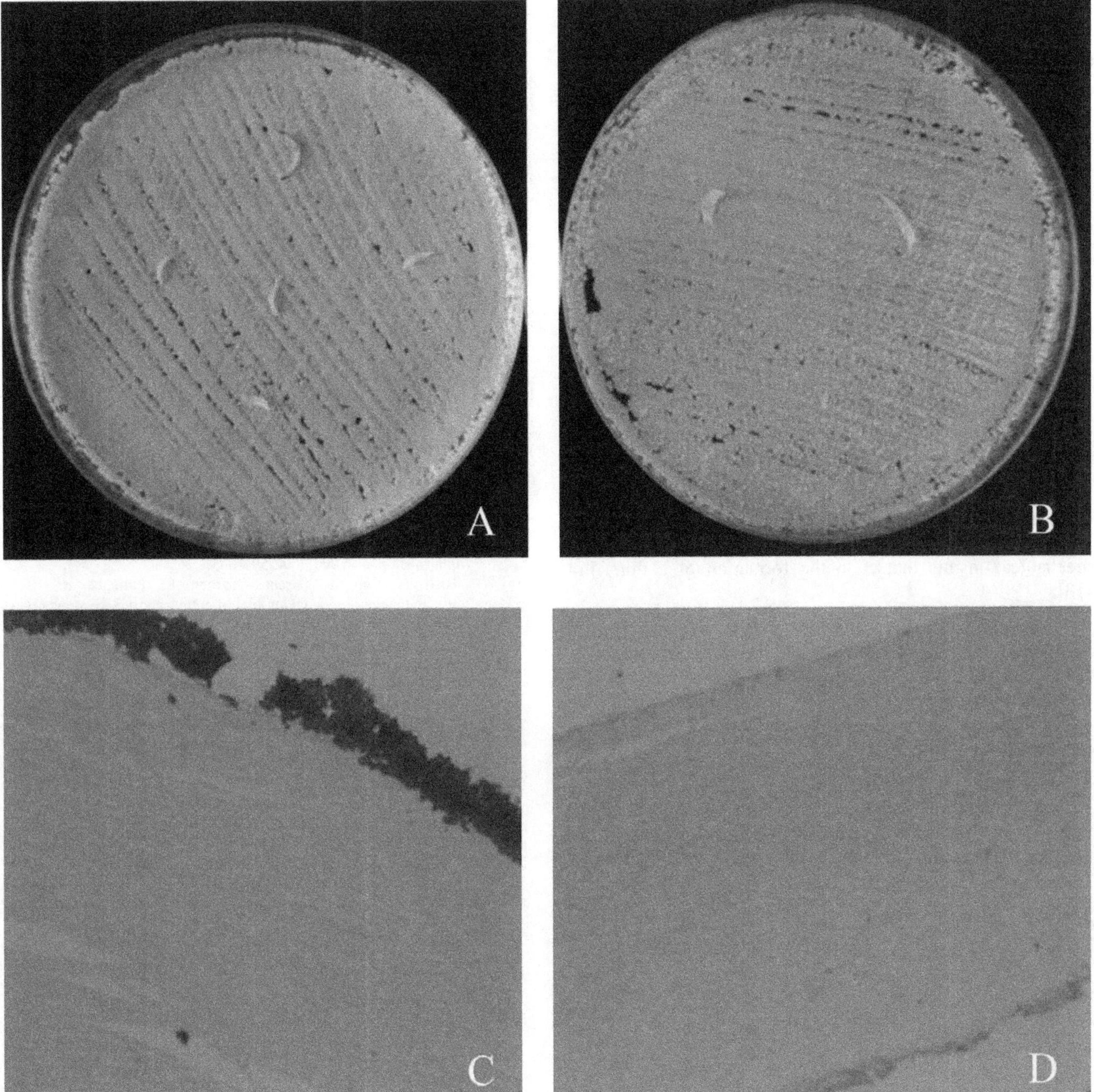

Fig. (4). *Candida parapsilosis,* following 7 days of incubation. Fungal growth on untreated (**A**) and treated nails (**B**). Fungal invasion of the nails of untreated (**C**) and treated (**D**) nails (100X; PAS stained).

pulverized nail clippings as the keratin source [5]. Lusiana *et al.* [5] reviewed the limitations of the current *in vitro* tests and proposed a novel model of infected nail plate using a keratin film made of human hair keratin, a largely available material, and compared it with bovine hoof, obtaining equivalent responses following treatment with antifungal preparations.

The method developed in this study uses intact human fingernail clippings and reflects more closely the natural physio-pathological conditions. This method proved simple, reproducible and representative of the *in vivo* human situation, although it was an *in vitro* study and as such it was not devoid of limitations. In particular, both sides of the nail were treated, thus not completely reflecting the actual *in vivo* treatment, but the treatment of one side would have resulted in the infection starting and progressing from the other side.

Our results in untreated nails are in good agreement with the known mechanisms of infection of the three tested fungal strains. The macroscopic and microscopic analyses of untreated nails showed that both dermatophytes were able to invade the whole thickness of the nail, while *S. brevicaulis* and *C. parapsilosis* remained limited to the surface. *T. rubrum* and *T. mentagrophytes* penetrated quickly into the nails and invaded them massively, the invasive process being completed within 7 days. *S. brevicaulis* invaded untreated nails rather slowly and only superficially. Analogously, *C.*

parapsilosis did not invade untreated nails and proliferated only on the nail surface, similarly to what is known in humans [4].

This *in vitro* model was used to test the ability of the HPCH-based medical device to prevent fungal infection of the nail. After a single treatment with the HPCH-based device, the nail fragments were protected from fungal colonization and this protection was long-lasting (over seven days). The results obtained in this study correlate with a recent publication in which HPCH treated bovine hoof slices were more resistant to penetration of dermatophytes with respect to untreated slices (e.g. penetration by *T. mentagrophytes* was < 25µm *versus* 275µm in the untreated control, at day 9) [12], while the application of commonly used aggressives, like isopropyl alcohol or urea, increased the ability of those pathogens to invade the nails. The results obtained in both studies can be attributed to the ability of the HPCH solution to form a barrier against the pathogens, as the product does not show any antifungal activity.

As previously reported the HPCH solution, applied to the surface of bovine hoof membranes, results, at scanning electron microscope, in smoother hooves, more resistant to mechanical insults thanks to the formation of a thin film [13].

These effects are of notable interest and indicate an additional potential beneficial role, in the prevention of onychomycosis in subjects at high risk or as a maintenance program following an efficacious antimycotic treatment, to avoid recurrences or reinfections, avoiding the risk to select resistant strains.

A recently published preliminary clinical trial reported significant benefits in the prophylaxis of onychomycosis in patients at risk [14]. Further studies may be needed to confirm those results.

ABBREVIATIONS

C.	=	*Candida*
DSM	=	Deutsche Sammlung von Mikrorganismen und Zellkulturen
HPCH	=	hydroxypropyl chitosan
PAS	=	Periodic acid-Schiff
S.	=	*Scopulariopsis*
SDA	=	Sabouraud Dextrose Agar
sp.	=	species singular
spp	=	species pluralis (multiple species)
T.	=	*Trychopyton*

CONFLICT OF INTEREST

The present work was funded by Polichem S.A. Authors are either employees (A.B. and L.F.) or former employee and/or consultant (F.M. and A.S.) of Polichem S.A.

ACKNOWLEDGEMENTS

We gratefully acknowledge the contribution of Giuseppe Togni and colleagues of IPAS laboratory (Ligornetto, Switzerland) for performing the microbiological work.

REFERENCES

[1] Murdan S. Topical nail products and ungual drug delivery. Boca Raton (USA), CRC Press 2013; pp. 1-35.

[2] Elewski BE. Onychomycosis: Pathogenesis, Diagnosis, and Management. Clin Microbiol Rev 1998; 11: 415-29.

[3] Daniel CR 3rd, Jellinek NJ. Commentary: the illusory tinea unguium cure. J Am Acad Dermatol 2010; 62: 415-7.

[4] Niewerth M, Korting HC. *Candida albicans* and the principle of opportunism: an assay. Mycoses 2002; 45: 253-8.

[5] Lusiana RS, Müller-Goymann CC. Infected nail plate model made of human hair keratin for evaluating the efficacy of different topical antifungal formulations against Trichophyton rubrum *in vitro*. Eur J Pharm Biopharm 2013; 84: 599-605.

[6] Tosti A, Hay R, Arenas-Guzmán R. Patients at risk of onychomycosis- risk factor identification and active prevention. J Eur Acad Dermatol Venereol 2005; 19 Suppl 1:13-6.

[7] Monti D, Saccomani L, Chetoni P, Burgalassi S, Saettone MF, Mailland F. *In vitro* transungual permeation of ciclopirox from a hydroxypropyl chitosan-based, water soluble nail lacquer. Drug Dev Ind Pharm 2005; 1: 11-7.

[8] National Committee for Clinical Laboratory Standards. Reference method for broth dilution antifungal susceptibility testing of conidium-forming filamentous fungi. Approved standard M38-A. Wayne, PA: NCCLS 2000.

[9] Osborne CS, Leitner I, Favre, Ryder NS. Antifungal drug response in an *in vitro* model of dermatophyte nail infection. Med Mycol 2004; 42: 159-63.

[10] Nowrozi H, Nazeri G, Adimi P, Bashashati M, Emami M. Comparison of the activities of four antifungal agents in an *in vitro* model of dermatophyte nail infection. Indian J Dermatol 2008; 53: 125-8.

[11] Schaller M, Borelli C, Berger U, *et al.* Susceptibility testing of amorolfine, bifonazole and ciclopiroxolamine against Trichophyton rubrum in an *in vitro* model of dermatophyte nail infection. Med Mycol 2009; 47: 753-8.

[12] Ghannoum MA, Long L, Isham N, *et al.* Ability of Hydroxypropyl Chitosan nail lacquer to protect against dermatophyte nail infection. AAC 2015; 59: 1844-8.

[13] Sparavigna A, Setaro M, Frisenda L. Physical and microbiological properties of a new nail protective medical device. J Plastic Dermatol 2008; 4: 5-12.

[14] Chimenti S, Difonzo E, Aste N, Frisenda L, Caserini M. The protective efficacy of a new Hydroxypropyl Chitosan -based product in subjects at risk of onychomycosis. J Plastic Dermatol 2013; 9: 185-9.

8

Psychodermatology: Past, Present and Future

Carmen Rodríguez-Cerdeira*[,1], José Telmo Pera-Grasa[2], A, Molares[3], Rafael Isa-Isa[4], Roberto Arenas-Guzmán[5]

[1]*Dermatology Department, CHUVI and University of Vigo, Vigo, Spain*

[2]*University of Vigo. Vigo. Spain*

[3]*FIDI Xeral-Calde, Hospital Lucus Augusti, Lugo, Spain*

[4]*Institute of Dermatology and Skin Surgery, Santo Domingo, Dominican Republic*

[5]*Dermatology Department, Hospital Dr, Manuel Gea González, D.F., México*

Abstract: A relationship between psychological factors and skin diseases has long been hypothesized. Psychodermatology addresses the interaction between the mind and the skin. Today, we know that it is essential to consider both biopsychosocial approaches and path physiological approaches to treatment, involving general practitioners, psychiatrists, dermatologists and psychologists. However, Psychodermatology is a relatively new discipline, and the body of literature addressing it is still scarce.

To obtain data, we consulted the archives of dermatological societies in Europe and America from the year of their founding until 2010. We also consulted other psychiatric and psychological societies and received responses from most of them.

Among the different stages in the historical evolution of Psychodermatology (the early, anecdotal phase; the methodological phase and the contemporary phase), it was only in the most recent phase that the European Society of Dermatology and Psychiatry was established. Other working groups and societies have emerged in several European countries: The German Working Group on Psychodermatology, French Society for Dermatology and Psychosomatics, Italian Society of Psychosomatic Dermatology, the Dutch Society of Psychosomatic Dermatology, the Spanish Society of Dermatology and Psychiatry etc.

More recently, a Psychodermatology two groups Psychodermatology were established first one within the Ibero Latin American College of Dermatology (CILAD) and the other one the Japanese Society of Psychodermatology (JSPD).

Summarize, this review details the historical evolution of the relationship between the skin and the mind. It also reveals the emergence of Psychodermatology as a discipline in its own right and describes the societies that have emerged worldwide as a result of collaboration between dermatologists and psychiatrists.

Keywords: Psychodermatology, European society of Dermatology and Psychiatry (ESDaP), Psychosomatic.

INTRODUCTION

The skin and central nervous system have common embryological origins; therefore, they also have common neuromodulators, peptides and biochemical systems of internal information. For this reason, the skin is an organ that is strongly reactive to emotion. Because the skin is the most accessible part of our body, it is not uncommon for many people to manifest aggressive impulses, anxiety, or self-destructive behavior through the skin, provoking dermatological symptoms. On the other hand, people with skin diseases that compromise their self-image may feel depressed, ashamed or anxious as a result of their illness. Psychodermatology is the result of the merger of these two seemingly unrelated disciplines. Dermatology pertains to the treatment of diseases of the skin, which are manifested externally. Psychology and Psychiatry pertain to the examination of mental processes, which are manifested internally.

Thus, these different approaches regarding the relationship between the psychic and the somatic are variations on a theme: the relationship between behavior, thought, and emotion and the biological body that sustains them.

An other important consideration is the link between inflammation and depression when depression is considered as a continuous dimensional variable rather than a categorical entity, as this allows one to take into consideration moderate and subclinical levels of depressed mood. For instance, a prospective study of 267, 85-year-old subjects with no psychiatric history revealed that elevated biomarkers of inflammation preceded the onset of depressed mood in an aged population with no psychiatric history; this

*Address correspondence to this author at the Dermatology Department, CHUVI and University of Vigo, Vigo, Spain;
E-mails: aristoteles_cerdeira@yahoo.es,
carmen.rodriguez.cerdeira@yahoo.es, crodcer@uvigo.es

Table 1. Inflammation and Depression

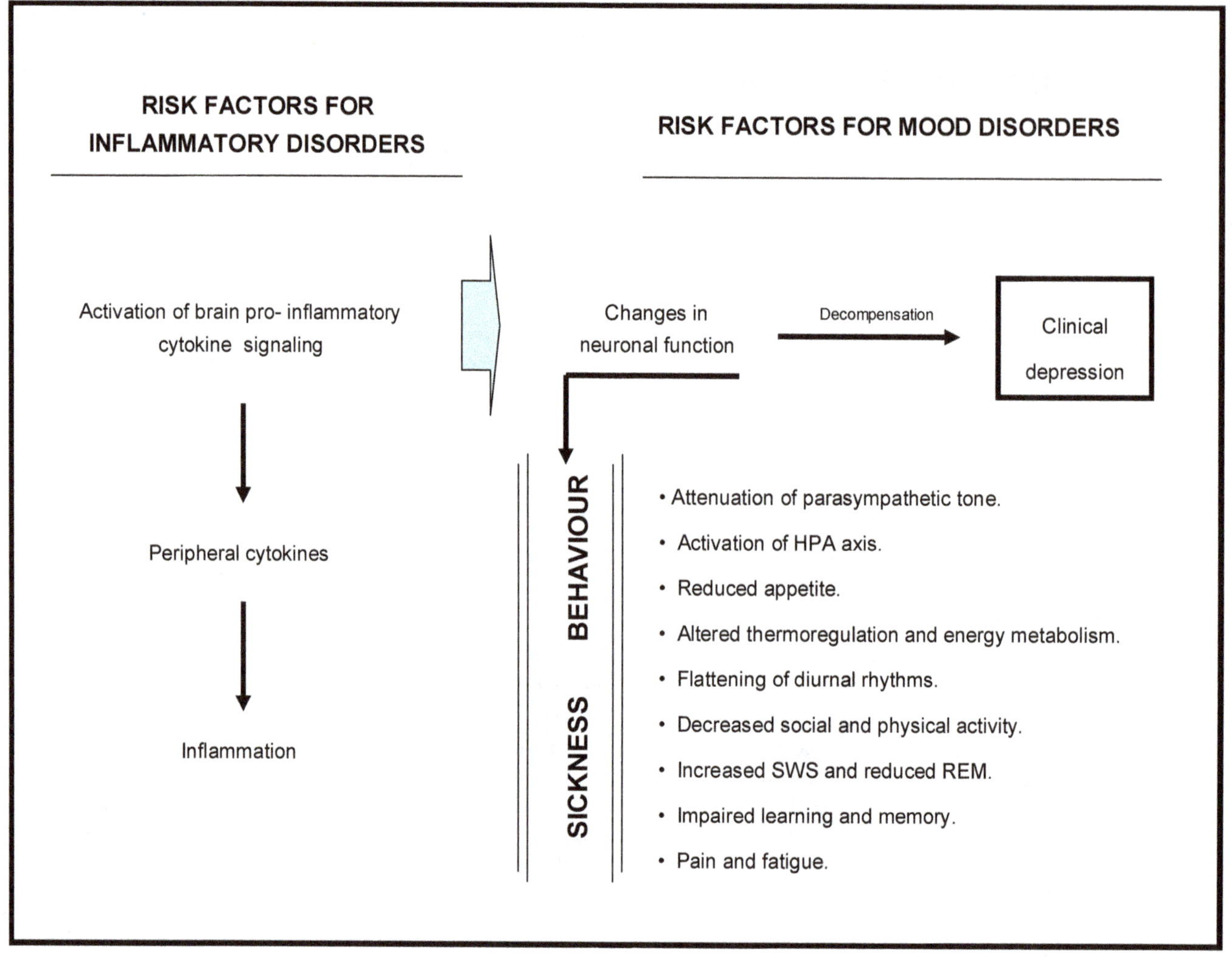

HPA: Hypothalamic-pituitary-adrenal, SWS: Slow-wave sleep, REM: Rapid eye movement.

must be taken into account in inflammatory conditions such as psoriasis (Table **1**) [1].

Today, we understand that Psychodermatology is a merger between Dermatology and Psychiatry that deals with the study of the influence of psychosocial stress in the exacerbation or chronicity of skin illness [2, 3]. Psychodermatology also analyses existing psychiatric co-morbidities in many dermatologic conditions and the role of adjuvant treatment, whether it be psychopharmacological, psychotherapeutic or social [4, 5]. However, clarifying this definition has not been easy. It would not have been possible without the dedication and effort of many health professionals. From its beginnings, in which there was hardly any knowledge about Psychodermatology, this discipline has now turned into an exciting field of study and source of support for patients with skin problems. Dermatologists, psychiatrists and psychologists, should create instruments to measure the incidence of:

- Stress, depression and skin disease
- Hypothalamic alterations and disease
- Classical conditioning and disease

Skin diseases such as psoriasis can profoundly influence a patient's self-image, self-esteem, and sense of well-being. Psoriasis is a multifactorial inflammatory condition with a disease burden that extends beyond the physical symptoms experienced by patients. Psoriasis affects all aspects of quality of life, including physical, psychological, social, sexual, and occupational elements. Data suggest that social stigmatization, high stress levels, physical limitations, depression, employment problems and other psychosocial co-morbidities experienced by patients with psoriasis are not always proportional to, or predicted by, other measurements of disease severity such as body surface area involvement or plaque severity [6].

The relation between psychological factors and psychiatric disorders in patients with skin diseases was discussed by researchers at different stages of the evolutionary process of building the Psychodermatology as a science with its own identity. The one hand psychological factors (stress, negative emotions) can influence the generation and aggravation of skin disorders (urticaria, atopic dermatitis, vitiligo), on the other hand psychological disorders can result in some skin diseases (psoriasis, atopic dermatitis). In the majority of cases the quality of life is poorly estimated by patients with skin problems.

We can say that Psychodermatology has a long history but a short past, which means that we can trace its history from the earliest texts related to skin disease with mental states. However, we cannot refer to psychodermatology as a discipline until the mid-twentieth century. This discipline, despite its youth, has an interdisciplinary character and, indeed, was built and continues to be built through the efforts of many professionals from different areas of medicine [7].

The Bible includes several episodes in which a relationship is established between the mind and the skin. The book of Genesis states "He put a sign Lord Cain, lest anyone find him hurt you..." The mark of Cain is a sign that he is "protected" from any attack, and his skin serves as a defense mechanism [4, 8].

Shortly thereafter, in Exodus, in the sixth plague in which Yahweh punishes the Pharaoh, there is another instance in which the skin acts as a signifier: "... take a handful of ashes from the furnace and Moses throw it toward the sky, the sight of Pharaoh, so that converted into a fine powder on all the land of Egypt and occurs in all the land of Egypt both men and animals and tumors eruptive pustules... " In other words, the pustules and tumors are an anticipated consequence of the conduct of the Pharaoh [9].

Hippocrates related the effects of fear on the skin. He noted that when our heart beats faster and with unusual force, we begin to sweat. In 1850, Erasmus Wilson wrote a book titled "Diseases of the skin." In his chapter on cutaneous neuroses, he speaks of alopecia areata, hypopigmented lesions, itching and parasitism mania, now known as delusions of parasitosis. This book is considered by many to be the starting point of Psychosomatic Dermatology [10].

The relationship between emotions and skin disorders has been recognized for decades. In 1925, Joseph Klauder noted the importance of psychotherapy in the evolution of skin diseases [11].

However, we must stress that, even in early texts, dermatological diseases are present and often associated with psychological states, meaning that Psychodermatology is alluded to in the earliest writings despite the fact that the rigorous and scientific study of the subject did not begin until the mid-twentieth century [12, 13, 14].

EARLY STAGE/ANECDOTAL

In this phase, simple relationships were sought between certain personality structures, states of emotional conflict (which were seen as causal phenomena), and something psychosomatic, which could be a dermatitis. It was assumed that this relationship was based on a detailed investigation of somatic, psychiatric and psychological behavior, the latter being based on a biographical history and results of psychological test batteries.

The pioneers in this phase were mainly psychiatrists trained in psychoanalysis or dermatologists who cooperated with psychiatrists.

At this stage, the concept of specificity arose: the hypothesis that a specific emotional conflict and a specific personality structure could be related to a certain psychosomatic disease or psychodermatitis [15].

Authors who are researching in this field thinking about the possibility of a linking with psychological stress to exacerbation of certain skin diseases. Both the clinical and the basic science evidence, however, can be hard to interpret in light of the difficulty of defining and quantifying psychological stress as well as the questions regarding the etiologic significance of neuroimmunological findings in skin diseases. Psychosomatic Dermatology is practiced in some manner by every dermatologist. In spite of this, there has been a virtual void in the literature from the middle 1950s until the present time.

METHODOLOGICAL PHASE

Around 1960, the field of psychology reacted to the anecdotal or initial phase. The material from which conclusions were drawn was considered insufficient and inadequate for statistical analysis and scientific assessment and prediction because it was often too selective and was not representative of the disease being studied. Control groups were few and the patient-doctor relationship was rarely noted.

Later, several other issues highlighting the defects of the anecdotal phase emerged in the literature: The motivation of the patient to receive treatment and the severity of emotional disturbance, regardless of the dermatitis, are essential. A specific set of symptoms of the disease, regardless of the dermatitis, can define the patient's behavior. The circadian rhythm of some metabolic processes, which have implications in the psychological and somatic behavior of the patient, have been sufficiently considered.

In this phase, the methodological approach takes into account the contributions of different disciplines to the scientific evaluation of psychodermatological phenomena. Therefore, conclusions that go beyond simple arguments, as occurred in the first anecdotal phase, can be drawn. At this stage, psychosomatic medicine and Psychodermatology were only an adjunct to psychoanalysis [16]. In that time clinicians trained in Dermatology and having submitted themselves to psychoanalysis have developed an original psychosomatic approach to skin disease at the Tarnier Hospital (Cochin-Port Royal University Hospital Center). Its main spring is detection and management of the patient's distress. They analyze the conditions under which it was possible to carry out this experiment and the implications of this approach which is directed at achieving a change in the way the department is run rather than adding one more specialized appendage to the outpatient care activity [17]

INTEGRATIVE PHASE

In this phase, the trend towards teamwork was more intense. The number of disciplines involved in increasing the awareness of psychological behavior was larger. The researcher and therapist were not only aware of the extent of the areas of contact with other biological sciences, but were also aware of the limits of their own contributions. Data pertaining to Psychodermatology requires not only thoroughness (such as psychoanalysis by trained people in the fifties), but also amplitude, so that increasing number of factors are taken into account [18].

The behavioral aspect of dermatitis goes beyond the individual. Dermatology has become aware of the fact that the pathology of skin diseases is part of the pathology of all humans.

It is obvious that in the formulation stage, the themes developed in the early stages remained significant, and the results of solid research contributed to knowledge. To provide the complete knowledge for monitoring patients with skin diseases, some factors, attitudes and variables were integrated, including some unmeasured factors resulting from the relationship with the patient (trying to change the patient's environment and goals) [19].

In this phase they considered that the most important theory for management of psycho-dermatological disorders requires evaluation of the skin manifestation and the social, familial and occupational issues underlying the problem. Once the disorder has been diagnosed, management requires a dual approach, addressing both dermatologic and psychological aspects. Even with self-induced skin problems, supportive dermatologic care is needed to avoid secondary complications, such as infection, and to ensure that the patient feel supported. Patients with psycho-dermatological disorders frequently resist referral to mental health professionals. Acceptance of psychiatric treatment or consultation may be enhanced through support from there family and friends [20].

CONTEMPORARY PHASE

In this phase they strongly believe that psycho-dermatological disorders can be broadly classified into some categories: psycho-physiological disorders, primary psychiatric disorders and secondary psychiatric disorders. The term "psycho-physiological disorder" refers to a skin disorder, such as eczema or psoriasis, that is worsened by emotional stress. "Primary psychiatric disorder" refers to a skin disorder such as trichotillomania, in which the primary problem is psychological; the skin manifestations are self-induced. "Secondary psychiatric disorders" affect patients with significant psychological problems that have a profoundly negative impact on their self-esteem and body image. Depression, humiliation, frustration and social phobia may develop as a consequence of a disfiguring skin disorder. This was the first step to building a European society that brings together all stakeholders in a new subspecialty that was the Psychosomatic Dermatology.

May 31, 1987 can be set as the starting point for this stage. Michael Musalek, with the invaluable help of Peter Berner and John Cotterill, organized the first International Congress on Psychosomatic Dermatology in Vienna. This was conceived as the first opportunity to provide the exchange of scientific and clinical information. It was a successful event, both in terms of the quality of the presentations and the number of participants, about 200 people from 20 countries worldwide.

Michael Musalek invested a great deal of time and attention to administrative details, and the European Society of Dermatology and Psychiatry (ESDaP) was formally established by decree of Vereinsbehörde, Sicherheitsdirektion für Wien, the Austrian Republic, on January 28, 1993. In 1989, John Cotterill held a second conference in Leeds. At the Third Congress, held in 1991 in Florence, Emiliano Panconesi held a meeting to formally discuss the creation of a stable association to organize periodic meetings to encourage contact between professionals and the exchange of scientific information (Table **2**). The meeting was attended by Peter Berner (Vienna), Marc Bourgeois (Bordeaux), Sylvie Consoli (Paris), John Cotterill (Leeds), Francesc Grimalt (Barcelona), John de Korte (Amsterdam), Uwe Gielen (Giessen), Caroline Koblenzer & Peter Koblenzer (Philadelphia), Michael Musalek (Vienna), Klaus Taube (Halle), Henriette Walter (Vienna) and Emiliano Panconesi (Florence) [17, 18]. After an intense meeting, which focused on issues such as the frequency of the Congress and standardizing terminology, the European Society of Dermatology and Psychiatry was created. Differences in terminology in each country, such as Psychodermatology, Psychocutaneous Medicine, and Psychosomatic Dermatology were superseded.

Table 2. **International Conferences in Psychosomatic Dermatology**

Chair	Year	Place
Michael Musalek	1987(1st)	Vienna (Austria)
Jonh Cotterill	1989 (2nd)	Leeds (UK)
Emiliano Panconesi	1991 (3rd)	Florence (Italy)
Peter & Caroline Koblenzer	1992 (4th)	Philadelphia (UE)

The creators and executive committee members of the first society were

- John Cotterill (Leeds), Chairman
- Marc Bourgeois (Bordeaux), Vice President
- Michael Musalek (Vienna), Secretary General
- John de Korte (Utrecht), Treasurer
- Peter Berner (Vienna), Counsellor
- Sylvie Consoli (Paris), Counsellor
- Francesc Grimalt (Barcelona), Counsellor
- Uwe Gielen (Linden), Counsellor
- Emiliano Panconesi (Florence), Counsellor
- Taube Klau (Halle), Counsellor
- Henriette Walter (Vienna), Counsellor

A fourth international conference was held in 1992 in Philadelphia. Several European colleagues were invited to participate, but for various reasons, they could not attend. The conference was organized by Peter and Caroline Koblenzer. They tried to promote collaboration between the ESDaP and the Psychocutaneous Medical Association of North America (APMNA) (Table **2**) [20-22].

The European Society for Dermatology and Psychiatry is a scientific society that was legally established in 1993 in Vienna under Austrian Law. It provides a forum for

European physicians and psychologists working in the fields of Psychodermatology, Psychosomatic Dermatology, and Dermatopsychiatry to foster the exchange of information and ideas. The organization also fosters networking among professionals in the field to improve the quality of scientific research in the area and recruit new members with expertise in the field.

The ultimate aim of the society is to foster the improvement of patient care by putting into practice insights gained through research in Psychodermatology.

ESDaP further aims

- To stimulate interest in Psychodermatology, particularly among European dermatologists, psychiatrists, psychologists, and other professionals in this field and in related ones.
- To promote interdisciplinary research and education on subjects connected with Dermatology, Psychology and Psychiatry in order to improve both understanding of pathology as well as clinical management of psychocutaneous diseases.
- To organize symposia and international congresses on Dermatology, Psychology and Psychiatry, aiming to provide both medical professionals as well as the general public with updated information on developments in the field of Psychodermatology.

Subsequent meetings have all been specifically ESDaP congresses, the fifth congress was held in Bordeaux (France) in 1993 and was organized by psychiatrist Marc Bourgeois. The sixth was held in Amsterdam (The Netherlands) in 1995 and was organized by the psychologist John de Korte. The seventh was held in Halle (Germany) and organized by dermatologist Klaus Taube. In the next congress in Paris in 1999, dermatologist and psychiatrist Sylvie Consoli introduced the journal *Dermatology & Psychosomatics*. There were also meetings in Holland and Germany. In 2001, Francesc Grimalt organized the ninth International Congress of ESDaP in Barcelona (Table **3**).

Table 3. International Conferences of the European Society of Dermatology and Psychiatry (ESDaP)

Chair	Year	Place
Marc Bourgeois	1993 (5th)	Bordeaux (France)
John de Korte	1995 (6th)	Amsterdam (The Netherlands)
Klaus Taube	1997 (7th)	Halle (German)
Sylvie Consoli	1999 (8th)	Paris (France)
Francesc Grimalt	2001 (9th)	Barcelona (Spain)
Françoise Poot	2003 (10th)	Brussels (Belgium)
Uwe Gieler	2005 (11th)	Giessen (German)
Francisco Tausk	2007 (12th)	Wroclaw (Poland)
Andrea Peserico	2009 (13th)	Venice (Italy)
Lucia Tomás-Aragonés	2011 (14th)	Zaragoza (Spain)

The chair of the ESDaP was occupied successively by the teachers John Cotterill, Emiliano Panconesi, Sylvie Consoli, Françoise Poot, John de Korte and the President Elect is Michael Dennis Linder [20, 21].

Moreover, the ESDaP organizes lectures and symposia at every EADV congress and an international congress every other year. Currently, most countries in the European Union have their own national work group on Psychodermatology (French Society for Dermatology and Psychosomatics, Italian Society of Psychosomatic Dermatology, The German group on Psychodermatology, the Dutch Society of Psychosomatic Dermatology, etc.) [22-25].

The number of participants in those meetings has been fairly constant over the years. The quality of presentations has remained high, and participants demonstrate increasing interest in the topics presented. In addition, interest in the field has been growing in younger physicians and psychologists.

According to Emiliano Panconesi *et al.* [18] relations between Association for Psychocuataneous Medicine of North America (APMNA) and ESDaP have much greatly improved over the last five years as participation in meetings organized by both associations maintains frequent individual contacts between them [26, 27].

In Spain, it was not until 1995 when the first meeting of the Spanish Group of Dermatology and Psychiatry was held. It was attended by 138 attendees, including psychologists, psychiatrists and dermatologists. However, the statutes that formed the Spanish Group for Dermatology and Psychiatry were not formally approved until 1999. The management committee consisted of two dermatologists and a psychiatrist, Antonio Rodríguez-Pichardo, Francesc Grimalt and Joaquim Pujol [24]

Later, in Madrid, the Spanish Group for Dermatology and Psychiatry (SGDaP) was established under the Spanish Academy of Medical-Surgical Dermatology and Venereology and chaired by Antonio Rodríguez-Pichardo. Annual meetings were held in different parts of Spain, always during February. In February 2006, the meeting was chaired by Dr. Carmen Brufeau in Murcia.

In Tenerife, the meeting was chaired by Marta Garcia-Bustinduy in February of 2007. During this meeting, Maria José Tribó coordinated the Spanish group of Dermatology and Psychiatry (SGDaP).

The next meeting took place in 2008 in Zaragoza. It was organized by Lucia Tomás-Aragones & Servando Marrón-Moya. The next meeting was held in Valladolid in 2009 and was chaired by Alberto Miranda.

The last meeting was held in February in 2010 in Palma de Mallorca. It was chaired by Joan Escales-Taberner. Currently, the SGDaP is coordinated by Aurora Guerra-Tapia.

The rest of Europe also formed working groups that contributed to improving training in Psychodermatology. For example, in The Netherlands, psychodermatologic clinicians receive training in Psychotherapy, Psychology or Psychiatry. In Germany, the German Working Group on Psycho-

Dermatology has developed training programs for basic psychosomatic dermatologists.

Most European countries have created their own working groups on Psychodermatology, such as the French Society for Dermatology and Psychosomatic, the Italian Society of Psychosomatic Dermatology, and the Dutch Society of Psychosomatic Dermatology, etc.

The German Working Group on Psychodermatology (APD = Arbeitskreis Psychosomatische Dermatologie) has developed an education program for dermatologists consisting of 80 hours of short-term medical education called psychosomatic basic knowledge. In 2005, they organized the 11th International Congress of the ESDaP with Uwe Gieler from the University of Giessen.

The Italian Society of Psychosomatic Dermatology (SIDEP) was developed on November 4, 1995 (under the name of the Italian Group of Dermatology Psychosomatics - GIDEP) in Venice on the occasion of the Residential Course of Psychosomatic Dermatology, held in Palazzo Giustiniani Lolin, home of the Fondazione Levi [24].

HISTORY OF PSYCHODERMATOLOGY IN THE CILAD

In October 2008, a group of dermatologists created a psychodermatology working group within the Ibero Latin College of Dermatology (CILAD). All dermatologists belonged to the CILAD. The working group was coordinated by Carmen Rodríguez-Cerdeira with the unconditional support of then-President of CILAD, Roberto Arenas Guzmán [28].

The founding members who proposed the creation of this group to the Board of the CILAD were as follows:

- Carmen Rodríguez-Cerdeira (Spain)
- Rafael Isa-Isa (Republica Dominicana)
- Roberto Arenas-Guzmán (México)
- Luna Azulay (Brasil)
- Antonio Guzman (Paraguay)
- Yolanda Ortiz (Mexico)
- Marcela Gaete (Chile)
- Mauricio Sandoval (Chile)
- Eduardo José Restifo (Argentina)
- William Andrés Romero (México)
- Hector Murakami (Perú)
- Eduardo Silva (Guatemala)

In April 2009, the board of the CILAD announced the acceptance of this group, and the coordination of the group was assumed by Carmen Rodríguez-Cerdeira (Spain) and the Secretary General Rafael Isa-Isa (Dominican Republic).

The purpose of this chapter is to promote and cultivate existing relationships among the three disciplines, namely, Dermatology, Psychiatry and Psychology. It also seeks to publicize the results of the efforts made in the study of diseases covered by the three specialties, with the aim of improving the treatment of patients. It aims to contribute to meetings and publications of high academic value that will be disseminated among the scientific community. Finally, it aims to promote good relations between the different Dermatology and Psychiatry societies all over the world to attempt to unify therapeutic protocols [24].

Finally, the 30th of September in 2011, Japan established the Japanese Society of Psychodermatology and held the 1st annual meeting in the Osaka, where the most prominent speakers as Eiichiro Ueda, Takashi Yamauchi, Yuko Higaki, Ritsuko Hosoya, Ryuzo Saito, among others, have been involved as it is reflected in the meeting web (http://www.jspd.org).

FUTURE PROSPECTS

This paper tries to highlight the importance of understanding psychosomatic problems and to develop a continuing medical education program (similar to that in other European countries). We hope that the dermatologists can appropriately counsel patients through better preparation and knowledge of the interaction between skin disorders and psychological problems.

We should try to establish ties that allow a working relationship between dermatologists, psychologists and psychiatrists. It is important for dermatologists to have basic knowledge about psychiatry. Doctors with less developed relation skills had more difficult consultations [29]. However, we cannot forget that in many cases, specialised psychiatric care is necessary (follow-up cases, psychotherapy, special prescription drugs) [30].

CONCLUSION

Until recently, when the link between the brain and skin was definitively proved in the field of psychoimmunology, the relationship between these two organs was largely unknown. It is likely that further psychodermatogical links will be revealed, and we will identify new relationships that will help us to better understand the association between Dermatology and Psychiatry.

Collaboration among dermatologists, psychiatrists and psychologists is evident throughout history, and the large number of scientific societies that have emerged in Europe and America reflect the continued growth of interdisciplinary research.

REFERENCES:

[1] Dantzer R, O'Connor JC, Freund GG, Johnson RW, Kelley KW. From inflammation to sickness and depression: when the immune system subjugates the brain. Nat Rev Neurosci 2008; 9: 46-56.

[2] Linthorst Homan MW, Spuls PI, de Korte J, Bos JD, Sprangers MA, van der Veen JP. The burden of vitiligo: patient characteristics associated with quality of life. J Am Acad Dermato 2009; 6: 411-20.

[3] Linthorst Homan MW, de Korte J, Grootenhuis MA, Bos JD, Sprangers MA, van der Veen JP. Impact of childhood vitiligo on adult life. Br J Dermatol 2008; 159: 915-20

[4] Cossidente A, Sarti MG. History and fundamentals of psychosomatic dermatology. Clin Dermatol 1984; 2: 1-16.

[5] Poot F, Sampogna F, Onnis L. Basic knowledge in psychodermatology. J Eur Acad Dermatol Venereol 2007:2 1: 227-34.

[6] Kimball AB, Jacobson C, Weiss S, Vreeland MG, Wu. The psychosocial burden of psoriasis. Am J Clin Dermatol 2005; 6: 383-92.

[7] Koblenzer CS. Psychosomatic concepts in dermatology. A dermatologist-psychoanalyst's viewpoint. Arch Dermatol 1983; 119: 501-12.

[8] Schwab JJ. Psychosomatic medicine: it's past and present. Psychosomatics 1985; 26: 583-5, 588-9, 592-3.

[9] Kanareĭkin KF, Bakhur VT. Evolution of psychosomatic medicine. Klin Med (Mosk) 1989; 67: 16-21

[10] Koo JYM. Pham CT. Psychodermatology. Practical guidelines on pharmacotherapy. Arch Dermatol 1992; 128: 381-8.

[11] Agustín M, Cotteril J, Gieler U, Zschocke I. Skin and the psyche: closing the gap. Dermatol Psichosom 2000; 1: 4-7.

[12] Koblenzer CS, Koblenzer PJ, Tausk FA. What is psychocutaneous medicine? Cutis. 2008; 81: 487.

[13] Tausk F, Elenkov I, Moynihan J. Psychoneuroimmunology. Dermatol Ther 2008; 21: 22-31.

[14] Cotterill JA. Dermatologic non desease. Dermatol Clin 1996; 14: 439-45.

[15] Panconesi E. Psychosomatic dermatology: past and future Int J Dermatol 2000: 39: 732-4.

[16] Musaph H. Psychodermatology. Psychother Pysychosom 1974; 24: 79-85.

[17] Escande JP. Institutional organization of a hospital dermatology service with a responsibility for psychosomatic care. Sem Hop 1984: 60: 916-9.

[18] Panconesi E. Psychosomatic factors in dermatology: special perspectives for application in clinical practice. Dermatol Clin 2005; 23: 629-33.

[19] Giovanni A, Nicoletta S. The Biopsychosocial Model Thirty Years Later. Psychother Psychosom 2008; 77: 1–2.

[20] Koblenzer CS. Psychocutaneous disease. Orlando: Grune & Stratton, 1987.

[21] Griesemer RD. Emotionally triggered disease in a dermatology practice. *Psychiatr Ann* 1978; 8: 49–56.

[22] Le Moal M, Battin J, Bioulac B, *et al.* Neurosciences in Bordeaux Bull Acad Natl Med 2008; 192: 817-31.

[23] Gieler U, Niemeier V, Kupfer J, Harth W. Psychosomatic dermatology Hautarzt. 2008; 9: 415-32.

[24] Grimalt F, Cotterill J. Dermatología y Psiquiatría: historias clínicas comentadas. Madrid: Aulamedica, 2002

[25] Gieler U, Harth W. Psychodermatology. Hautzart 2008; 59: 287-8.

[26] Gieler U, Taube K. Comment on the continuing education article by R. Hoffmann and R. Happle "Alopecia areata". Position of the Psychosomatic Dermatology Professional Circle of German Dermatology Society. Hautarzt 1999; 50: 816-9.

[27] Koo J, Lebwohl A. Psychodermatology: The Mind and Skin Connection. Am Fam Physician 2001; 64: 1873-8.

[28] Rodríguez-Cerdeira C. Fundamentos básicos en Psicodermatología. Tresctres: Santiago de Compostela (Spain), 2010.

[29] Poot F. Doctor-patient relations in dermatology: obligations and rights for a mutual satisfaction. J Eur Acad Dermatol Venereol 2009; 23: 1233-9

[30] Moffaert M. Psychodermatology: an overview. Psycother Psychosom 1992; 58:125-36.

9

Trichoscopy Simplified

Ebtisam Elghblawi*

Dermatology OPD, STJTL, Tripoli, Libya

Abstract: It has been a long while since skin surfaces and skin lesions have been examined by dermoscopy. However examining the hair and the scalp was done again recently and gained attention and slight popularity by the practical tool, namely trichoscopy, which can be called in a simplified way as a dermoscopy of the hair and the scalp. Trichoscopy is a great tool to examine and asses an active scalp disease and hair and other signs can be specific for some scalp and hair diseases. These signs include yellow dots, dystrophic hairs, cadaverized (black dots), white dots and exclamation mark hairs.

Trichoscopy magnifies hair shafts at higher resolution to enable detailed examinations with measurements that a naked eye cannot distinguish nor see.

Trichoscope is considered recently the newest frontier for the diagnosis of hair and scalp disease.

Aim of this paper. The aim of this paper is to simplify and sum up the main trichoscopic readings and findings of hair and scalp disorders that are commonly encountered at clinic dermatology settings.

Keywords: Dermoscopy, diagnosis, hair, hair loss, scalp dermoscopy, trichoscopy.

INTRODUCTION

Any dermatology clinic will be quite busy and in many instances faced with many patients mostly women complaining of hair loss, which can have significant effects on their self-esteem and quality of life. A normal terminal hair is identical in thickness and colour right through its length (Fig. **1**). The width of normal hairs is usually more than 55 mm. Trichoscopy of normal scalp illustrates follicular units composing of 2-4 terminal hairs and 1 or 2 vellus hairs (less than 0.03 mm in width).

Trichoscopy can be either performed with a handheld dermoscope or a videodermoscope (with software equipped). Trichoscopy works similar to the skin surface and at right angles to the histological plane; like the histopathology [1]. It should examine hair and scalp in all locations namely frontal, occipital, and temporal areas. The choice of fluid immersion is individual choice. Water, ultrasound gels, aqueous gels, liquid paraffin, alcohol, and oil can be used to enhance clarity and visualization. However air bubbles or paraffin can impede or blurs vision and also gels [2].

Trichoscopy aids in visualizing hair at a working magnifications of 20-fold to 70- fold, and some higher up to 160 [3, 4]. Trichoscopy is a quick, easy, priceless, novel, efficient, and a non-invasive device, which can save time and money to achieve a clear-cut diagnosis and enable treatment to start [4]. It assists visualization of the surface and beneath constitutions and colour outlines of scalp and hair [5]. It offers rapid appreciation of scalp and hair disorders, and advances diagnostic accuracy. It predicts the course of the disease and lessens the needless need for biopsies. It can be generally alienated into hair signs, vascular patterns, pigment patterns and interfollicular patterns, all of which can denote specific disease and aid in making the proper diagnosis.

Fig. (1). Normal scalp and hair (uniform shaft and colour).

Likewise recently, its function extended to aid in diagnosing some inflammatory scalp conditions like lichen planopilaris (LPP), scalp psoriasis, and discoid lupus erythematosus (DLE).

TRICHOSCOPIC MAIN AND SPECIAL FINDINGS

Starting off with the main clinical appreciations and then the main trichoscopic main findings and recognitions are shown (Table **1**).

*Address correspondence to this author at the Dermatology OPD, STJTL, Tripoli, Libya; E-mail: ebtisamya@yahoo.com

Table 1. Types of alopecia.

Non-Cicatricial Alopecias	Cicatricial Alopecias
Female pattern hair loss (FPHL) Telogen effluvium (TE) Androgenetic alopecia (AGA) Alopecia areata (AA) Alopecia areata incognita (AAI) Scalp psoriasis and seborrheic dermatitis Tinea capitis Trichotillomania (TTM) Syphilitic alopecia	Lichen planopilaris (LPP) Discoid lupus erythematosus (DLE) Frontal fibrosing alopecia (FFA) Folliculitis decalvans and tufted folliculitis. Dissecting cellulitis (DC) Pseudopelade Brocq

NON-CICATRICIAL ALOPECIAS

Female Pattern Hair Loss (FPHL): FPHL typically presents with noticeable patterns of hair loss, thus making a bedside diagnosis possible [6, 7].

Trichoscopic Findings

According to Bhamla *et al.* [8], the presence of hair with different calibre is classic of FPHL and imitates progressive hair miniaturization due to the disease (about 75% showed anisotrichosis on trichoscopy) (Fig. **2**).

Telogen Effluvium (TE): TE is a self-limiting, abrupt generalized hair loss and thinning process, with premature development of catagen and telogen follicles with premature termination of anagen follicles, and almost never causes apparent baldness; however patients panic and complain of handful hair shedding as its severe at earlier stages.

Trichoscopic Findings

Presence of empty hair follicles and decreased hair density, one follicular hair unit dominance (Fig. **3**) and perifollicular discolouration (perpilar sign) and upright short hair re-growth [5, 9]. TE is a diagnosis of exclusion.

Androgenetic Alopecia (AGA): AGA is the most common form of hair loss both in men and women, and is featured by a progressive loss of hair diameter, length, and pigmentation and over time may become cosmetically undesirable [10].

FAGA was clinically alleged in cases of frontal accentuation (Christmas-tree pattern), with sparing of the occiput [3] (Fig. **4**). It can be examined properly by parting the frontal and occipital hair line.

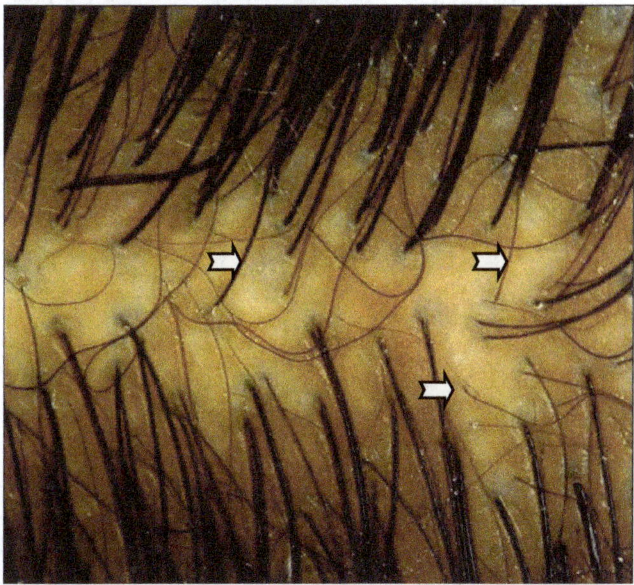

Fig. (2). Anisotrichosis [8, 19].

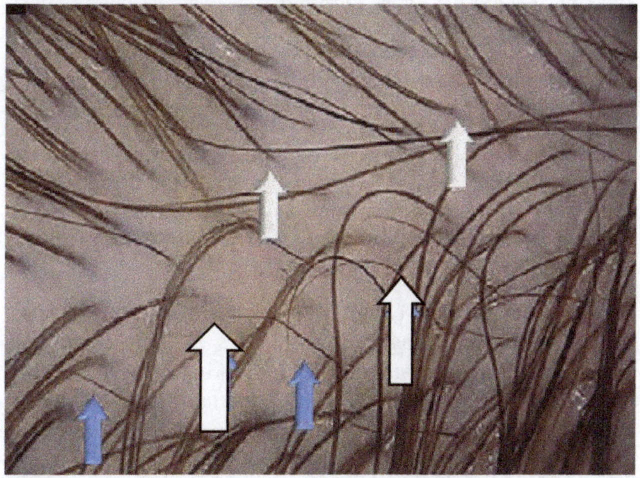

Fig. (3). Upright hair in blue arrow and one follicular hair unit in white arrow [13].

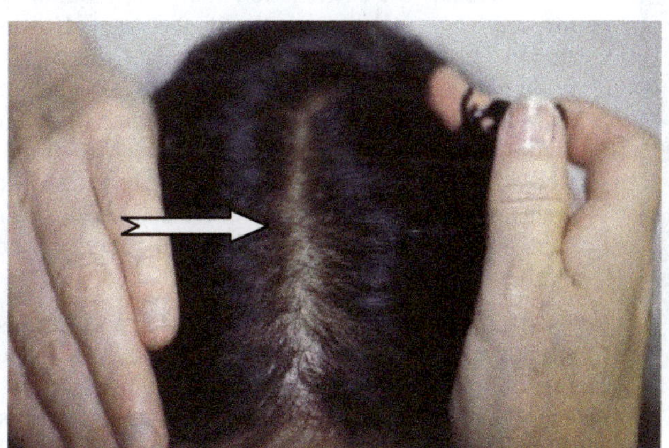

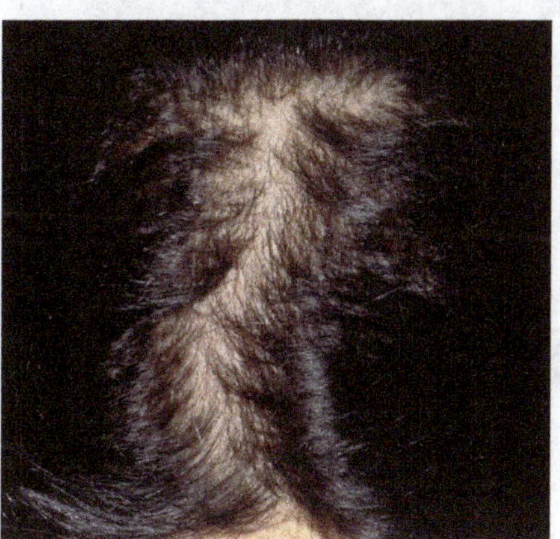

Fig. (4). Frontal accentuations, Christmas tree pattern [26].

Trichoscopic Findings

Increased proportion of thin and vellus hairs, anisotrichosis due to miniaturization of the hair follicles (Fig. **5**), empty follicle [10], perifollicular discoloration and the presence of a variable number of yellow dots (YD) and decline in one follicular hair unit (Figs. **5**, **6**).

It has been suggested that a diversity of 20% is diagnostic of FAGA [3, 5, 10].

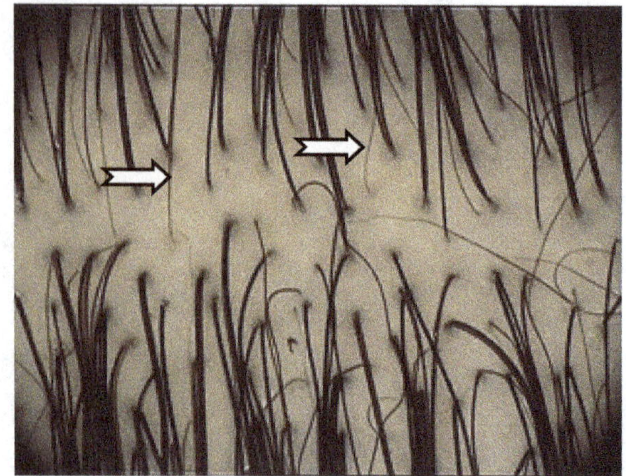

Fig. (5). Anisotrichosis, due to miniaturization of the hair follicles; more than 20% of hair shafts [5, 6, 20].

White dots were seen and are suggested to be related to severe disease stage. They signify empty follicular opening which replaced by fibrosis in advanced phase of the disease (Fig. **7**).

There are certain diagnostic criteria for FAGA. Moreover, in FAGA the number of yellow dots, pilosebaceous units with only one hair and with PFP was signifycantly increased in androgenic alopecia.

Alopecia Areata (AA): AA is an autoimmune disease that is disturbing anagen hair follicles [11]. It is an area which is devoid of hair with smooth skin in the scalp. The hair starts to fall out suddenly, often in clumps.

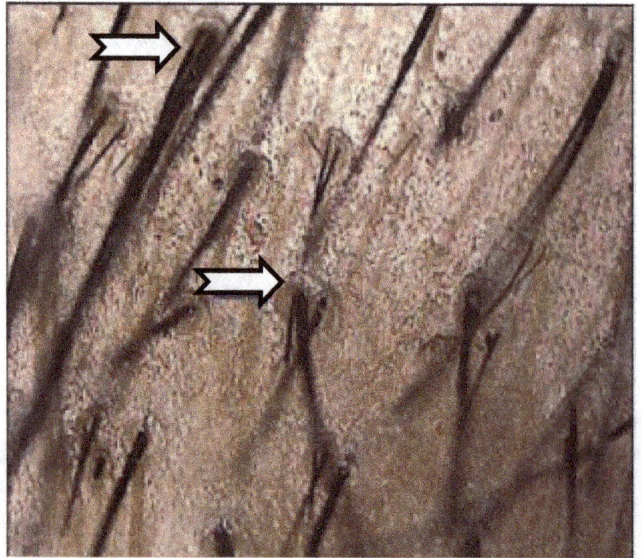

Fig. (6). Peripilar halo [13].

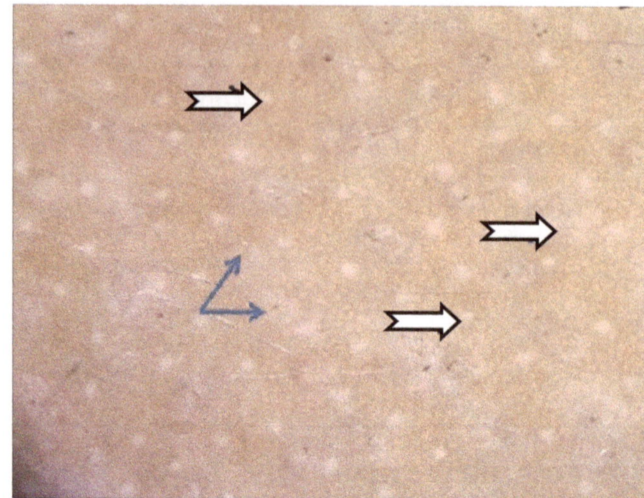

Fig. (7). White dots [5, 6, 20].

Trichoscopic Findings

In active AA patients, the hallmark trichoscopic specific features were yellow dots, uniform cadaverized (black dots), dystrophic broken hair (micro-exclamation, tapered hairs which is a marker of active disease), trichoptilosis, pig tail, and short vellus hairs and upright re-growing hair [12-14] (Figs. **8-11**).

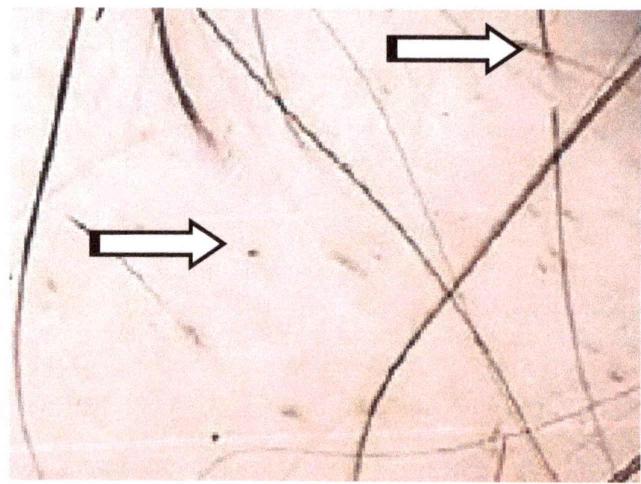

Fig. (8). Black dots, micro exclamation hair mark [13].

Previously the exclamation mark was thought to be a sign for recovery and re-growth of the hair. However some studies had contradicted the concept of active disease findings, as a Turkish study by Kibar *et al.* [15] concluded that white dots and black dots were related to severe disease, while exclamation mark hairs related to mild disease. According to Tosti and Estrada [16], yellow dots, short vellus are sensitive marker of AA and black dots, tapering hairs and broken hairs are most specific marker, and the only markers of AA activity.

Alopecia Areata Incognita (AAI): AAI is considered as a diversity of alopecia areata, featured by acute diffuse shedding of telogen hairs and trichodynia, and it stimulates androgenetic alopecia and telogen effluvium with occurrence of disperse and severe hair thinning in short time. Molina *et* *al.* [17] stated AAI affects mostly women below forty however there is some disagreement.

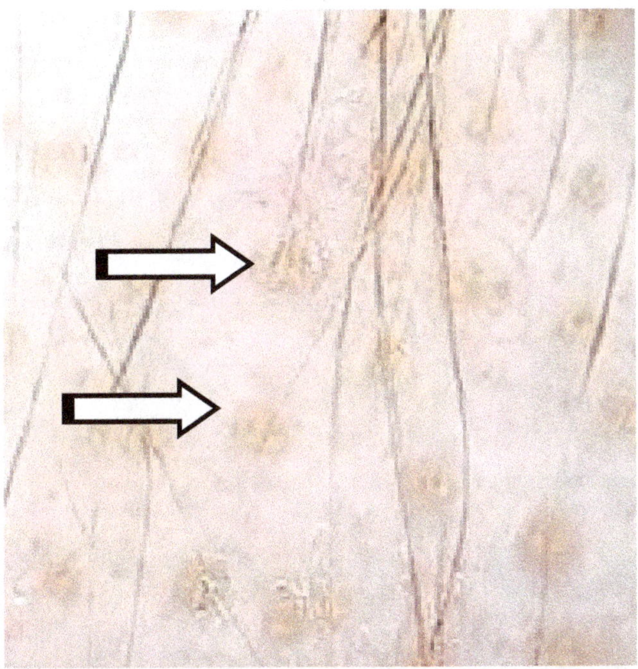

Fig. (9). Yellow dots [13].

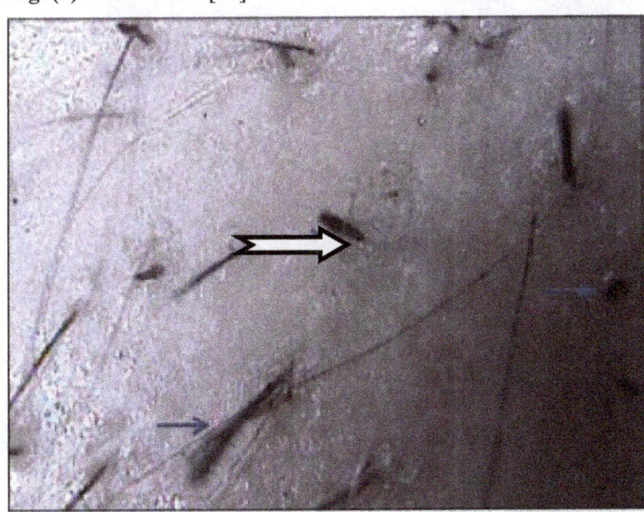

Fig. (10). Exclamation mark hair [13].

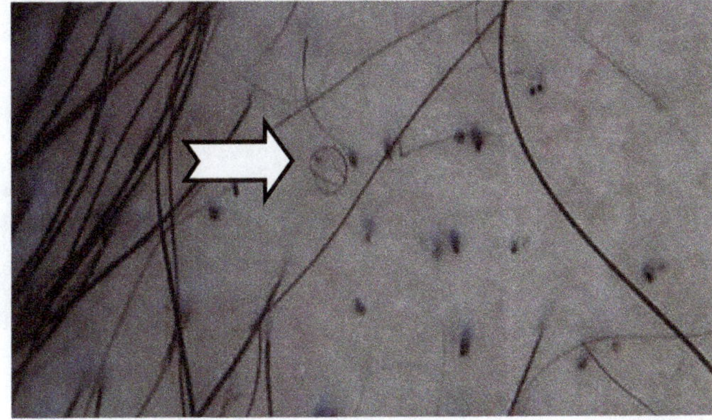

Fig. (11). Pig tails [14].

Trichoscopic Findings

According to Tosti and Estrada [16], there are numerous, diffuse yellow dots of different size and uniform colours within the follicular orifices of both empty and hair-bearing with a large number of re-growing of tapered terminal hairs in the entire scalp (Fig. **12**).

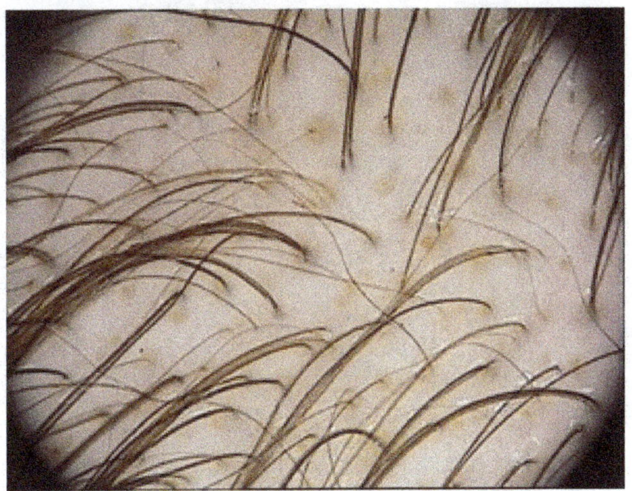

Fig. (12). YD in whole scalp; hairy and none hairy areas.

Scalp Psoriasis and Seborrheic Dermatitis: Psoriasis and seborrheic dermatitis are equally chronic erythemato-squamous dermatoses that can involve the scalp. It may be hard to distinguish between both clinically when it affects only the scalp [18] and thus it poses a diagnostic challenge, however involvement of frontal hair lines is distinctive for scalp psoriasis.

Trichoscopic Findings

Atypical red vessels (ARV), red dots and globules (RDG), signet ring vessels (SRV), structureless red areas (SRA), glomerular vessels (GV), twisted red loops (TRL), perifollicular pigmentation (PP) and hidden hairs (HH) were seen mostly in favour of psoriasis while twisted red loops (TRL) and comma vessels (CV) were specific for seborrheic dermatitis [18, 19] (Figs. **13-16**).

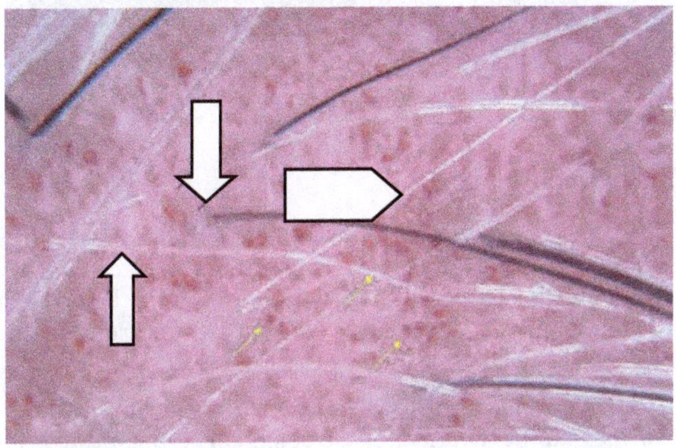

Fig. (13). RDG top and arborsing vessels bottom [23].

Tinea Capitis: A common condition, of superficial fungal infection of the scalp, which is seen in children. The disease is primarily caused by dermatophytes, namely the *Trichophyton* and *Microsporum* genera that invade the hair shaft.

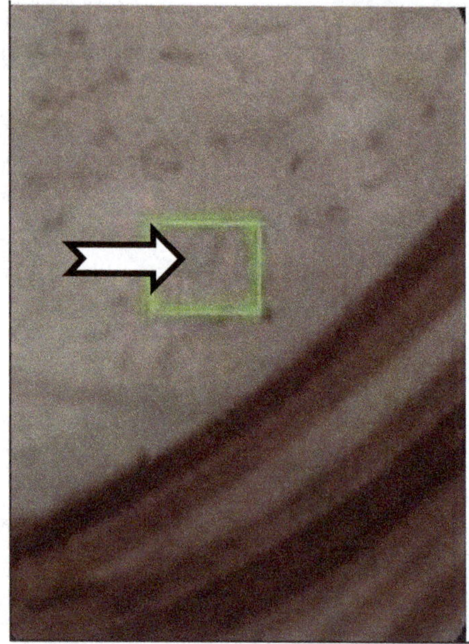

Fig. (14). Comma vessels [23].

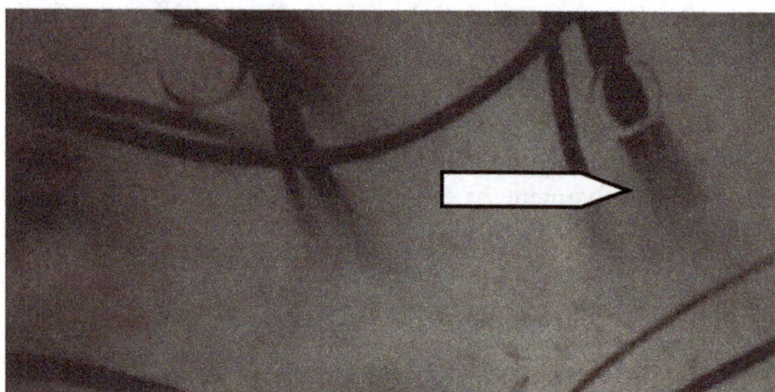

Fig. (15). HH [23].

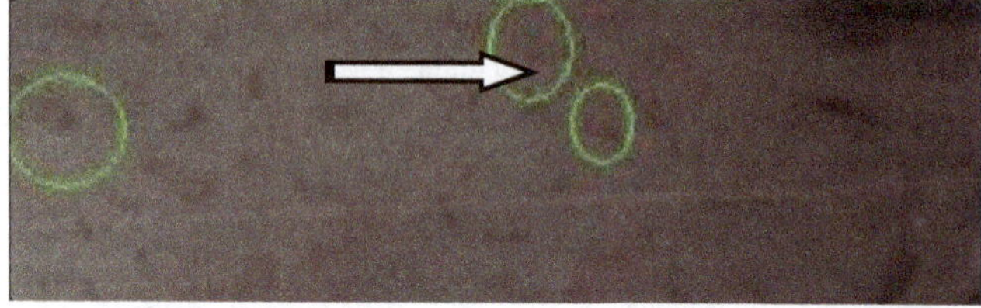

Fig. (16). Singlet ring vessel [22].

Trichoscopic Findings

In tinea capitis patients, trichoscopic readings include the followings namely; comma shaped hairs (Figs. **12**, **14**), corkscrew hairs, black dots, and short broken hairs, and zigzag shaped hairs (Figs. **17-19**) are the diagnostic trichoscopic features of tinea capitis [1].

The zigzag shaped hairs or corkscrew (twisting -coiled) hair looks to be a variant of the comma hair, manifesting in black patients.

Trichotillomania (TTM)/Trichotillosis: Trichotillomania (TTM)/Trichotillosis is self-inflicted injury and distinguished by patchy alopecia of hair bearing areas.

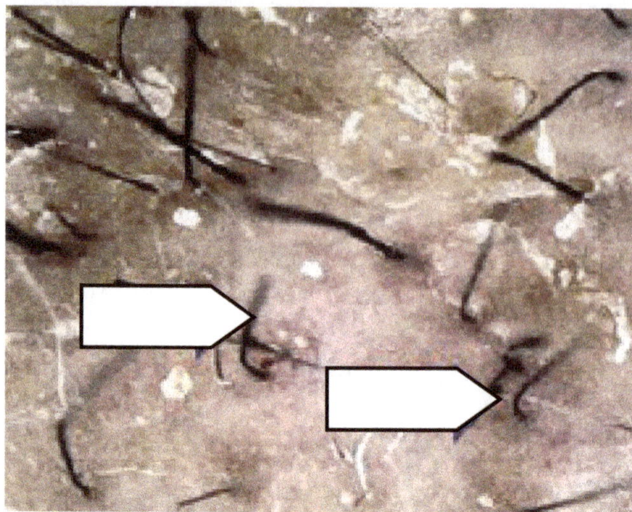

Fig. (17). Comma hairs [14].

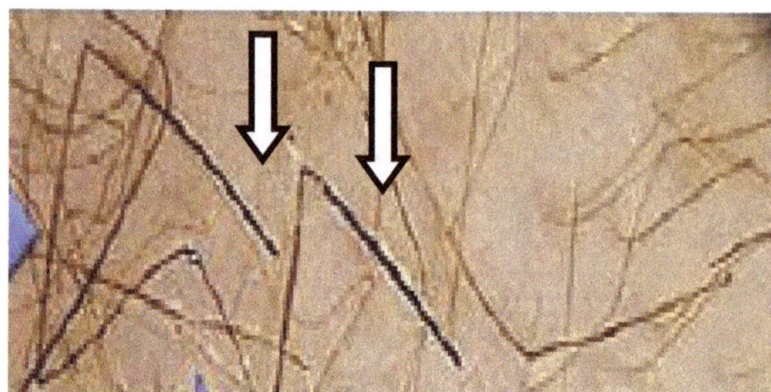

Fig. (18). Zigzag hairs [14].

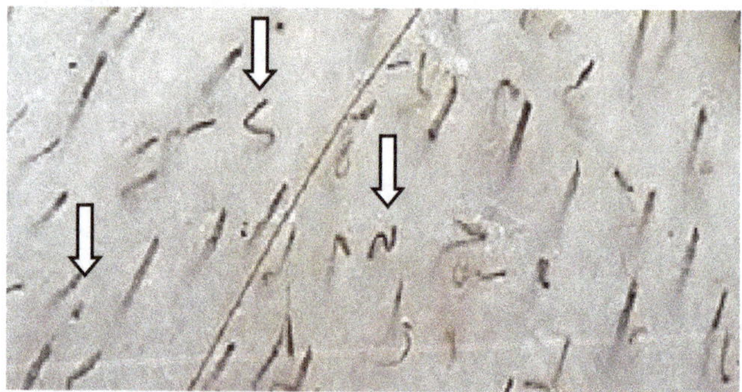

Fig. (19). Comma and Zigzag and black dots [13].

It factually means dismal urge and craving to pull out hair repeatedly, with a sense of pleasure, gratification, or relief after the hair is plucked. The pulling behaviour serves as a coping mechanism for anxiety, stress, and other difficult emotions.

It is considered amongst the psycho-cutaneous diseases as it to be associated with psychiatric comorbidity, social, and functional hurt.

Trichoscopic Findings

Short hair with trichoptilosis “split ends" and irregular coiled hairs, upright re-growing hairs, and black dots. Additionally some other findings, flame hair, v-sign, follicular hemorrhages, decreased hair density, broken hairs at different levels, and absence of exclamation signs [11] (Figs. **15**, **16**). Recently, Tulip hair (Fig. **16**), flame hair, v-sign and hair powder were observed as well in some cases [11, 14, 20].

According to Ahu Yorulmaz, *et al.* [21], recent trichoscopic findings demonstrated decreased hair density, vellus hairs, broken hairs, hair with trichoptilosis, coiled hairs, flame hairs, tulip hairs, V-sign, black dots, and broom fibers.

The follicular micro-hemorrhage has a diagnostic sign in TTM. It appears as a red dot corresponding follicular ostia that is swollen with the blood clot due to traumatic forceful hair plucking (Fig. **20**).

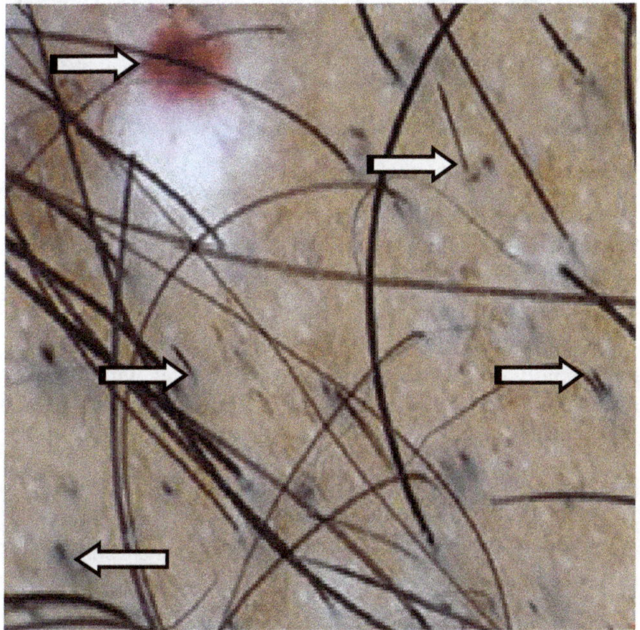

Fig. (20). Follicular hemorrhage, black dots, V shape, flame hair and tulip hair [10, 11, 21, 22].

Newly suggested, the flame hairs, v-sign, tulip hairs, and hair powder are added, and Abu emphasize these signs are explicit only for TTM. Flame hairs are semi-transparent, wavy and cone-shaped hair remains, that occurs due to strict mechanical hair pulling and tears up (Figs. **20**, **21**).

Syphilitic Alopecia: Syphilitic alopecia is unusual in patients with secondary syphilis. However it is known to be moth-eaten alopecia.

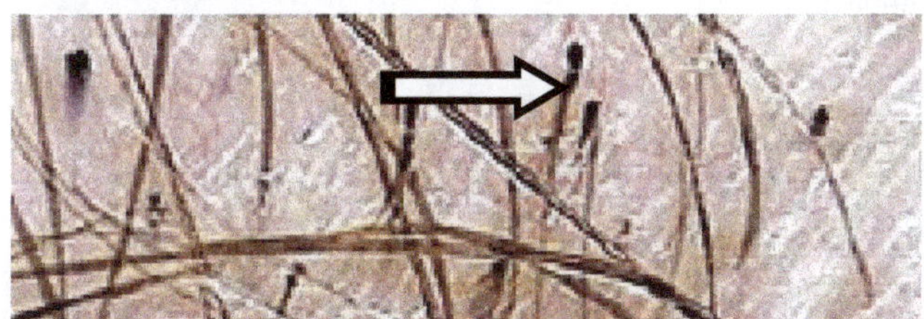

Fig. (21). Tulip hairs [10, 11, 21, 22].

Trichoscopy Findings

Previously the trichoscopic features of syphilitic alopecia have not been looked into. According to Ye *et al.* [22], there are black dots, focal atrichia, hypopigmentation of hair shaft, empty ostia of hair follicle and yellow dots (Fig. **22**).

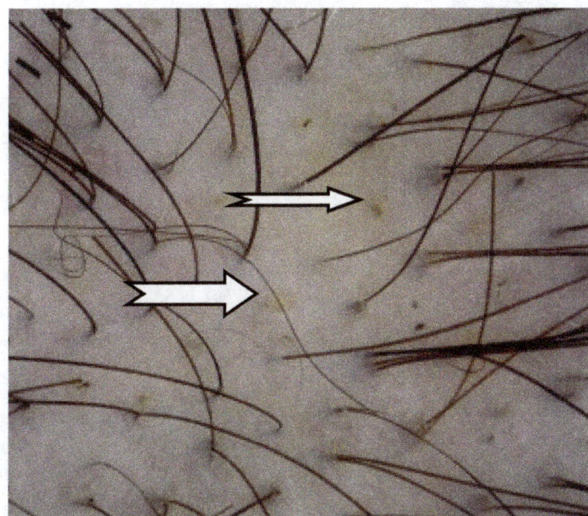

Fig. (22). Black and yellow dots [16].

CICATRICIAL ALOPECIAS

Recently it has been discovered that the scarring incurred are due to irreversible insult of the stem-cell-rich bulge area of the hair, which is required for the cyclic regeneration of the lower follicle [16]. Thus in any trichoscopy we can expect no hair follicle orifice and a fibrous white band.

Lichen Planopilaris (LPP): LPP clinically manifest as purplish plaques affecting the central scalp, and then ending up at later stages with atrophy and permanent alopecia of the scalp [23].

Trichoscopic Findings

Tubular perifollicular scaling (peripilar casts), and perifollicular erythema (arborizing vessels around the follicular ostia) due to perifollicular inflammation (Figs. **23**, **24**) with elongated blood vessels [24].

Frontal Fibrosing Alopecia (FFA): FFA is a clinical variant of lichen planopilaris, and is distinguished by the recession of the frontotemporal hairline (FTHL) [25].

Trichoscopic Findings

Trichoscopic findings are loss of follicular opening, follicular hyperkeratosis, follicular plugs and erythema. And according to Toledo *et al.* [25] the presence of perifollicular erythema will be a direct marker of FFA activity (Fig. **25**).

Discoid Lupus Erythematosus (DLE): DLE clinically appears as erythematous scaly follicular plaques in the early stages, which then get thickened with adherent scales and follicular plugging [23]. In late stage, lesions become depressed (atrophy), depigmented, with telengiectasia, and the follicular openings is completely lost. DLE may show hair re-growth if promptly treated and thus early treatment is important [16].

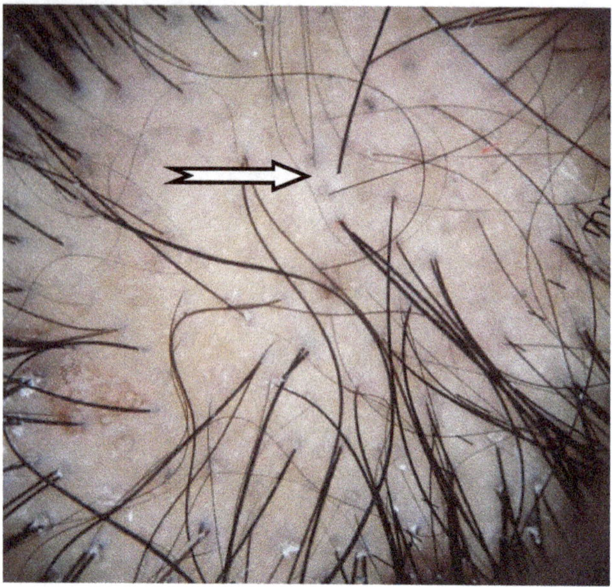

Fig. (23). White dots of LPP [1].

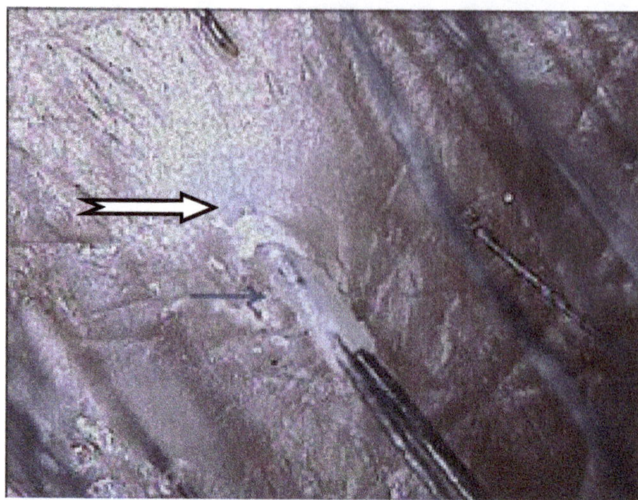

Fig. (24). Perifollicular scales/ casts [1].

Trichoscopic Findings

Scattered dark-brown discoloration of the skin, large yellow dots and thick arborizing vessels [24] (Figs. **26**, **27**).

According to Tosti and Estrada [16] scalp atrophy is appreciated by a diffuse white colour of the scalp. Arborizing and tortuous vessels are seen inside DLE plaques. Red to pinkish-red, round and polycyclic dots of uniform size are often distributed around follicular openings and may be a peculiar finding as well.

Folliculitis Decalvans (FD) and Tufted Folliculitis (TF): Folliculitis decalvans (baldheadedness with scarring) is a variety of alopecia that associated with scarring. It is distinguished by redness, swelling and pustules oozing pus around the hair follicle which leads to inflammation of the hair follicle (folliculitis) with damage of the hair follicle and thus permanent hair loss with scaring. It is also called tufted folliculitis (TF) [26].

Trichoscopic Findings

Multiple upright tufted hairs of 5-20 hair shafts per follicle ostia (polytrichia) with starburst pattern perifollicular hyperplasia in folliculitis decalvans [23] (Figs. **28**, **29**).

Dissecting Cellulitis (DC): Is an uncommon condition that affects the scalp vertex and posterior neck, commonly seen in black males (skin type 5&6) aged 20-40 years, and called doll hair (Fig. **30**).

It starts clinically as simple folliculitis or perifolliculitis then rapidly erupts as multiple painful nodules with purulent discharge that coalesce to form interconnecting abscesses and sinuses.

Trichoscopic Findings

It is seen "3D" yellow dots imposed over dystrophic hairs in dissecting cellulitis [24].

Pseudopelade Brocq: Pseudopelade of Brocq is an unusual form of enduring alopecia of the scalp and mostly affects middle aged and older women. The cause of which is unknown. Its diagnosis by exclusion of LPP and DLE, and described as 'foot print in snow'.

Trichoscopy Features

According to Rudnicka *et al.* [27], the trichoscopy features of classic pseudopelade of Brocq are nonspecific. It appears as white areas with no follicular openings. Also some solitary dystrophic hairs can be seen at the periphery of the lesion.

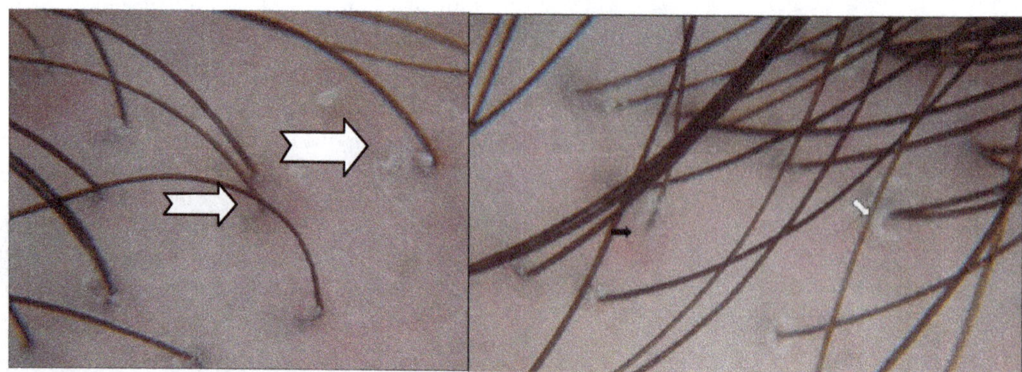

Fig. (25). Perifollicular scales, follicular hyperkeratosis, follicular plugs and erythema [3].

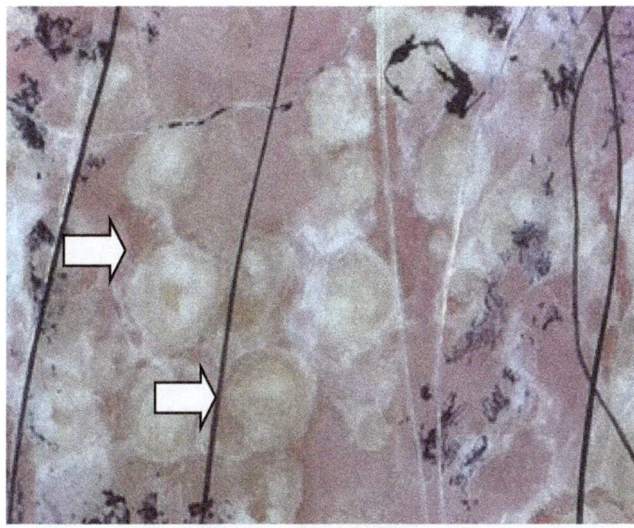

Fig. (26). Numerous yellow Follicular keratotic plugging [25].

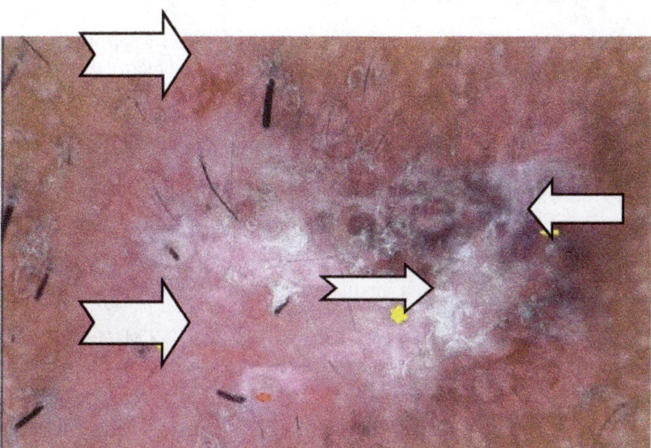

Fig. (27). Thick arborizing blood vessels, and red follicular dots interspersed with scar areas [1].

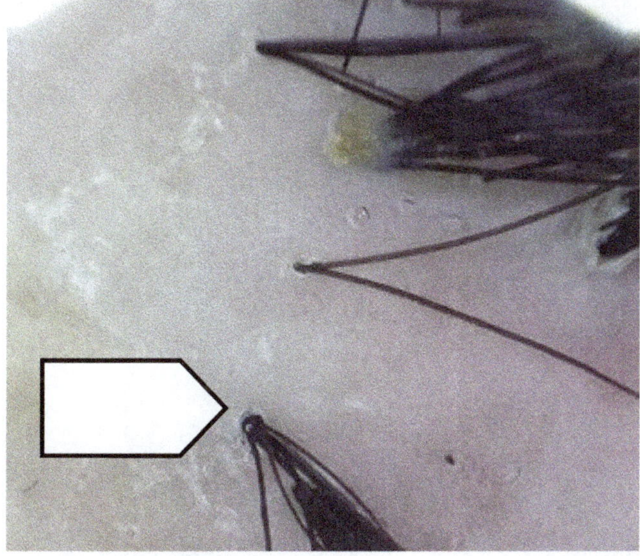

Fig. (28). Tufted hair [13].

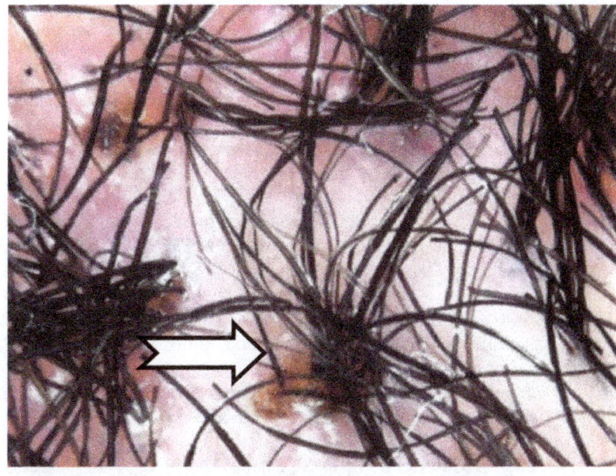

Fig. (29). Polytrichia and redness [17].

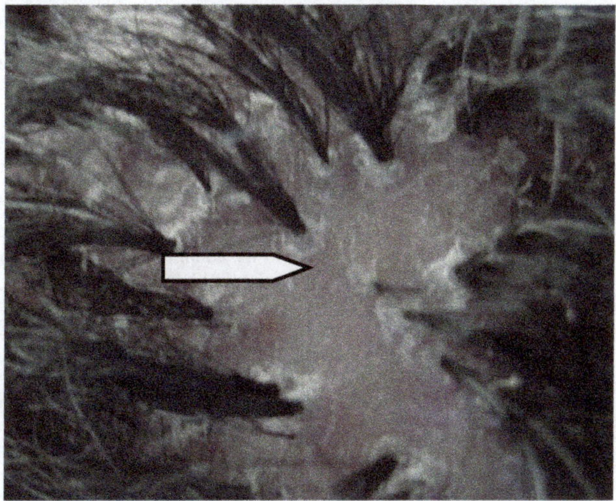

Fig. (30). DC Doll hairs.

In closing, diffuse hair loss of different intensity is a frequent complaint, in particular among women. Trichoscopy is a very useful handy and non-invasive tool in the armamentarium of dermatologist for the clinical evaluation and diagnosis of hair and scalp disorders. It enhances diagnostic potential, and revealed new novel features to advance our understanding. Nonetheless, the diagnosis cannot be made without a clinical case approach, available data, and histology reading in some cases. All are complement to each other.

CONFLICT OF INTEREST

The author confirms that this article content has no conflict of interest.

ACKNOWLEDGEMENTS

A special thanks goes to my lovely Liverpool diploma tutor, Dr. Olive Clara, for her believe on me and kind support always for editing my English.

REFERENCES

[1] El-Taweel AE, El-Esawy F, Abdel-Salam O. Different trichoscopic features of tinea capitis and alopecia areata in pediatric patients. Dermatol Res Pract 2014; 2014: 848763.

[2] Rudnicka L, Olszewska M, Rakowska A, Oledzka E, Slowinsja M. Trichoscopy: a new method for diagnosing hair loss. J Drugs Dermtol 2008; 7(7): 651-4.

[3] Rakowska A. Trichoscopy (hair and scalp videodermoscopy) in the healthy female. Method standardization and norms for measurable parameters. J Dermatol Case Rep 2009; 3(1): 14-9.

[4] Rakowska A, Slowinska M, Kowalska-Oledzka E, Olszewska M, Rudnicka L. Dermoscopy in female androgenic alopecia: method standardization and diagnostic criteria. Int J Trichol 2009; 1(2): 123-30.

[5] Pedrosa AF, Morais P, Lisboa C, Azevedo F. The importance of trichoscopy in clinical practice. Dermatol Res Pract 2013; 2013: 986970.

[6] Zhang X, Caulloo S, Zhao Y, Zhang B, Cai Z, Yang J. Female pattern hair loss: clinico-laboratory findings and trichoscopy depending on disease severity. Int J Trichol 2012; 4(1): 23-8.

[7] Herskovitz I, de Sousa IC, Tosti A. Vellus hairs in the frontal scalp in early female pattern hair loss. Int J Trichol 2013; 5(3): 118-20.

[8] Bhamla SA, Dhurat RS, Saraogi PP. Is trichoscopy a reliable tool to diagnose early female pattern hair loss? Int J Trichol 2013; 5(3): 121-5.

[9] Jain N, Doshi B, Khopkar U. Trichoscopy in alopecias: diagnosis simplified. Int J Trichol 2013; 5(4): 170-8.

[10] Galliker NA, Trüeb RM. Value of trichoscopy *versus* trichogram for diagnosis of female androgenetic alopecia. Int J Trichol 2012; 4(1): 19-22.

[11] Peralta L, Morais P. Photoletter to the editor: the friar tuck sign in trichotillomania. J Dermatol Case Rep 2012; 6(2): 63-4.

[12] de Moura LH, Duque-Estrada B, Abraham LS, Barcaui CB, Sodre CT. Dermoscopy findings of alopecia areata in an African-American patient. J Dermatol Case Rep 2008; 2(4): 52-4.

[13] Jain N, Doshi B, Khopkar U. Trichoscopy in alopecias: Diagnosis simplified. Int J Trichol 2013; 5(4): 170-8.

[14] Thakur BK, Verma S, Raphael V, Khonglah Y. Extensive tonsure pattern trichotillomania-trichoscopy and histopathology aid to the diagnosis. Int J Trichol 2013; 5(4): 196-8.

[15] Kibar M, Aktan S, Lebe B, Bilgin M. Trichoscopic findings in alopecia areata and their relation to disease activity, severity and clinical subtype in Turkish patients. Australas J Dermatol 2015; 56(1): e1-6.

[16] Tosti A, Duque-Estrada B. Dermoscopy in hair disorders. J Egypt Women Dermatol Soc 2009; 7(1): 1-4.

[17] Molina L, Donati A, Valente NS, Romiti R. Alopecia areata incognita. Clinics (Sao Paulo) 2011; 66(3): 513-5.

[18] Kibar M, Aktan S, Bilgin M. Dermoscopic findings in scalp psoriasis and seborrheic dermatitis; two new signs; signet ring vessel and hidden hair. Indian J Dermatol 2015; 60: 41-5.

[19] Kim G, Jung H, Kim B, *et al.* Dermoscopy can be useful in differentiating scalp psoriasis from seborrhoeic dermatitis. Br J Dermatol 2011; 164(3): 652-6.

[20] Ankad BS, Naidu MV, Beergouder SL, Sujana L. Trichoscopy in trichotillomania: A useful diagnostic tool. Int J Trichol 2014; 6(4): 160-3.

[21] Yorulmaz A, Artuz F, Erden O. A case of trichotillomania with recently defined trichoscopic findings. Int J Trichol 2014; 6(2): 77-9.

[22] Ye Y, Zhang X, Zhao Y, *et al.* The clinical and trichoscopic features of syphilitic alopecia. J Dermatol Case Rep 2014; 8(3): 78-80.

[23] Ankad BS, Beergouder SL, Moodalgiri VM. Lichen planopilaris *versus* discoid lupus erythematosus: a trichoscopic perspective. Int J Trichol 2013; 5(4): 204-7.

[24] Rakowska A, Slowinska M, Kowalska-Oledzka E, *et al.* Trichoscopy of cicatricial alopecia. J Drugs Dermatol 2012; 11(6): 753-8.

[25] Toledo-Pastrana T, Hernández MJ, Camacho Martínez FM. Perifollicular erythema as a trichoscopy sign of progression in frontal fibrosing alopecia. Int J Trichol 2013; 5(3): 151-3.

[26] Fabris MR, Melo CP, Melo DF. Folliculitis decalvans: the use of dermatoscopy as an auxiliary tool in clinical diagnosis. An Bras Dermatol 2013; 88(5): 814-6.

[27] Rudnicka L, Rakowska A, Kerzeja M, Olszewska M. Hair shafts in trichoscopy: clues for diagnosis of hair and scalp diseases. Dermatol Clin 2013; 31(4): 695-708.

Pyoderma Gangrenosum Following the Revision of a Breast Reconstruction and Abdominoplasty

Mio Nakamura*,[1], Amir M. Ghaznavi[2], Vigen Darian[2] and Aamir Siddiqui[2]

[1]*Wayne State University School of Medicine, Detroit, MI, USA*

[2]*Division of Plastic and Reconstructive Surgery, Department of Surgery, Henry Ford Health System Detroit, MI, USA*

Abstract: Pyoderma gangrenosum (PG) is a rare ulcerative dermatologic disease and little is known about its etiology and pathogenesis. Recent reports show that there have been limited but increasing number of cases of PG following aesthetic surgeries. Post-surgical PG is often misdiagnosed, which can have serious clinical consequences. The following case report describes a young woman who underwent a cosmetic breast augmentation and abdominoplasty which was complicated by post-operative necrotizing fasciitis. She was presented one year later for surgical correction of her acquired breast and abdominal deformities. Post-operatively she developed a severe inflammatory skin response presumed to be a wound infection. However, after repeated surgical debridements, the wounds persisted without a defined bacterial or fungal organism. After clinical exclusion of all other etiologies, PG was diagnosed and confirmed with histopathology. The patient was subsequently treated with aggressive immunosuppressive therapy, and the lesions resolved without any signs of residual PG. This case report attempts to increase awareness for the rare post-surgical complication of PG in aesthetic surgery and to improve future diagnosis and management of such cases.

Keywords: Abdominoplasty, breast reconstruction, neutrophilic dermatoses, post-operative complication, pyoderma gangrenosum, wound complication.

INTRODUCTION

Pyoderma gangrenosum (PG) is a rare ulcerative dermatologic disease in which little is known about its etiology and pathogenesis. PG is characterized by inflammatory skin lesions without evidence of infection. PG is commonly associated with systemic diseases such as inflammatory bowel disease, hematologic disorders, arthritis, and psoriasis, suggesting a possible autoimmune process. When manifesting outside of this context, PG can go largely unrecognized. An extensive Medline search from 1980-2012 shows that there have been limited but increasing number of reported cases of PG as a post-operative complication following aesthetic surgeries [1-3]. Pathergy, a process in which cutaneous tissue antigens become altered or exposed following trauma and subsequently become vulnerable to host-mediated immune responses, is thought to be involved [4].

Post-surgical PG is often misdiagnosed as a wound infection, which can have serious clinical consequences. Clinical manifestations of PG vary and contribute to the difficulty of diagnosis. Its similarity in presentation to necrotizing fasciitis and other soft tissue infections can delay diagnosis of PG [5]. The following case report attempts to increase awareness for the rare post-surgical complication of PG in aesthetic surgery and to improve future diagnosis and management of such cases.

*Address correspondence to this author at the Wayne State University School of Medicine, 540 E. Canfield St., Detroit, MI 48201, USA;

E-mail: mnakamur@med.wayne.edu

CASE REPORT

A 31-year-old female presented in septic shock at post-operative day 13 following a bilateral breast augmentation, mastopexy, and abdominoplasty. She was promptly taken for debridement of the infected surgical sites and removal of the implants. She underwent a prolonged hospital course undergoing a series of debridements and washouts of the wounds. Over the course of five months the surgical wounds healed.

She returned one year later with a chronic draining sinus from her abdomen and an acquired deformity to her abdominal and chest walls. She requested operative revision of the deformities and excision of the sinus tract (Fig. **1**). The procedure entailed repositioning the umbilicus, removing the abdominal wall scarring and sinus tract, and concentric resection of skin around the nipple-areolar complex bilaterally. There were no operative complications, and the patient was discharged from the hospital a few days following the operation.

She returned two days following discharge with fever and bloody drainage from her abdominal incision. She was mildly tachycardic with acute blood loss anemia. She was taken for evacuation of a 250 cc hematoma. The wound was left open and managed post-operatively with negative pressure therapy. She subsequently went for serial debridements of the abdominal and breast wounds, which continued to appear necrotic with drainage of murky fluid. No microbial organisms could be isolated from any operative cultures or drained fluid; however, she continued to spike fevers and have an elevated white blood cell count.

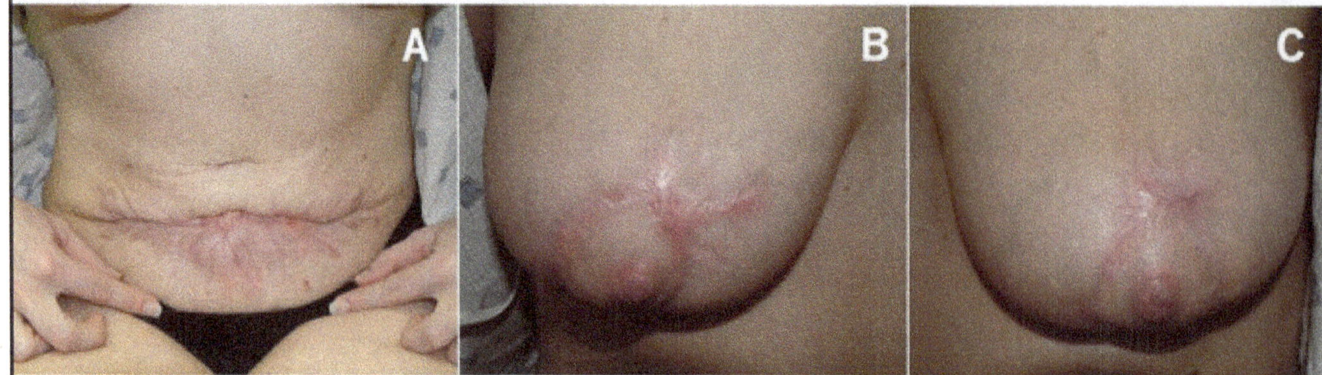

Fig. (1). (**A-C**). Abdominal sinus tract and contracted breast scars from complications of initial breast reconstruction and abdominoplasty.

Over the course of her hospital stay, two small violacious papules in the suprapubic area developed near the abdominal wound edge. Tissue samples were obtained for histopathology and staining for fungal and bacterial organisms. Histopathology of the tissue demonstrated dense neutrophilic infiltrate consistent with PG (Fig. **2**). She was started on immunosuppressive therapy with cyclosporine 175 mg/day (3 mg/kg). When the tissues stains came back negative for fungal and bacterial organisms, the cyclosporine was increased to 275 mg/day (5 mg/kg); however, new lesions continued to develop over the next few days. She was subsequently given a dose of infliximab 300 mg (5 mg/kg). Within 48 hours she became afebrile, the white blood cell count trended down, and her pain decreased significantly. Examination four days later showed some active areas of PG; therefore pulse solumedrol 1 g/day for five days was added. After completing the regimen, she was started on oral prednisone 60 mg/day while on cyclosporine 275 mg/day. At discharge from the hospital, the areas of PG were almost completely re-epithelialized without new active areas (Fig. **3**). She was discharged home on cyclosporine 175 mg/day and an eight-day taper dose of prednisone.

During the course of five months, skin grafts were placed over all wounds. There were no residual sign of PG. She was seen at a two-year post-operative visit with complete resolution of PG and well healed scars of her breast and abdomen (Fig. **4**).

DISCUSSION

It has been eighty years since Brunsting made the first description of PG in 1930 [6], yet little progress has been

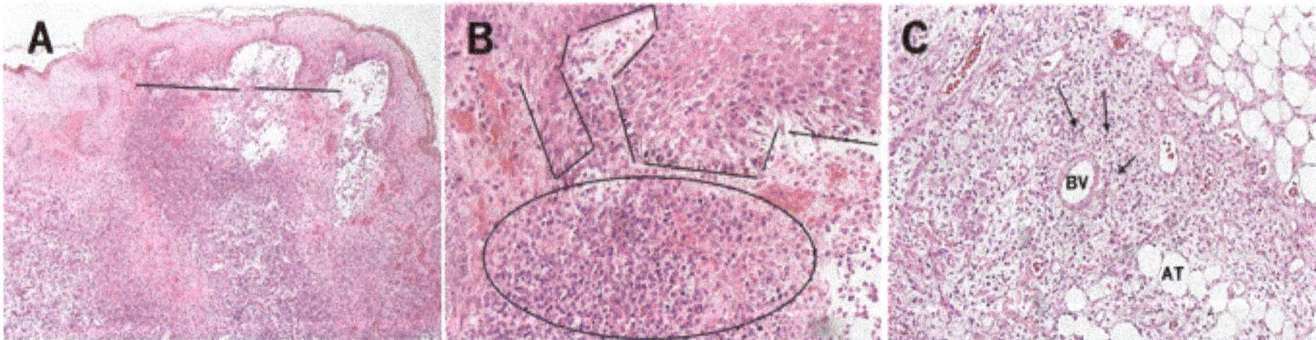

Fig. (2). (**A**) Hematoxylin and eosin stain of ulcerations, with disruption of the dermal-epidermal junction (black lines), 40x; (**B**) Disruption of dermal epidermal junction (black lines) with an aggregation of neutrophils in the dermis with infiltration into the epidermis (black circle), 200x; (**C**) Aggregation of neutrophils (arrows) surrounding blood vessels (BV) and adipose tissue (AT) 200x.

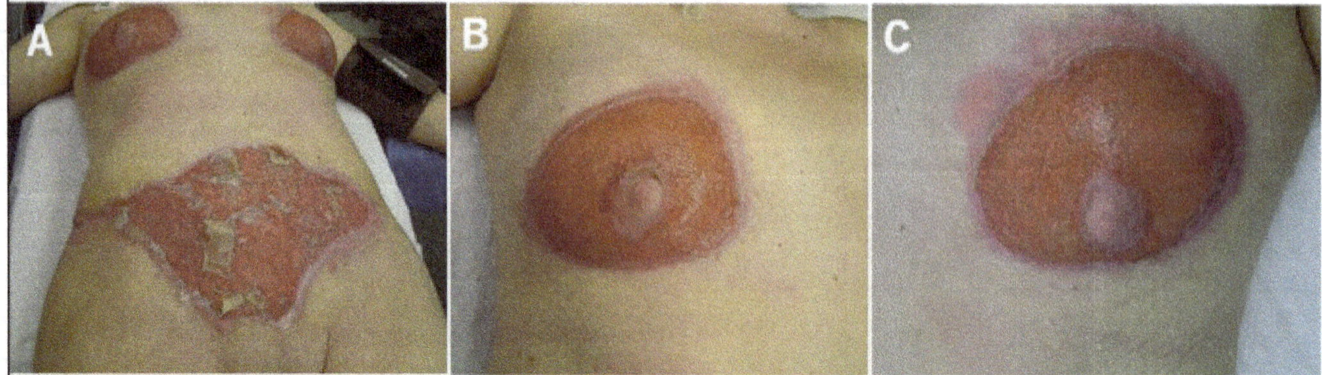

Fig. (3). (**A-C**). Wounds after initiation of immunosuppressive therapy.

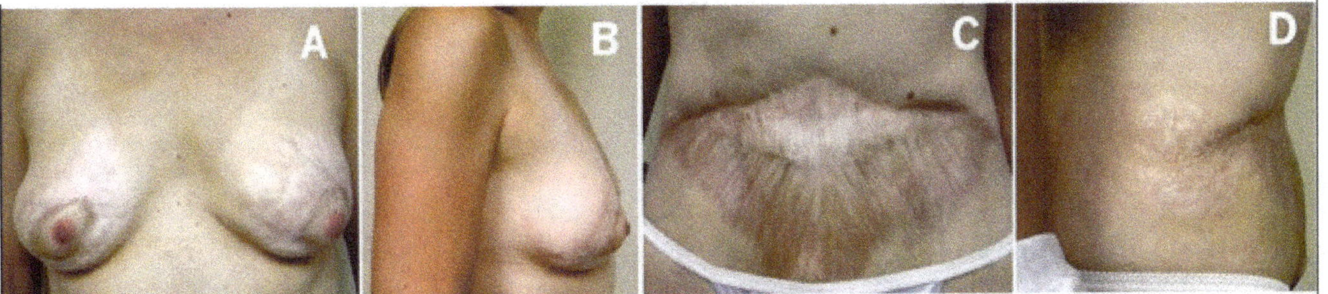

Fig. (4). (A-D). At the two-year post-operative visit with complete resolution of PG and well healed scars of her breast and abdomen.

made in defining the etiology and pathogenesis. There are increasing reports of PG as a post-surgical complication in patients with no known autoimmune diagnosis. Awareness of such a presentation of PG is lacking, which ultimately leads to significant disfigurement and impairment for the patient.

Inquiring about the patient's medical history will reveal diseases that may be associated with PG, such as inflammatory bowel disease, hematologic disorders, arthritis, and psoriasis. Laboratory values such as antinuclear antibody titer and rheumatoid factor can be useful to rule out possible underlying autoimmune diseases. Other findings are nonspecific, such as leukocytosis and elevated erythrocyte sedimentation rate and C-reactive protein. In our case, the patient had no known history or abnormal labs that could be associated with her subsequent diagnosis of PG.

Histopathology of PG will show nonspecific neutrophilic infiltrate. Wound culture and staining for bacteria and fungi should be negative in PG; however, it is possible to have colonization or secondary infection of PG lesions. In our case, we began to suspect PG when histopathology showed dense neutrophilic infiltrates. At that time, we did not have the final results of the bacterial and fungal staining and therefore could not initiate full treatment with immunosuppressant therapy.

There are many types of post-surgical wound complications, many of which have similar presentations. This contributes to the difficulty in diagnosis and management of post-surgical wound complications. A simple wound infection can develop into more severe soft tissue infections such as necrotizing fasciitis. Skin color will change from red-purple to blue-grey, followed by bullae and gangrene formation. In necrotizing fasciitis, the infection will have spread down to the muscle fascia and can later be anesthetized [7]. Although four variants of PG have been described, PG is most often characterized by rapid development of painful and necrolytic ulcers with irregular, violaceous, and undermined borders [8]. In our case, the patient initially presented with a hematoma. It is unknown whether PG was present at this time or if it manifested following the hematoma evacuation; it is possible that PG does not always present in its classical forms.

Ultimately, clinical diagnosis of PG should be entertained when there is evidence of an overabundant inflammatory response despite the absence of microorganisms on culture or histopathological staining. In PG, repeated irritation of the lesions worsens the condition. There should be high suspicion for PG when a suspected wound infection spreads or worsens with serial debridemnts.

Once diagnosis of PG is established, prompt treatment is indicated with pain management and local and/or systemic immunosuppressant therapy. Local wound care is important for protecting the site from further trauma. Surgical debridement should be avoided but may not be contraindicated when there is a need for removal of necrotic borders [9]. Although immunosuppressant therapy will quickly arrest progression, providers should be aware that it increases vulnerability to infection [10].

Attempts to increase awareness for post-surgical PG and its complex clinical manifestations are beneficial for decreasing the disease burden. In our case, early consideration of PG would have made a significant difference in the outcome for the patient. Further studies are indicated to discover how to provide a beneficial wound-healing environment for patients with PG on immunotherapy to avoid opportunistic infections. Since PG has a tendency to recur, the role of prophylactic immunosuppressive therapy with future surgical intervention will be a topic of interest for future research.

CONFLICT OF INTEREST

The authors confirm that this article content has no conflict of interest.

ACKNOWLEDGEMENTS

We thank Dr. Juan Gomez-Gelvez for his assistance and interpretation of pathology slides.

REFERENCES

[1] Rajapakse Y, Bunker CB, Ghattaura A, *et al.* Case report: Pyoderma gangrenosum following Deep Inferior Epigastric Perforator (Diep) free flap breast reconstruction. J Plast Reconstruct Anesthet 2010; 63: e395-6.

[2] De Felice E, Bronwen A. Pyoderma gangrenosum; a rare complication of sclerotherapy. Phlebology 2009; 5: 213-4.

[3] Bonamigo RR, Behar PR, Bellar C, Bonfia R. Pyoderma gangrenosum after silicone prosthesis implant in the breasts and facial plastic surgery. Int J Dermatol 2008; 47: 289-91.

[4] Powell FC, Su WP, Perry HO. Pyoderma gangrenosum: a review of 86 cases. Q J Med 1985; 55: 173-86.

[5] Barr KL, Chatwal HK, Wesson SK, Bhattacharyya I, Vincek V. Pyoderma gangrenosum masquerading as necrotizing fasciitis. Am J Otolaryng 2009; 30: 273-6.

[6] Brunsting LA, Goeckerman WH, O'Leary PA. Pyoderma gangrenosum: clinical and experimental observations in five cases occurring in adults. Arch Dermatol and Syph 1930; 22: 655-80.

[7] Schwartz MN, Pasternack MS. Cellulitis and subcutaneous tissue infections. In: Mandell GL, Bennett JE, Dolin R, editors. Principles and Practice of Infectious Diseases. 6th ed. Philadelphia: Churchill Livingstone; 2005. p. 1172.

[8] Dabade TS, Davis MDP. Diagnosis and treatment of the neutrophilic dermatoses (pyoderma gagrenosum, Sweet's syndrome). Dermatol ther 2011; 24: 273-84.

[9] Shadt CR, Callen JP. Management of neutrophillic dermatoses. Dermatol ther 2012; 25: 158-72.

[10] Schintler MV, Grohman M, Donia C, Aberer E, Scharnagl E. Management of an unfortunate triad after breast reconstruction: pyoderma gangrenosum, full-thickness chest wall defect and Acinetobacter Baumannii infection. Reconstr Aesthet surg 2010; 63: e564-7.

Main Allergens Observed in Patients with Contact Dermatitis in a Brazilian Population Group

Zamir Calamita*, Ana Cristina Rizzo Alonso, Lorena Carla Oliveira da Costa and Andrea Bronhara Pelá Calamita

Marília Medical School (FAMEMA), São Paulo, Brazil

Abstract: *Background*: The skin contact test or patch test is considered to be a fundamental tool for investigating allergic contact dermatitis (ACD). Better knowledge on the prevalence of allergens in the environment is a good strategy for enabling a better approach towards contact dermatitis (CD) cases.

Objective: The objective of the present study was to evaluate the prevalence of the main allergens of ACD in a population group in the interior of the state of São Paulo, Brazil.

Methods: The results from 368 patch tests on adult patients with CD were evaluated through a retrospective study under the supervision of the Discipline of Allergy and Clinical Immunopathology and the Discipline of Dermatology at the Marília Medical School.

Results: Mean age was 41.2 (±_17.2) years, with predomination of women (71.5%). The majority of the patients (91.3%) presented reactivity to at least one substance. Nickel sulfate and the perfume mix stood out as the most allergenic substances.

Conclusion: Among the variety of substances to be tested in an etiological investigation for CD, perfumes and nickel are especially likely to be allergens in this population group.

Keywords: Allergic contact dermatitis, contact dermatitis, fragrance, nickel, perfume, patch test, skin test.

INTRODUCTION

Contact dermatitis (CD) is a highly prevalent disease in the Brazilian environment and is responsible for a large proportion of occupational dermatosis and 4 to 7% of dermatological consultations [1].

It is caused by external agents that, when in contact with the skin, trigger an inflammatory reaction. It usually manifests clinically as eczema. The disease is classified as: primary-irritant contact dermatitis; allergic contact dermatitis; phototoxic contact dermatitis; or photoallergic contact dermatitis. Allergic contact dermatitis (ACD) is a consequence of an immune reaction mediated by T cells against substances named haptens, which generally have low molecular weight [2].

The skin contact test or patch test is the most efficient method for confirming the etiological diagnosis of ACD [3]. This test may be influenced by genetic factors and factors related to the ethnicity of the individuals analyzed [4]. Brazil has continental dimensions, important regional differences and highly diversified population characterized by a high rate of miscegenation between Caucasians, Amerindians and Africans.

The British guidelines for CD recommends the patch test for patients with persistent eczema-like eruptions, either when ACD is suspected or when it cannot be ruled out (evidence level II/ recommendation degree A), with sensitivity and specificity of between 70% and 80% [1].

METHODS

This was a retrospective study, in which the medical files of 368 adult patients with CD were evaluated. These patients were seen between August 2000 and January 2012 at the Allergy outpatient service of the Marília Medical School (FAMEMA) and at a private Allergy and Dermatology clinic in the municipality of Marília, which is located in the interior of the state of São Paulo, Brazil. The study was supervised by the Discipline of Allergy and Clinical Immunopathology and the Discipline of Dermatology of FAMEMA. All the patients who underwent the patch test during this period were included in the study.

The following data were analyzed: age, sex, profession and history of other allergies. The patch tests results were first read 48 hours after the patches had been placed and then 72 hours after placement. The tested substances were listed in Table **1**. They were produced by Alergofar (an allergen product laboratory), a Brazilian company registered with the National Sanitation Surveillance Agency (*Agência Nacional de Vigilância Sanitária* - ANVISA). The substances were applied to the patient's back by means of rectangular patches made of hypoallergenic adhesive tape with filter paper disks

*Address correspondence to this author at the Marília Medical School (FAMEMA), Vicente Ferreira, 648, Marília, São Paulo, Brazil;
E-mails: calamita@unimedmarilia.com.br,
zcalamita@hotmail.com

of area 1.0 cm², which were duly identified. The reading criteria used were adapted from those of the Brazilian Workgroup for Contact Dermatitis (*Grupo Brasileiro de Estudo em Dermatite de Contato*, GBEDC) [5]:

Negative: no reaction

Doubtful: poorly defined mild erythema

Weakly positive: defined erythema, infiltration and papules

Strongly positive: erythema, infiltration, papules and vesicles

Very strongly positive: erythema, infiltration, papules and coalescent vesicles forming blisters

The present study was approved by the Research Ethics Committee of FAMEMA.

RESULTS

The mean age found was 41.2 (±_17.2) years with a median of 38 years. The patients were predominantly female (71.5%).

Regarding professional occupation, 22.3% worked in commerce, 16% were either housewives or worked as cleaners, 8.2% were teachers, 7.3% were healthcare professionals, 6.3% had retired, 5.7% were factory workers, 1.6% were policemen, 1.4% were farm workers, 0.5% worked in construction, 0.5% were hairdressers and the remaining 30.2% had other occupations.

The great majority of patients, i.e. 336 (91.3%), demonstrated reactivity in the patch test, of whom 34.2% reacted to only one substance, while 57.1% reacted to two or more substances. In total, 1,097 reactions were detected, of which 108 were doubtful and 989 were positive. A mean of 2.94 or almost three positive substances was found for each reactive patient. Among the positive results, 212 were very strongly positive, 495 strongly positive and 282 weakly positive.

Regarding the substances tested, we observed that nickel sulfate was the most allergenic substance, followed by the perfume mix. Table **1** presents the percentages of allergenic reactions observed for each of the tested substances, along with their concentrations.

Regarding other allergies, 14.6% reported having rhinitis, 11.6% had a history of drug hypersensitivity, 6.2% reported having chronic hives and 3.8% had asthma. Only 16 patients out of the 368 evaluated had histories of atopic dermatitis (0.04%).

DISCUSSION

Contact dermatitis is one of the main complaints within the specialties of allergy and dermatology. It is an important cause of morbidity, occupational incapacity and diminished quality of life for the people affected.

The importance of monitoring this condition is demonstrated by the fact that, every two years, the North American workgroup on contact dermatitis presents the results of their patch test assessments, carried out using a standardized series of allergens [6-8].

Table 1. Substances tested with their respective concentrations and sensitization percentages.

Substances and Concentrations Tested	Percentages of Sensitization
Nickel sulfate 5%*	36.70%
Perfume mix 8%*	27%
Thimerosal 0.05%*	23.60%
Hydroquinone 1%*	14.10%
Balsam of Peru 25%*	12.20%
Benzoic acid 5%*	11.90%
PPD mix 0.4%*	11.70%
Imidazole derivatives 7%*/**	10.60%
Paraben mix 15%*	9.20%
Potassium bichromate 0.5%*	8.20%
Promethazine 1%*	7%
Carba mix 3%*	6.80%
Colophony 20%*	6.20%
Thiuram mix 1%*	5.70%
Benzocaine 5%*	5.40%
Epoxy resin 1%*	5.20%
Neomycin 20%*	4.60%
Aniline 1%*	4%
Toluene 0.5%*	4%
Ethylenediamine 1%*	3.50%
Lanolin 30%*	3.50%
Turpentine 10%*	3.20%
Mercuric chloride 0.1%*	3%
Chloramphenicol 2%*	3%
Latex in natura	3%
Sulfanilamide 5%*	3%
4-tert-butylphenol 1%*	2.70%
Imidazolidinyl urea 2%	2.70%
Kathon CG 0.01%*/***	2.70%
Nitrofurazone 1%	2.40%
Vioform 6%*	2.40%
Sodium lauryl sulfate 2%****	2.20%
Quinoline mix 6% *	2.20%
Propylene glycol 5%*	1.90%
Anthraquinone 2%*	1.60%
Para-aminobenzoic acid 10%*	1.60%
Boric acid 1%****	1.40%
Cobalt chloride 2%*	1.40%
Triclosan 1%*	1.40%
Quaternium-15 0.5%*	1%
Mercapto mix 2%*	0.80%
Formaldehyde 2%****	0.50%
Sodium hypochlorite 5%****	0.50%
Eosin 50%*	0.30%
Polyethylene glycol 4%*	0.30%
Chlorhexidene 1%****	0%
Phenol 0.5%****	0%
Pyrogallol 1%****	0%
Resorcinol 1%*	0%

*Diluted in petrolatum ** miconazole, ketoconazole and tioconazole, in equal parts ***mixture of methylchloroisothiazolinone and methylisothiazolinone ****Diluted in water.

The present study involved 49 substances that are potentially present in the Brazilian environment, thus encompassing more than 30 substances from the standard set established by the GBEDC [5], which therefore enables broader evaluation of probable allergens.

Demographically, as observed in the present study, other Brazilian studies also found greater predominance among young female adults [5, 9, 10].

Test results that were positive for at least one substance were observed among 91.3% of the patients evaluated, while other Brazilian studies found this result among 62% to 62.8% [5, 6]. The higher percentage of reactors in this study probably occurred because the population studied had a high degree of suspicion to present contact dermatitis. This happened because the group was composed of selected patients in a specialized clinic in allergy area.

The main allergen found was nickel sulfate (36.7%), and this was similar to the findings from other Brazilian studies: (25.1%) [5] and 31,4% [9], and foreign studies [6-8, 11]. The second most prevalent allergen in the present study was the perfume mix (27%), as also observed in a study carried out in Germany [11], although different to two other Brazilian studies [5, 9]. These studies found that thimerosal was the second most prevalent substance, while in the present study this substance was the third most prevalent. The fact that 87.3% of the tests in the present investigation were positive for these substances is highly relevant. Moreover, among the ten main positive substances found in Brazilian studies, four match those found in the present assessment: nickel, thimerosal, perfume mix and potassium bichromate [5, 9].

Nickel contact dermatitis (NCD) gives rise to important loss of quality of life and can lead to occupational damage, as well as significant expense on healthcare. Although such conditions may be related to occupational diseases, most are in fact related to non-occupational cases [12].

NCD occurs when metallic objects are in contact with the skin, especially when they are corroded by sweat, saliva or other body fluids, thereby releasing nickel ions that act like hapten and induce sensitization.

The amount of exposure to nickel according to area can be quantified in $\mu g/cm^2$ and may vary depending on the amount of nickel released and the duration of contact. European legislation established limits for the nickel concentration and the amount released from products that are in touch with the skin, which were 0.05% and 0.5 $\mu g/cm^2$/week, respectively [12, 13]. Subsequently, decreased prevalence of nickel allergy in Denmark and Germany was observed [12]. Stainless steel and gold usually release less than 0.5 $\mu g/cm^2$/week, while other materials covered by nickel generally release more than this amount and are therefore important triggers and causes of worsening of NCD among previously sensitized patients.

Earrings are one of the main triggers of NCD, particularly among women. Moreover, in addition to the ears, the neck and eyelids are frequently areas of sensitization due to the use of necklaces and through polished fingernails that come into contact with the region of the eyes and neck. Nickel can also be found in makeup products, hair dyes and various metallic objects such as bracelets, buttons, clothes, cloth dyes, coins, etc.

Regarding occupational exposure, nickel is also a central issue. A Brazilian study demonstrated that occupational exposure had occurred among 39% of the 404 patients with positive reactions to any of the three metals that were studied (nickel, cobalt and chrome). Nickel was shown to be the most allergenic among the three, either alone or associated with others [14]. A British study observed nickel sensitization in 12% of the 1,190 cases of occupational dermatitis that were evaluated [15]. Sensitization usually occurs through non-occupational exposure, which worsens after exposure at work. However, occasionally, sensitization occurs at the workplace, especially in humid environments where there is contact with nickel [13]. In general, these workers develop chronic eczema, especially on their hands.

Regarding perfumes, these are known to be the most common cause of contact dermatitis due to cosmetics [16]. The composition of the perfume mix consisted of cinnamic aldehyde, cinnamic alcohol, alpha-amyl cinnamic alcohol, geraniol, eugenol, isoeugenol, oakmoss absolute and hydroxycitronellal. Reactions can occur through contact with perfumes, cosmetics, soaps, detergents, medications, papers, hygienic wipes or even the perfumed items from other people.

Contact dermatitis due to perfumes may occur in a generalized or localized manner, such as on the hands, face, neck, trunk, axillae and legs, and may or may not be associated with occupational risk [17]. Regarding occupational issues, dermatitis has been especially associated with physical therapists, masseuses, nurses for elderly people, etc.

A multicenter study encompassing Europe, the United States and Japan, which had the objective of identifying possible new chemical components (other fragrances) for researching with regard to contact dermatitis due to perfumes, showed that 76% of the individuals evaluated presented a reaction to the perfume mix. Allergy due to perfumes preferentially affected women, on their faces and hands, and many patients reporting a personal history of rhinitis, asthma or atopic dermatitis. Regarding the other ingredients that were tested, it was found that 60% to 70% of the patients who were allergic to perfumes reacted to the total set of fragrances of the mix studied [18].

Use of perfumes in areas previously injured by eczema seems to favor new sensitizations. Moreover, if the fragrances are contained within mixtures with irritants such as soaps, detergents or other possible primary irritants, these could act as coadjuvants for precipitating the allergy. This may also happen through use of deodorants or other perfumes in recently depilated and irritated areas, such as the axillae [19].

In conclusion, there was a high positivity rate among the patients tested. Nickel sulfate and the perfume mix acted as the most sensitizing substances, corresponding together to 63.7% of the positive tests.

CONFLICT OF INTEREST

The authors confirm that this article content has no conflict of interest.

ACKNOWLEDGEMENTS

Declared none.

REFERENCES

[1] Bourke J, Coulson I, English J. Guidelines for the management of contact dermatitis: an update. Br J Dermatol 2009; 160: 946-54.

[2] Martins LEAM, Reis VMS. Imunopatologia da dermatite de contato alérgica. An Bras Dermatol 2011; 86(3): 419-33.

[3] Duarte I, Lazzarini R, Buense R, Pires MC. Dermatite de contato. An Bras Dermatol 2000; 75(5): 529-48.

[4] Deleo VA, Taylor SC, Belsito DV, *et al.* The effect of race and ethnicity on patch test results. J Am Acad Dermatol 2002; 46(Suppl 2): S107-12.

[5] Grupo Brasileiro de Estudo em Dermatite de Contato; Sociedade Brasileira de Dermatologia. Departamento Especializado de Alergia. Estudo multicêntrico para elaboração de uma bateria-padrão brasileira de teste de contato. An Bras Dermatol 2000; 75(2): 147-56.

[6] Zug KA, Warshaw EM, Fowler JF Jr, *et al.* Patch-test results of the North American Contact Dermatitis Group 2005-2006. Dermatitis 2009; 20(3): 149-60.

[7] Fransway AF, Zug KA, Belsito DV, *et al.* North American Contact Dermatitis Group patch test results for 2007-2008. Dermatitis 2013; 24(1): 10-21.

[8] Warshaw EM, Belsito DV, Taylor JS, *et al.* North American Contact Dermatitis Group patch test results: 2009 to 2010. Dermatitis 2013; 24(2): 50-9.

[9] Rodrigues DF, Neves DR, Pinto JM, Alves MFF, Fulgêncio ACF. Results of patch-tests from Santa Casa de Belo Horizonte Dermatology Clinic, Belo Horizonte, Brazil, from 2003 to 2010. An Bras Dermatol 2012; 87(5): 800-3.

[10] Minelli L, Swenson AM. Estudo de 70 casos de eczema de contato: alérgenos observados. Rev Bras Alerg Imunopatol 1997; 20(5): 173-8.

[11] Schäfer T, Böhler E, Ruhdorfer S, *et al.* Epidemiology of contact allergy in adults. Allergy 2001; 56: 1192-6.

[12] Torres F, Graças M, Melo M, Tosti A. Management of contact dermatitis due to nickel allergy: an update. Clin Cosmet Investig Dermatol 2009; 2: 39-48.

[13] Kim YY, Kim MY, Park YM, Kim HO, Koh CS, Lee HK. Evaluating the nickel content in metal alloys and the threshold for nickel-induced allergic contact dermatitis. J Korean Med Sci 2008; 23: 315-9.

[14] Duarte I, Amorim JR, Perázzio EF, Junior RS. Metal contact dermatitis: prevalence of sensitization to nickel, cobalt and chromium. An Bras Dermatol 2005; 80(2): 137-42.

[15] Shum KW, Meyer JD, Chen Y, Cherry N, Gawkrodger DJ. Occupational contact dermatitis to nickel: experience of the British dermatologists (EPIDERM) and occupational physicians (OPRA) surveillance schemes. Occup Environ Med 2003; 60: 954-7.

[16] Scheinman PL. Allergic contact dermatitis to fragrance: a review. Am J Contact Dermat 1996; 7(2): 65-76

[17] Uter W, Schnuch A, Geier J, Pfahlberg A, Gefeller O. Association between occupation and contact allergy to the fragrance mix: a multifactorial analysis of national surveillance data. Occup Environ Med 2001; 58: 392-8.

[18] Larsen W, Nakayama H, Fischer T, *et al.* Fragrance contact dermatitis - a worldwide multicenter investigation (part III). Contact Dermatitis 2002; 46(3): 141-4

[19] Guin JD, Berry VK. Perfume sensitivity in adult females: a study of contact sensitivity to a perfume mix in two groups of student nurses. J Am Acad Dermatol 1980; 3: 299-302.

12

Knowledge of HIV and HPV Infection, and Acceptance of HPV Vaccination in Spanish Female Sex Worker

C. Rodríguez-Cerdeira[*,1], E. Sánchez-Blanco[2], A. Gutierrez[2], A. Rodriguez-Rodriguez[2] and B. Sánchez-Blanco[3]

[1]*Department of Dermatology, CHUVI/ University of Vigo, Vigo, Spain*

[2]*University of Vigo, Vigo, Spain*

[3]*Department of Emergency, CHUVI· Vigo, Spain*

Abstract: *Objective*: To examine the socioeconomic variables, lifestyles, and sexual behaviors of female sex workers; their knowledge about the risk of HIV and human papillomavirus (HPV) infection; the HPV vaccine, and their attitudes toward it.

Methods: 168 female sex workers (18-49 years old) filled out a questionnaire consisting of 5 parts with a total of 19 items.

Results: Knowledge of Pap smears was moderate; 47% of the participants had undergone at least one. Most respondents (52.4%) had never heard of HPV. Most (88%) recognized HIV as a virus that can be acquired sexually. For most women, recommendations from non governmental organizations (NGOs) (68.5%) were the major influences in deciding to be vaccinated and learning how to take care of their health.

Conclusion: The cost-effectiveness ratios for HPV control and vaccination strategies would be more favorable if younger women are targeted and initial catch-up efforts are targeted to female sex workers by revising screening policies. Healthcare workers and volunteers in NGOs should be educated and trained about HIV, HPV infection, and HPV vaccination and its relationship with genital cancer.

Keywords: Female sex worker, HIV, HPV vaccination, sexual behavior.

INTRODUCTION

Prostitution (commercial sex work) is commonly regarded as “the oldest profession.” The United Nations defines sex work as “the exchange of money or goods for sexual services, either regularly or occasionally, involving female, male, and transgender adults, young people, and children where the sex worker may or may not consciously define such activity as income-generating” [1]. The term covers a broad range of transactions, and the context in which these transactions occur has implications for assessing those at risk. While some may freely choose sex work as their occupation, others are coerced into it through violence, trafficking, or debt bondage [2].

The concept of commercial sex workers is rarely investigated, perhaps because of the often-informal nature of the workplace, associated stigma, and frequent illegality of the activity. We reviewed the literature on health, occupational risks, and safety among female sex workers (FSW) and identified cultural and local variations, and commonalities [3].

In a comment in *The Lancet*, Groneberg *et al.* [4] mention the following occupational hazards that need to be taken into account in the lives of commercial sex workers: violence, harassment, infections, bladder problems, stress, depression, alcohol and drug addiction, latex allergy, and death. Legal regulations play extremely important roles in harm-reduction strategies. Alexander [5] adds musculoskeletal injuries to this list. Other occupational hazards include having money stolen by clients, being forced to have unprotected sex, and pregnancy [6].

Immigration status may further disempower sex workers. It is assumed that FSW who are migrants are at higher risk, although this may be due to the fact that some women are lured or sold across national borders specifically for the purposes of what is basically sexual slavery. Bautista *et al.* [7, 8] studied immigrant and non-immigrant FSW in Argentina and found that syphilis and hepatitis C were more common among Argentinean sex workers, whereas hepatitis B was more common among migrant FSW. Regression analysis indicates that the distinguishing factors among migrant FSW are being single, no occupation, and that low-paid bar and cabaret workers are more likely to engage in anal sex.

Sex work involves specific interactions between the worker and client, and it is difficult to separate these 2 players in any attempt to improve and promote safe sex work

*Address correspondence to this author at the Servicio Dermatología. CHUVI. Hospital do Meixoeiro, 36200 Vigo. Spain;

E-mails: carmen.rodriguez.cerdeira@sergas.es; crodcer@uvigo.es

encounters. Any attempt to demonize or justify the health and safety of one player over the other is not only philosophically challenging, but is likely to undermine the benefits of any effective health promotion approach in this industry, where risk to workers and clients is a dynamic interaction [9, 10]. Recently, Langanke & Ross [11] studied internet forums that serve to promote sexual safety and where clients of FSW share experiences; they highlight the potential importance of the internet as a medium not only as a marketplace for sexual services, but also for health and safety information for both clients and commercial sex workers [12].

There is evidence that effective interventions targeted at FSW involve health promotion approaches that are created by FSW themselves and their organizations. Furthermore, such approaches are the most effective and accepted by workers and clients [13-15].

Over the last few years, an increasing proportion of FSW in Spain are immigrants. This phenomenon is particularly prevalent in Northwestern Spain, where a very large proportion of FSW originate from other countries, the majority of which come from Latin America. It is likely that migrant FSW differ from others in terms of sociodemographic characteristics as well as their sexual and health-seeking behaviors. Although the HIV epidemic in Northwestern Spain has been driven predominantly by injection drug use, sexual transmission is playing an increasing role in the process. Findings revealed that FSW have knowledge about transmission of HIV infection and AIDS. However, they had misconceptions as to how HIV infection is transmitted, as they believed that poor nutrition and sharing facilities play a role. Knowledge of mechanisms of protecting themselves against infection, such as use of a condom during coitus was also evident [16]. On the other hand, screening programs in Spain are distributed unequally and have poor coverage. The target populations are heterogeneous and the criteria for their identification are unclear. Cytology laboratories frequently use their own terminology when issuing reports. It is difficult to determine the screening cost of cervical cancer in Spain, as no standardized procedure exists for cost analysis. Not all population censuses of tumors record in situ cervical carcinomas. The average screening coverage in Spain is 75%, with large differences between communities. Around 35% of Spanish women have limited access to preventative follow-ups; this group is comprised of women older than 55 years, with low socioeconomic status, those living in rural areas, and FSW. According to this information, screening should be mixed. Women who do not attend health centers within an established time should be actively contacted. Thus, screening should commence at 25 years of age or within the first 3 years after starting sexual relationships. The diagnosis of high grade-cervical intraepithelial neoplasia (HG-CIN) should be incorporated into the population tumor records. Cost-benefit analysis programs should be initiated for the implemented screening programs [17, 18].

Awareness of sexually transmitted infections (STIs) and the virus that causes genital cancer is relatively low among FSW. In the present study, we surveyed FSW to examine their knowledge and behaviors regarding genital cancer screening and Pap smears, human papilloma virus (HPV), and the HPV vaccine, as well as their attitudes toward vaccination. We also examined their health status and its potential impact on the public health of the community in which they work.

MATERIALS AND METHODS

Sample Size

The estimated population of FSW in the provinces of Ourense and Pontevedra in Northwestern Spain is 1500, and the expected prevalence of HPV infection is 50%; assuming a 95% confidence level and 7% error, it indicates that a sample of 168 women is required.

Data Collection

A descriptive, cross-sectional study was conducted on a sample of one hundred sixty-eight FSW aged 18-49 years involved in this project were recruited over the years 2010-2011 from different areas of prostitution (e.g., clubs, spas, the neighborhood, and the streets) in Pontevedra and Ourense through a mobile unit belonging to a related NGO and taken to health services, where they were interviewed and examined.

The participants who attended our clinic were asked to participate in the study. Their knowledge about cervical cancer screening, Pap smears, HIV, HPV, the HPV vaccine, and their attitudes toward vaccination were examined. An adhoc questionnaire (approximately 15 minutes long) was designed to collect information through face to face interviews conducted by a trained health worker in a confidential setting during or after the clinical examination. Participants signed an informed consent prior permission and the Ethics Committee of Galicia request.

The questionnaire consisted of 5 parts with a total of 19 items as follows:

1. Age (years)
    a. 18-25
    b. 26-33
    c. 34-41
    d. 42-49
2. Country
    a. Spain
    b. Eastern Europe
    c. Latin America
    d. Africa
3. Level of education
    a. Primary school
    b. Secondary school
    c. High school
    d. University
4. Marital status
    a. Single
    b. Married

c. Separated/divorced
d. Widow
e. Unknown

5. Smoking habit
   a. Never
   b. Occasionally
   c. Frequently
6. Drinking habit
   a. Never
   b. Occasionally
   c. Frequently
7. Parity
   a. One child
   b. Two children
   c. Three or more
8. Knowledge of one's health
   a. Poor
   b. Medium
   c. Good
9. Hormonal pill contraception use
   a. Never
   b. Occasional
   c. Frequent
10. Condom use during vaginal sex with current partner
   a. Never
   b. Sometimes
   c. Always
11. Condom use during vaginal sex with clients
   a. Never
   b. Sometimes
   c. Always
12. Have you ever had a Pap smear?
   a. Never
   b. Sometimes
   c. Always
13. Have you ever had an STI?
   a. Yes
   b. No
14. Do you know that viruses may cause some types of cancer?
   a. Yes
   b. No
15. Have you heard about HIV infection?
   a. Yes
   b. No
16. Have you heard about HPV infection?
   a. Yes
   b. No
17. Have you heard about the HPV vaccine?
   a. Yes
   b. No
18. Would you like to receive an HPV vaccine?
   a. Yes
   b. No
19. Who informs you about how you should care for your health?
   a. NGOs
   b. Friends
   c. Internet or media

The first part included 7 questions involving the participants' sociodemographic background. Demographic questions included age, country, education, marital status, smoking habit, drinking habit, and parity. The second part included 4 items examining the subjects' knowledge of their own health, hormonal contraception, condoms, and Pap smears. In this part, the subjects answered whether they had ever had a Pap smear. In the third part, knowledge about HPV was assessed using a 3-item scale. In addition, this part included questions about previous STIs, as well as their connection with cervical cancer, and transmission. The fourth part of the survey examined both knowledge about HIV, HPV, and attitudes toward HPV vaccination. Finally, the participants were asked about their source of health information.

In addition, we obtained the participants' complete medical histories, including weight, height, and previous and current diseases.

Statistical Analysis

The proportions of HPV and HIV awareness were determined by age and country. Multiple logistic regression analysis was used to study the relationship between HPV and HIV awareness and the explanatory variables, which were selected based on the current literature. Interactions between geographic origin and all variables entered in the regression were examined.

We used likelihood ratio tests and Wald tests to calculate the *p*-values. A multiple logistic regression model was built incorporating all variables from univariate analyses. A backward approach was chosen, and the variables included in the final regression models were those that maximized the likelihood values. We tested linear relationships between ordered categorical variables and the log odds of knowledge of HIV and HPV infection. The relationships were assessed by comparing the models, assuming either the absence or presence of a linear relationship between the variable and the log odds of knowledge of HIV and HPV infection through likelihood ratio tests.

Analyses were conducted using PASW Statistics 18 by estimating odds ratios (OR) and their corresponding 95% confidence intervals (CI). Multivariate analyses for HIV and HPV were initially performed separately for the different variables.

RESULTS

The survey was conducted between July 2010 and July 2011. One hundred fifty-three women (aged 18-49 years) agreed to participate in the survey. Their mean (SD) age was 28.2 (7.41) years (range, 18-49 years); 10% of participants were younger than 20 years, and 75% were younger than 35 (Fig. **1**). They were predominantly from Latin America (35.1%), followed by Spain (23.08%), Eastern Europe (24.52%), and Africa (17.31%). Regarding education, 57.5% of the participants were illiterate (although they could read and write as different NGOs teach them), 33.5% had graduated from primary school, 7.8% had finished high school, and 1.2% (only women from Eastern Europe) had a university degree or more (Table **1**). Regarding smoking status, 49.1% and 29.3% of the women were occasional and habitual smokers, respectively. Most (53.6%) had at least 1 child, and 14.9% had 2 or more.

The majority of participants (79%) were occasional drinkers. The women were asked whether they had ever had a Pap smear; 52.7% (n = 88) indicated that they had never had one. Regarding self-rated health, 49.1% reported poor knowledge, 47.3% moderate, and 3.6% had no idea.

Over 90% of the women reported penetrative vaginal sex with either regular partners or clients. Although condom use was high with clients — only 11.3% did not use condoms with clients — 70% did not use them with regular partners (Fig. **2**).

Condom use with clients was lower among women from other countries than women from Spain (p = 0,001, OR,

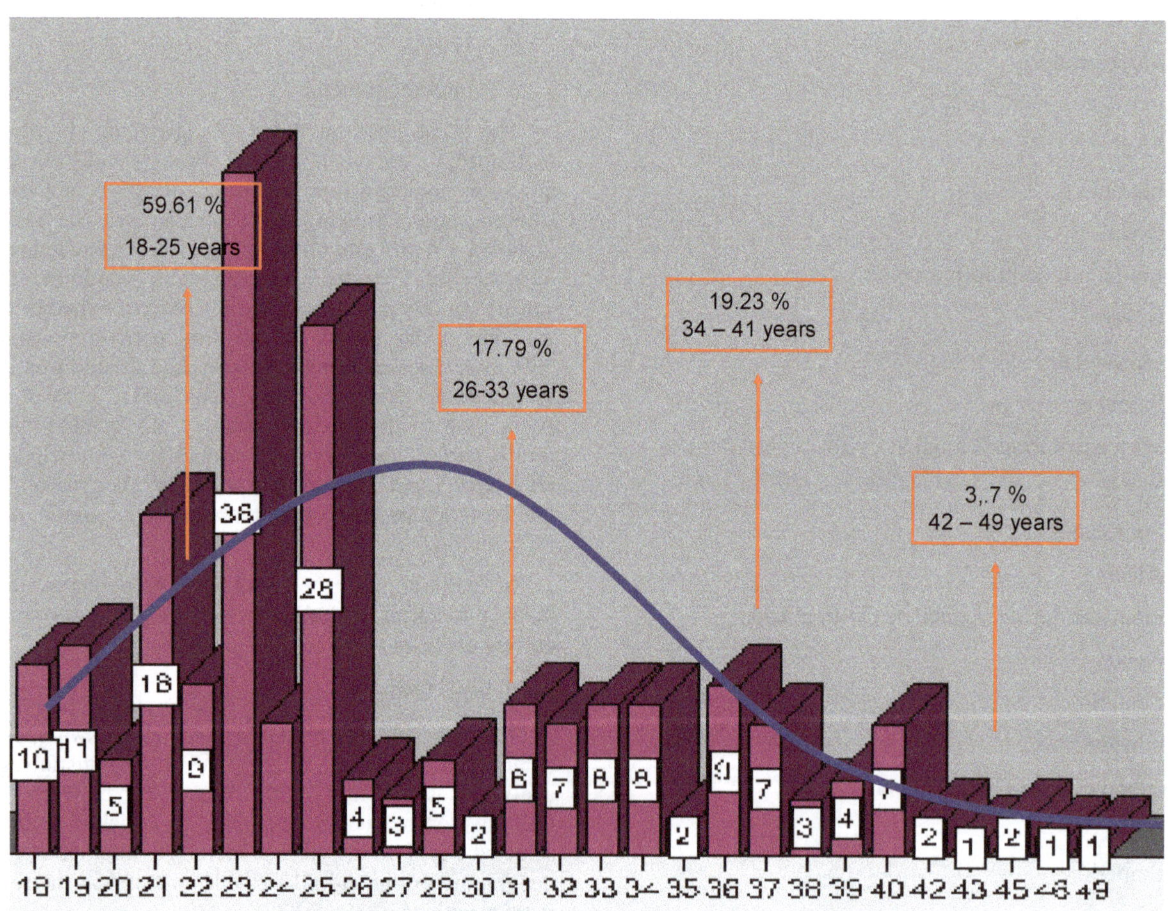

Fig. (1). Their mean (SD) age was 28.2 (7.41) years (range, 18-49 years).

Table 1. The largest group of female sex worker participating in our study consists of immigrant women.

AGE	18-25	26-33	34-41	42-49	Total
Spain	16 (7,69%)	9 (4,33%)	16 (7,69%)	7 (3,37%)	**23,08%**
Eastern Europe	38 (18,27%)	8 (3,85%)	5 (2,40%)	0 (0%)	**24,52%**
Latin America	48 (23,08%)	12 (5,77%)	13 (6,25%)	0 (0%)	**35,1%**
Africa	22 (10,58%)	8 (3,85%)	6 (2,88%)	0 (0%)	**17,31%**
Total	59,61%	17,79%	19,23%	3,37%	**100%**

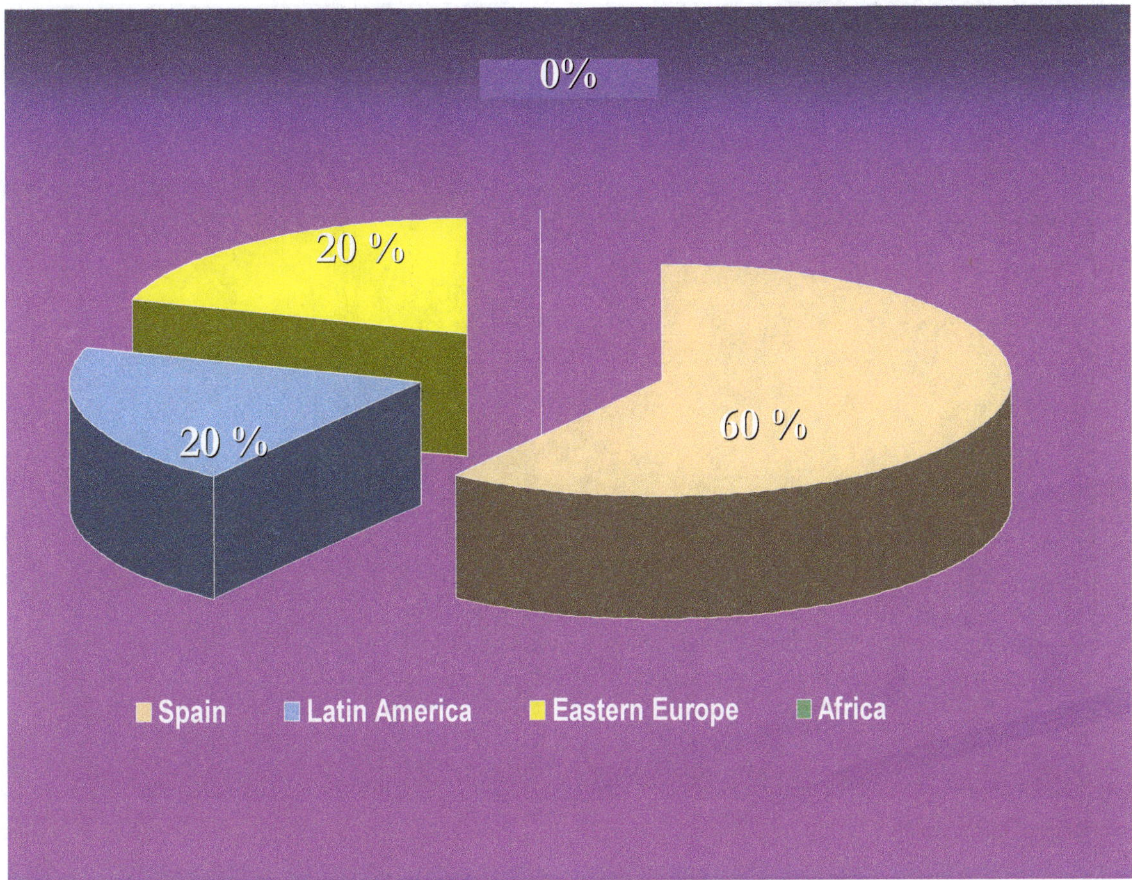

Fig. (2). The male condom use both vaginal intercourse with clients and in the private sphere is highly significant in relation to country of origin.

0.136; 95% CI, 0.049-0.381), whereas condom use with regular partners was more frequent (p = 0,005, OR, 0.36; 95% CI, 0.049-0.381) among Spanish women. Condom breakeage with clients in the month before the survey were high (~45%). Eastern European women had a risk that was 2.941-fold higher than that of Spaniards of not knowing about HPV vaccines.

There was no relationship between country or age and knowledge about HIV (Fig. **3**). Eastern European women knew less (OR, 2.941; 95% CI, 1.071-8.074). Regarding vaccines, women who had been tested for HIV and had a history of Pap smears knew more HPV. These findings are useful for future HPV vaccination campaigns and may be particularly useful for developing intervention programs for individuals with the largest deficits in HPV knowledge.

Participants who always used condoms with their clients knew significantly more about vaccines (95% CI, 0.115-0.790) than those who never used condoms with clients (95% CI, 0.036-0.623) (p = 0.009). In addition, the participants with a history of any STI knew significantly more about the existence of HPV vaccines (80%; 95% CI, 0.103-0.473) (p = 0.000). In all, 10.3% of participants were HIV-positive. Information on the HIV status of current partners was available for 100% of the women who were HIV-positive; 89.4% of their current partners were HIV-positive as well. There were no differences in HIV prevalence between women who had engaged in sex work for 1-3 years (31.1%), 3-5 years (44.9%), and >5 years (23.4%).

When the participants were asked if they knew viruses might cause some types of cancer, 42.9% of respondents answered correctly, whereas 56.5% did not know. Most (88%) of the women responded correctly to the question about HIV infection and their consequences. Moreover, 41% of the respondents had heard of a vaccine for cervical cancer. Most had heard about caring for themselves from NGOs (68.3%) and the internet or mass media (13.8%) (Fig. **3**). The majority (56%) of respondents had never heard of HPV. Among the women who had never heard of HPV (46.1%), 99% knew about vaccines and had a positive attitude toward them.

Although 82.7% of the participants were willing to be vaccinated, only 3% of them were vaccinated at that time. On the other hand, 21% of the subjects unwilling to be vaccinated had doubts about the new vaccine or did not have enough money. For most of the women (65.4%), recommendations from NGO volunteers were the major influences for deciding to be vaccinated.

DISCUSSION

The main goal of this study was to guide future HIV prevention efforts in this high-risk population in Northwestern Spain by assessing the current knowledge of FSW on HIV, determining the role of injection drug use in the epidemic, and determining other risk factors for HIV

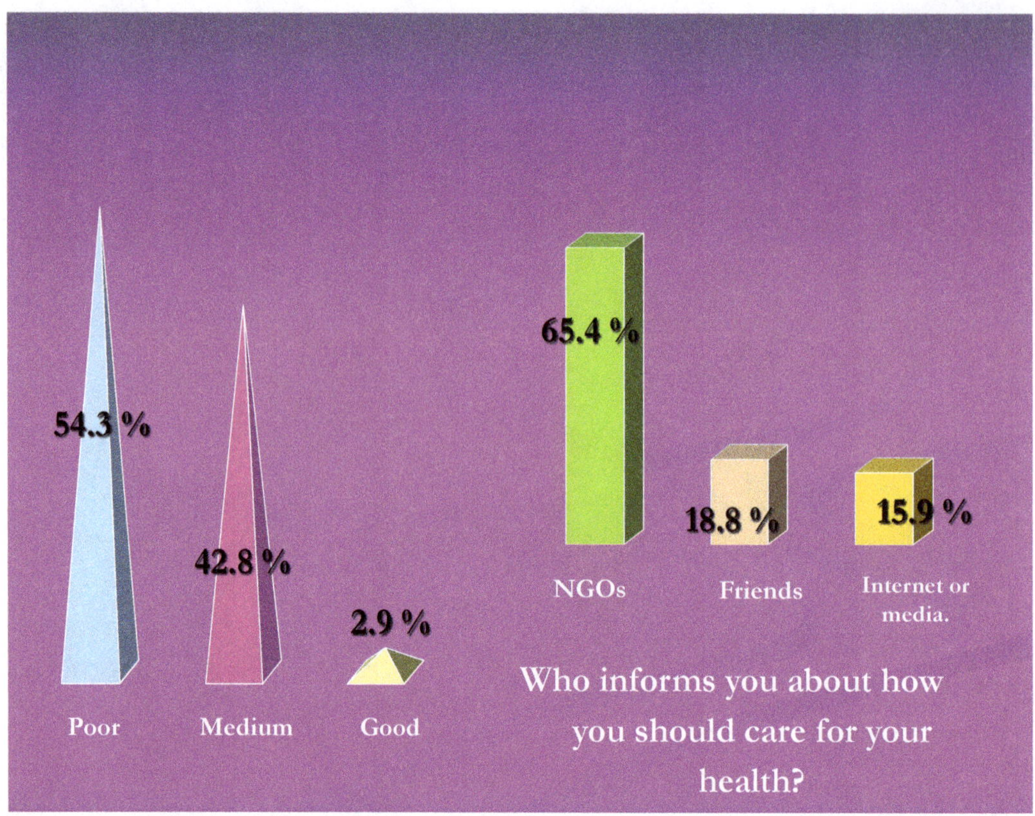

Fig. (3). Knowledge of one's health.

infection. The most frequent transmission route in cases of AIDS in Galicia, Spain, is associated with injected drugs, which corresponded to 43.4% of all cases in 2008 [16]. On the other hand, heterosexual transmission is the second most frequent route, corresponding to 30.1% (48% in women) of cases in 2008. Nonetheless, recent data from other Spanish communities should be taken into account. It is also possible that AIDS incidence will increase over the coming years in this group. The most common geographic area from which the immigrants originate is Latin America (48% of cases; 33 men and 28 women) followed by Europe (32%), and sub-Saharan Africa (15%). The most common mode of transmission of HIV, in this group, is heterosexual transmission, which comprises 44% of cases (56 of 127), followed by shared syringe use among injection drug users, comprising 29% of cases. In Europeans, the most common mode of transmission is unsafe sexual behavior, involving 27 of 41 cases (66%) in total; homo- and bisexuals represent 17% of these cases [16].

When asked, "Have you ever heard of HIV?" Spaniards and Africans knew significantly more than Eastern Europeans and Latin Americans did (Fig. **2**).

On the other hand, the prevalence of HPV in the female lower genital tract in Northwestern Spain is still high; infection was prevalent in young women, indicating a decrease in infection in middle age. However, postmenopausal women exhibited higher infection rates. The HPV-16 serotype was the most prevalent (27%), followed by HPV-31 (11%), HPV-52 (7%), HPV-56 (5%), and HPV-58 (2%). Multiple infections were present in 38% of the participants and decreased with age. The HPV-16 and HPV-31 serotypes exhibit similar behavior in both single and multiple infections [17, 18]. This study presents the first data on the incidence of HPV in FSW. With the use of vaccines against HPV — especially the tetravalent vaccine — there will be a lower rate of abnormal cytological results in vaccinated women in the short- or medium-term; this is based on the vaccine's expected preventive potential, which may range 50-70%. Furthermore, with the use of the vaccine in combination with present screening programs, we could reduce the annual number of cases of cervical cancer and other associated pathologies in Spain by 92%. We obtained these data in a study in a normal population [17].

In order to assess the public's understanding of HPV vaccination and testing, it is important to evaluate knowledge of HPV and its relationship with genital cancer. In the current population-based study that included 153 women who were 18-45 years old, we found that, overall, 46% reported having heard of HPV. This proportion ranged from 30.4% in Latin Americans to 19.6% in Africans. The results of this study corroborate the findings of other studies in that many women in the general population still do not know about HPV. Moreover, even fewer FSW know about HPV. Less is known about the existence of HPV than of HIV.

In a major Catalonian study of over 350 immigrant FSW from Eastern Europe, Latin America, and Africa, Folch *et al.* [19] found that younger age and unprotected sex were associated with gonorrhea and chlamydia. They note that over 70% of FSW in Spain now are immigrants and that precarious legal (70% are illegal immigrants), working, and family situations, as well as poor access to social services may make these women more vulnerable to STIs. However, they found that the prevalence of STIs among migrant FSW in Spain is lower than that in other European countries. Furthermore, they also found that the rates of chlamydia and gonorrhea are consistent with those in other sexually active young people in Catalonia. None of the women in this study were injection drug users, which may also account for the low prevalence of health problems and HIV, although there was no direct comparison with non-immigrant FSW. We found a very low rate of HIV among the FSW, and STIs data did not differ greatly from the normal population.

FSW from Eastern Europe (who were also the youngest) knew the most about HPV, whereas those from Africa knew the least. Although these differences were of borderline statistical significance due to the small number of women in some groups, they were maintained in age-adjusted analyses. Therefore, the country of origin must reflect differences in either past or current sexual behaviors. Unfortunately, no detailed data were available for all women [14].

The fact that no differences were observed for acute STIs by geographic origin suggests that past exposure to HPV may be a determinant of current HPV epidemiology.

There is strong evidence that FSW have unsafe sex, as highlighted by the high prevalence of terminated pregnancies (78.5%) and other STIs (50.3%).

Furthermore, unsafe sex took place more frequently with regular partners than clients [20].

The prevalence of STIs was neither related to age nor in the patients from different geographic areas.

Multivariate analysis revealed that knowledge about the association between HIV and its consequences and the relationship between education and condom use with partners were strongly associated. Related to the knowledge of the association between HPV and cervical cancer, knowledge of the routes of HPV transmission and awareness about vaccines among the FSW was strongly associated with education, knowledge of one's health, parity, and condom use with clients [21].

Moreover, previous knowledge about HPV and the HPV vaccine; personal beliefs about vaccination; many sexual partners; perceived support of providers, partners, and parents; endorsement of universal HPV vaccination; low vaccine cost; and vaccine safety were all significantly associated with the acceptance of HPV vaccination [22-24].

Alcohol and drug use are frequently associated with sex work either because the nature of the work leads to self-medication, or because sex work is a relatively easy way to obtain money to finance a drug habit. However, the specific context of sex work may also require sex workers to consume alcohol. In a classic study, Fernández-Esquer [25] studied *cantineras*, Latinas working in lower-class bars (*cantinas*) in North and Central America who earn a sales commission from every beer they get clients to buy for them.

In Northwestern Spain, drinking is virtually obligatory for FSW and is paid for by men who expect sexual favors in exchange. A female sex worker may consume up to 8 beers during a "normal" working day. In such cases, alcohol use is an integral part of the work and is not a precursor or consequence of the work; however, it is still a female sex worker issue. Similar concerns are warranted for other sex workers in bars, where they also work as waitresses and are expected to encourage alcohol consumption by patrons and potential clients. The health consequences of high and onsistent alcohol consumption — apart from the immediate safety issues of unsafe sex and poor judgment in the selection of clients who may be abusive — may include long-term liver disease, heart disease, obesity, and depression, among others [26, 27]. In the present study, 79% of the participants were casual drinkers, 48% presented liver disease, and 2.4% had heart disease; height ranged 1.50-1.68 m and weight was 57-75 kg with an average BMI of 30% [28].

Finally, the time spent in commercial sex work was significantly associated with HIV knowledge. However, information on the time spent in commercial sex work is often missing, and past history of STIs is also susceptible to recall bias. It is likely that a certain random misclassification may have taken place, which could explain the lack of an observed association [29].

CONCLUSION

In conclusion, this study confirms that more education about HIV, HPV, and HPV vaccination is urgently needed for women. This is the first study to assess what FSW in Northwestern Spain know about HIV, HPV, and HPV vaccines; it provides useful information for further research and policy makers. Social care professionals should advise FSW about care and vaccines. It is important to convey preventative messages to the personal sphere of FSW (i.e., their private partners and clients) and to facilitate the access of FSW to the health system. Since women may feel uncomfortable talking about STIs, it is important to be mindful of this when explaining HIV, HPV, HPV vaccination, and genital cancer. The important findings of the present study highlight the need for effective education for practitioners, social workers, and NGO volunteers. It is also important to remember that the government should support such programs, including assistance and vaccines, for this low-income group.

CONFLICT OF INTEREST

The authors confirm that this article content has no conflict of interest.

ACKNOWLEDGEMENTS

Declared none.

REFERENCES

[1] Seib C, Fischer J, Najman JM. The health of female sex workers from three industry sectors in Queensland, Australia. Soc Sci Med 2009; 68 (3): 473-8.

[2] Zhang C, Li X, Hong Y, Chen Y, Liu W, Zhou Y. Partner violence and HIV risk among female sex workers in China. AIDS Behav 2011; (16)4: 1020-30.

[3] Hong Y, Li X. Behavioral studies of female sex workers in China: a literature review and recommendation for future research. AIDS Behav 2008;12(4): 623-36.

[4] Groneberg DA, Molliné M, Kusma B. Sex work during the world cup in Germany. Lancet 2006; 368: 840-1.

[5] Alexander P. Sex work and health: A question of safety in the workplace. J Am Med Women's Assoc 1998; 53: 77-82.

[6] Montano SM, Hsieh EJ, Calderón M, Ton TG, Quijano E, Solari V, Zunt JR. Human papillomavirus infection in female sex workers in Lima, Peru. Sex Transm Infect 2011; 87 (1): 81-2.

[7] Bautista CT, Pando MA, Reynaga E, *et al.* Sexual practices, drug use behaviors, and prevalence of HIV, syphilis, hepatitis B and C, and HTLV-1/2 in immigrant and non-immigrant female sex workers in Argentina. J Immigr Minor Health 2009; 11: 99-104.

[8] Plumridge L, Abel G. A "segmented" sex industry in New Zealand: Sexual and personal safety of female sex workers. Aust NZ J Public Health 2001; 25: 78-83.

[9] Sanders T. A continuum of risk? The management of health, physical and emotional risks by female sex workers. Soc Health Ill 2004; 26: 557-74.

[10] Farley M, Cotton A, Lynne J, *et al.* Prostitution and trafficking in nine countries: an update on violence and posttraumatic stress disorder. J Trauma Pract 2003; 3: 3374.

[11] Langanke H, Ross MW. Web-based forums for clients of female sex workers: development of a German internet approach to HIV/STD-related sexual safety. Int J STD AIDS 2009; 20 (1): 4-8.

[12] Hong Y, Li X, Fang X, Lin X, Zhang C. Internet use among female sex workers in China: Implications for HIV/STI prevention. AIDS Behav 2011; 15(2): 273-82.

[13] Nguyen NT, Nguyen HT, Trinh HQ, Mills SJ, Detels R. Clients of female sex workers as a bridging population in Vietnam. AIDS Behav 2009; 13. (5): 881-91.

[14] Barrington C, Latkin C, Sweat MD, Moreno L, Ellen J, Kerrigan D. Talking the talk, walking the walk: social network norms, communication patterns, and condom use among the male partners of female sex workers in La Romana, Dominican Republic. Soc Sci Med 2009; 68 (11): 2037-44.

[15] Yang C, Latkin C, Luan R, Nelson K. Peer norms and consistent condom use with female sex workers among male clients in Sichuan province, China. Soc Sci Med 2010; 71 (4): 832-9.

[16] Rodriguez-Cerdeira C, Cruces MJ, Taboada JA. A quarter century with AIDS. Open AIDS J 2011; 1: 1-8

[17] Rodríguez-Cerdeira MC, Guerra-Tapia A, Alcantara CR, Escalas J. Human Papilloma Virus (HPV) and genital cancer. Open Dermatol J 2009; 3: 111-22.

[18] Rodríguez-Cerdeira C, Chillón R, Díez-Moreno S, Guerra-Tapia A. Prevalence and genotypic identification of human papillomavirus infection in a population from northwestern Spain. Open Dermatol J. 2009; 3: 18-21.

[19] Folch C, Esteve A, Sanclemente C *et al.* Prevalence of HIV, *Chlamydia trachomatis*, and *Neisseria gonorrheae* and risk factors for sexually transmitted infections among immigrant female sex workers in Catalonia, Spain. Sex Transm Dis 2008; 35: 178-83.

[20] Hoffman L, Nguyen HT, Kershaw TS, Niccolai LM. Dangerous subtlety: relationship-related determinants of consistency of condom use among female sex workers and their regular, non-commercial partners in Haiphong, Vietnam AIDS Behav. 2011;15: 1372-80.

[21] Sanders T. Protecting the health and safety of female sex workers: the responsibility of all. BJOG 2007; 114 (7): 791-3.

[22] Gonik B. Strategies for fostering HPV vaccine acceptance. Infect Dis Obstet Gynecol 2006; 36797: 1-4.

[23] Kahn JA, Rosenthal SL, Hamann T, Bernstein DI. Attitudes about human papillomavirus vaccine in young women. Int J STD AIDS 2003; 14: 300-6.

[24] Boehner CW, Howe SR, Bernstein DI, Rosenthal SL. Viral sexually transmitted disease vaccine acceptability among college students. Sex Transm Dis 2003; 30: 774-8.

[25] Fernández-Esquer ME. Drinking for wages: Obligatory alcohol abuse among Cantineras. J Stud Alcohol. 2003; 64: 160-6.

[26] Parks KA, Hsieh YP, Lorraine CR, Levonyan-Radloff K. Daily assessment of alcohol consumption and condom use with known and casual partners among young female bar drinkers. AIDS Behav. 2011; 15(7): 1332-41.

[27] Samet JH, Pace CA, Cheng DM, *et al.* Alcohol use and sex risk behaviors among hiv-infected female sex workers and HIV-infected male clients of female sex workers in India. AIDS Behav. 2010; 14(Suppl 1): S74-83.

[28] Kershaw TS, Arnold A, Lewis JB, Magriples U, Ickovics JR. The skinny on sexual risk: the effects of bmi on sti incidence and risk. AIDS Behav. 2011; 15 (7): 1527-38.

[29] Belza MJ, Clavo P, Ballesteros J, *et al.* Social and work conditions, risk behavior and prevalence of sexually transmitted diseases among female immigrant prostitutes in Madrid (Spain) Gac Sanit. 2004; 18 (3): 177-83.

13

Characterization of Adult-Type IgA Vasculitis (Henoch-Schönlein Purpura)

Katsuhiro Hitomi*, Seiichi Izaki, Yuichi Teraki, Yuko Aso, Megumi Yokoyama, Saori Takamura, Yumiko Inoue and Yoshiki Sato

Department of Dermatology, Saitama Medical Center, Saitama Medical University, Kawagoe, Saitama, Japan

Abstract: The clinical features of adult-type IgA vasculitis have not been well characterized. To analyze the characteristics of IgA vasculitis in adults, patients diagnosed with IgA vasculitis based on EULAR/PRINTO/PRES criteria (2012) in our institution between 2003 and 2012 were studied, comprising 85 adults (age ≥ 21 years) and 37 pediatric patients (≤ 20 years). Compared with pediatric cases, adult disease showed significantly higher serum C-reactive protein and IgA values, a lower percentage of cases was associated with infections (56.5% *vs* 89.2%, $P < 0.001$) but there was a greater range of infections affecting different tissues and organs, and there was occasional cases with malignancy (8.2%) including four cases of lung carcinoma and three with hematological disorders. The skin lesions in adults tended to be widely distributed on the abdomen and waist (15.3% *vs* 2.7%, $P = 0.045$). Adult cases were associated with greater renal involvement, as evidenced by proteinuria, hematuria and/or urinary casts, compared with the pediatric group (76.2% *vs* 48.6%, $P = 0.003$) and disease recalcitrance was also significantly higher (38.8% *vs* 18.9%, $P = 0.031$). Examination of the serum levels of immunoglobulins in adults showed that a sole increase in IgA was associated with renal and gastrointestinal manifestations, but this was not seen in cases with concurrent increases of IgA and IgG or IgA, IgG and IgM. Although the retrospective nature of the study is a limitation, it identified possible associations with the wide range of infections, more severe renal damage, and malignancy in adult IgA vasculitis.

Keywords: Adult, anaphylactoid purpura, Henoch–Schönlein purpura, immunoglobulin A, malignancy, renal damage, vasculitis.

INTRODUCTION

Henoch–Schönlein purpura (HSP) and anaphylactoid purpura was renamed immunoglobulin A (IgA) vasculitis in the 2012 revised International Chapel Hill Consensus Conference Nomenclature of Vasculitides [1]. Immune complexes of IgA and unidentified antigens are thought to be pathogenic in this condition [2], and immunofluorescence studies demonstrate deposition of IgA on the vessel walls. Skin involvement manifests as palpable purpura due to the extravasation of cellular and liquid components of the blood from inflamed dermal vessels. Vascular damage is caused by activation of the complement cascade that results in the production of complement membrane attack complex [3], and proteolytic enzymes and oxidants released by neutrophils. Previously, we proposed that the interrupted apoptosis of neutrophils leads to vascular damage in leukocytoclastic vasculitis (LCV), based on ultramicroscopic immunolabeling findings [4]. IgA immune complexes also contribute to nephritis [5] and gastrointestinal symptoms [6]. Arthralgia and arthritis also occur in this disease.

IgA vasculitis primarily affects the pediatric population [7, 8]. The diagnostic criteria established by the American College of Rheumatology (ACR) in 1990 include patient age ≤ 20 years as one of its four criteria [9]. Typically, the onset of disease in pediatric patients is preceded by an upper respiratory infection [8]. IgA vasculitis is known to occur in adult and elderly patients with similar manifestations, but the adult disease has not been fully characterized. Blanco *et al.* [10] in 1997 summarized 46 adult (> 20 years) cases compared with 116 cases in children (≤ 20 years), reporting that renal involvement and joint symptoms are more common in adult cases with a lower occurrence of abdominal pain and fever. Tancrede-Bohin *et al.* [11] investigated predictive factors for renal involvement in adult patients and showed that a recent history of infection, pyrexia, the spread of purpura to the trunk, and elevated biological markers of inflammation are predictive factors for IgA glomerulonephritis. García-Porrúa *et al.* [12] reported that renal insufficiency is more frequent in adults (> 20 years) than in children (< 14 years). Diehl *et al.* [13] described IgA vasculitis in eight elderly patients aged between 64–85 years and concluded that renal involvement is relatively common and more severe in the elderly. From their experience of three adult cases of IgA vasculitis associated with malignancy and their review of 31 similar cases in the literature, Zurada *et al.* [14] suggested that IgA vasculitis may be associated with malignancy and that malignancy may cause IgA vasculitis in adults.

In this study, the clinical features of IgA vasculitis in adult patients were characterized, and compared with those in pediatric patients.

*Address correspondence to this author at the Department of Dermatology, Saitama Medical Center, Saitama Medical University, 1981 Kamoda, Kawagoe, Saitama 350-8550, Japan;
E-mail: k-hitomi@js4.so-net.ne.jp

METHODS

The departmental records of patients diagnosed with IgA vasculitis in our institution between 2003 and 2012 were retrospectively analyzed. This study was approved by the Institutional Review Board of Saitama Medical Center (No. 696) in February 2013. Patients were separated into two groups based on the ACR age-related IgA vasculitis diagnostic criterion [9]: pediatric (≤ 20 years) and adult (≥ 21 years) groups. The accuracy of the diagnosis of all cases was reviewed against the criteria of the European League Against Rheumatism/Paediatric Rheumatology International Trials Organisation/Paediatric Rheumatology European Society (EULAR/PRINTO/PRES) [15], which requires the presence of purpura or petechiae predominantly on the lower limbs, plus one of the following features: 1) abdominal pain, 2) LCV or proliferative glomerulonephritis with IgA-dominant deposits, 3) arthritis or arthralgia, or 4) proteinuria, hematuria or urinary casts. Furthermore, evidence of IgA deposition in immunofluorescence studies of skin biopsies was required for the diagnosis in the adult group but this was not strictly applied in the pediatric group because of the relatively low biopsy rate in this group. Of 187 cases (144 and 43 in the adult and pediatric groups, respectively), 122 were studied in detail, consisting of 85 and 37 in the adult and pediatric groups, respectively. The number of patients in the pediatric group was low, since pediatric patients who voluntarily consulted the pediatricians in the same hospital were not involved in the present analysis.

The clinical features of IgA vasculitis, association with infection and malignancy, clinical course, laboratory parameters and histological findings were compared between the pediatric and adult groups. Fisher's exact test and Student's t-test were used for statistical analysis.

RESULTS

Patient Characteristics

Fig. (**1**) shows the age distribution of patients in the study. The mean ages (± S.D.) of the pediatric and adult groups were 9.8 ± 5.0 years and 51.7 ± 17.4 years, respectively (Table **1**), and the male-to-female ratio was 1.18 and 1.24, respectively, with a slight male predominance in both groups. All adult patients (100% [85/85]) had IgA deposition in the biopsied skin lesions. Although the number of biopsies was relatively low (37.8% [14/37]) in the pediatric group, IgA positivity was high (100% [14/14]). The mean values (± S.D.) of serum C-reactive protein (CRP) (2.62 ± 3.73 mg/dl in adults *vs* 0.92 ± 0.99 mg/dl in pediatric group; $P < 0.001$) and IgA (405.1 ± 129.6 mg/dl *vs* 232.5 ± 89.1 mg/dl, respectively; $P < 0.001$) were higher in adult than in the pediatric group.

Association with Infection and Malignancy

As shown in Table **2**, signs/symptoms of infection were significantly lower in the adult group than those in the pediatric group (56.5% [48/85] *vs* 89.2% [33/37], $P < 0.001$). The presence of elevated levels of anti-streptolysin O (ASO) and/or anti-streptokinase (ASK) antibodies was consistently lower in the adult group compared with the pediatric group (25.4% [18/71] *vs* 47.1% [16/34], $P = 0.026$). Throat bacterial cultures were less likely to be positive in the adult

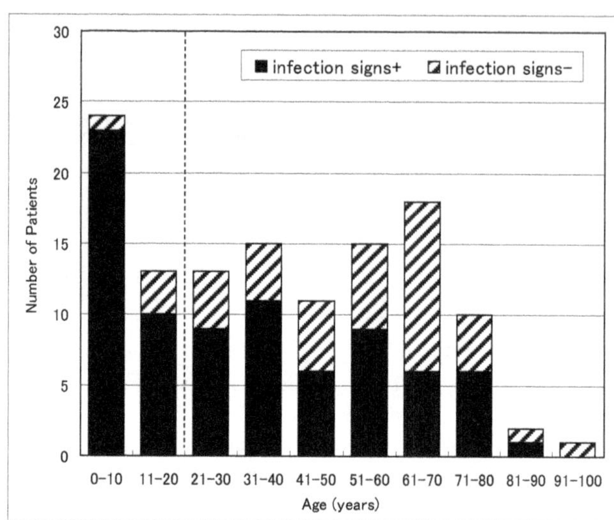

Fig. (1). The age distribution of patients with IgA vasculitis, with and without signs of infection. Patients were separated into ten age groups as shown on the abscissa. Patients presenting with signs of infection are represented by solid bars and those without signs of infection by hatched bars.

Table 1. Patient characteristics and laboratory data.

		Age ≤ 20 (n = 37)	Age ≥ 21 (n = 85)	*P*
Sex	Male: Female	20: 17	47: 38	*0.899*
Age (years)	Mean ± SD	9.8 ± 5.0	51.7 ± 17.4	
	Range	4–20	21–91	
Biopsy	Performed	14/37 (37.8)	85/85 (100)	
	IgA positivity	14/14 (100)	85/85 (100)	
Serum levels	CRP (mg/dl)	0.92 ± 0.99 (0–4.1)	2.62 ± 3.73 (0–24.7)	*< 0.001***
	IgA (mg/dl)	232.5 ± 89.1 (56.8–445.7)	405.1 ± 129.6 (155.0–785.2)	*< 0.001***

**$P < 0.02$.

group than in the pediatric group (45.3% [24/53] *vs* 74.2% [23/31], $P = 0.010$). The percentage of positive cultures for *Staphylococcus aureus* and *Streptococcus species* was not significantly different between the two groups, while *Haemophilus influenzae* was significantly less common in the adult group than in the pediatric group (4.2% [1/24] *vs* 30.4% [7/23], $P = 0.017$). A range of infections were present in the preceding four weeks or at the time of diagnosis of IgA vasculitis in the adult group, including pneumonia (n = 1), pyelonephritis (n = 1), epididymitis (n = 1), cellulitis (n = 1) and fever of unknown origin (n = 3); these preceding or concurrent infections were not observed in the pediatric group except for one case of fever of unknown origin. In addition, palmoplantar pustulosis and acrodermatitis

Table 2. Infection and malignancy associated with IgA vasculitis.

	Age ≤ 20 (n = 37)		Age ≥ 21 (n = 85)		*P*
	n	(%)	n	(%)	
Recent signs of infection[1]	33/37	(89.2)	48/85	(56.5)	< 0.001**
Questionnaire					
Recent symptoms of infection	19/37	(51.4)	29/85	(34.1)	0.073
Upper respiratory infection	18/19	(94.7)	22/29	(75.9)	0.086
Others	1/19	(5.3)	7/29	(24.1)	0.086
Laboratory examination					
Increased serum levels of					
ASO[2] and/or ASK	16/34	(47.1)	18/71	(25.4)	0.026*
Throat bacterial culture positivity	23/31	(74.2)	24/53	(45.3)	0.010**
Bacterial strains					
MSSA[3]	12/23	(52.2)	12/24	(50.0)	0.882
MRSA[4]	1/23	(4.3)	2/24	(8.3)	0.576
Haemophilus influenzae	7/23	(30.4)	1/24	(4.2)	0.017**
Streptococcus spp.	6/23	(26.1)	11/24	(45.8)	0.159
Others	3/23	(13.0)	2/24	(8.3)	0.601
Association of malignancy	0/37	(0)	7/85	(8.2)	0.072
MALT[5] lymphoma	0	(0)	1/7	(14.3)	
Multiple myeloma	0	(0)	1/7	(14.3)	
Myelodysplastic syndrome	0	(0)	1/7	(14.3)	
Lung carcinoma	0	(0)	4/7	(57.1)	

[1]Signs of infection include fever, sore throat, cough, redness, swelling and tenderness.
[2]Reference levels: ASO, 0–140 (IU/ml) and ASK, less than × 320.
[3]Methicillin-sensitive *Staphylococcus aureus*.
[4]Methicillin-resistant *Staphylococcus aureus*.
[5]Mucosa-associated lymphoid tissue.
*$P < 0.05$, **$P < 0.02$.

continua of Hallopeau affected two adult patients with IgA vasculitis.

Notably, in 7 of 85 adult patients (8.2%), malignancies were found at presentation, during hospitalization or in the follow-up period (18.1 ± 25.8 months [mean ± SD]). These included four cases of advanced lung carcinoma (n = 4; two cases with stage IV adenocarcinoma, one with stage III small cell carcinoma and one with stage IV squamous cell carcinoma), and hematological malignancies including myelodysplastic syndrome (n = 1), mucosa-associated lymphoid tissue (MALT) lymphoma (n = 1), and multiple myeloma (n = 1). The patient with MALT lymphoma was 36 years old, while other patients with malignancies were ≥ 56 years of age. Serum IgA levels of four adult patients with lung carcinoma were higher than adult patients without malignancy (613.5 ± 86.2 mg/dl *vs* 394.1 ± 126.0 mg/dl, $P = 0.038$). With persistent cough as an initial symptom, two lung carcinomas were found during hospitalization of IgA vasculitis patients. In patients with MALT lymphoma and multiple myeloma, IgA vasculitis repeatedly improved and relapsed, associated with the state of malignancy. However, regardless of the presence or absence of malignancy, there was no significant difference in other clinical features and laboratory data. Malignancies in the pediatric group were not found at presentation and during the follow-up period (6.1 ± 6.3 months).

Distribution Pattern of Purpura and Morphology of Skin Lesions

All patients in both groups had palpable purpura on the lower extremities (Table **3**). Lesions on the abdomen and waist were statistically more common in the adult group than in the pediatric group (15.3% [13/85] *vs* 2.7% [1/37], $P = 0.045$). Hemorrhagic bullae and erosions more commonly affected adult than pediatric patients (14.1% [12/85] *vs* 5.4% [2/37]), but this was statistically insignificant ($P = 0.165$).

Renal, Gastrointestinal and Joint Manifestations

The proportion of patients with signs of renal manifestations was higher in the adult group compared with the pediatric group (76.2% [64/84] *vs* 48.6% [18/37], $P = 0.003$). Compared with pediatric patients, a significantly higher proportion of adult patients had proteinuria (52.4% [44/84] *vs* 27.0% [10/37], $P = 0.010$) and hematuria (56.0% [47/84] *vs* 29.7% [11/37], $P = 0.008$) (Table **3**). Furthermore, urinary casts including granular, waxy, fatty, red blood cell,

Table 3. Cutaneous signs and renal, gastrointestinal and joint manifestations in IgA vasculitis.

Clinical Manifestations	Age ≤ 20 (n = 37)		Age ≥ 21 (n = 85)		P
	n	(%)	n	(%)	
Purpura	37/37	(100)	85/85	(100)	-
Distribution					
Trunk	8/37	(21.6)	19/85	(22.4)	0.929
Chest/back	0	(0)	2/85	(2.4)	0.347
Abdomen/waist	1/37	(2.7)	13/85	(15.3)	0.045*
Genital area/buttocks	8/37	(21.6)	13/85	(15.3)	0.395
Upper extremities	14/37	(37.8)	38/85	(44.7)	0.481
Lower limbs	37/37	(100)	85/85	(100)	-
Morphology					
Hemorrhagic bullous lesions/erosions	2/37	(5.4)	12/85	(14.1)	0.165
Renal manifestations	18/37	(48.6)	64/84	(76.2)	0.003**
Proteinuria	10/37	(27.0)	44/84	(52.4)	0.010**
Hematuria	11/37	(29.7)	47/84	(56.0)	0.008**
Abnormal urinary sediment					
Urinary casts[1]	13/37	(35.1)	60/84	(71.4)	<0.001**
Red blood cell deformity	4/37	(10.8)	20/84	(23.8)	0.099
Renal biopsy	1/37	(2.7)	8/84	(9.5)	0.188
Gastrointestinal symptoms	12/36	(33.3)	38/84	(45.2)	0.270
Abdominal pain	12/36	(33.3)	36/84	(42.9)	0.329
Hematochezia/fecal occult blood	2/3	(66.7)	7/16	(43.8)	0.466
Arthralgia	19/36	(52.8)	33/84	(39.3)	0.172
Elbow	1/36	(2.8)	6/84	(7.1)	0.350
Wrist	3/36	(8.3)	5/84	(6.0)	0.632
Knee	6/36	(16.7)	23/84	(27.4)	0.209
Ankle	13/36	(36.1)	20/84	(23.8)	0.167
Hip	0	(0)	2/84	(2.4)	0.350
Shoulder	0	(0)	1/84	(1.2)	0.511
Finger	0	(0)	3/84	(3.6)	0.251
Toe	0	(0)	2/84	(2.4)	0.350
Not described	0	(0)	1/84	(1.2)	-

[1]Urinary casts include granular, waxy, fatty, red blood cell, white blood cell and epithelial cell casts but not hyaline casts.
$*P < 0.05$, $**P < 0.02$.

white blood cell and epithelial cell casts but not hyaline casts were more frequently found in adults than in pediatric patients (71.4% [60/84] *vs* 35.1% [13/37], $P < 0.001$). The presence of red blood cell deformity was not significantly different between the two groups. Severe renal disease requiring a renal biopsy occurred in eight cases in the adult group (one case had rapidly progressive glomerulonephritis), but only one renal biopsy was performed in the pediatric group. Gastrointestinal symptoms were present in 45.2% (38/84) and 33.3% (12/36) of patients in the adult and pediatric groups, respectively, but the difference was statistically insignificant ($P = 0.270$). Arthralgia affected more than half (52.8% [19/36]) of the pediatric patients. Although this was relatively less in the adult group (39.3% [33/84], $P = 0.172$), various joints including the hip, shoulders, fingers and toes were affected.

Therapy and Outcome

Table **4** shows the admission rate, use of prednisolone, antibiotics and dapsone, and clinical outcome. Admission was recommended when patients had renal, abdominal or joint manifestations in addition to skin lesions. More than two thirds of adult patients were hospitalized for treatment and bed rest. The rate of admission was significantly higher in the adult group than in the pediatric group (68.2% [58/85]

Table 4. Admission rate, medical therapy and outcome of IgA vasculitis.

		Age ≤ 20 (n = 37)		Age ≥ 21 (n = 85)		P
		n	(%)	n	(%)	
Admission rate		16/37	(43.2)	58/85	(68.2)	*0.009***
Medical therapy						
	Prednisolone	15/37	(40.5)	41/85	(48.2)	*0.433*
	Antibiotics	20/37	(54.1)	26/85	(30.6)	*0.140*
	Dapsone	8/37	(21.6)	34/85	(40.0)	*0.050*
Prognosis						
	Recurrence	4/37	(10.8)	15/85	(17.6)	*0.338*
	Recalcitrance	7/37	(18.9)	33/85	(38.8)	*0.031**
	Renal sequelae	3/37	(8.1)	11/85	(12.9)	*0.441*

*$P < 0.05$, **$P < 0.02$.

vs 43.2% [16/37], P = 0.009). Prednisolone was given to approximately half of adult patients, which was higher than that in the pediatric group, but the difference was insignificant (48.2% [41/85] *vs* 40.5% [15/37], P = 0.433). Antibiotic use was greater in the pediatric group (54.1% [20/37]), which may reflect the association of IgA vasculitis with infection. Dapsone was sometimes used to treat adult patients (40.0% [34/85]). Recurrence of skin lesions and/or other manifestations one month or more after initial resolution was more common in the adult group, but the difference was insignificant (17.6% [15/85] *vs* 10.8% [4/37], P = 0.338). Recalcitrant cases that did not show improvement despite treatment for more than one month were more common in the adult group compared with the pediatric group (38.8% [33/85] *vs* 18.9% [7/37], P = 0.031). Eleven adults (12.9% [11/85]) and three teens (8.1% [3/37]) had renal sequelae. Because of persistent proteinuria (n = 8) and/or hematuria (n = 12), they still needed outpatient nephrology care on December 2013. But the renal disease did not lead to chronic renal failure.

Aggressive medical therapy consisting of steroid pulse therapy, half-dose pulse steroid therapy and/or immunosuppressants such as cyclophosphamide, mizoribine or cyclosporine was required for renal disease in five adult patients, whereas such therapy was not required in the pediatric group. With respect to severe gastrointestinal involvement, a 29-year-old male patient required oral prednisolone and factor XIII infusion. He had complained of an uncomfortable feeling in the abdomen, and had decreased plasma factor XIII activity (41%) that was below the lower limit of 70%. Another 64-year-old male patient had severe abdominal pain, bloody diarrhea and rapidly progressive anemia. His factor XIII activity was 46%. Upper gastrointestinal endoscopy showed multiple duodenal ulcers. Intravenous infusion of prednisolone at 60 mg/day completely resolved those abdominal involvements except for decreased factor XIII activity. However, during tapering of prednisolone to 40 mg/day, he had sudden severe bloody stools followed by acute respiratory distress syndrome. The jejunal artery bleeding was found on angiography. Unfortunately, the patient died six months after disease onset because of peritonitis despite aggressive therapy including partial jejunectomy. Although factor XIII activity was not always examined in our hospital, there were significant differences in the prevalence of gastrointestinal involvement between normal or high factor XIII activity (≥70%) and low activity groups (<70%) (44.4% [8/18] *vs* 100% [8/8], P = *0.007*) in adults. In contrast, all pediatric patients had an uneventful recovery.

Relationship Between Renal Involvement and Other Clinical Characteristics in the Adult Group

Adult patients with IgA vasculitis were separated into those with and without renal involvement, which was indicated by the presence of proteinuria, hematuria and/or urinary casts, for further analysis (Table **5**). The proportion of patients suffering from purpura on the trunk and upper extremities was significantly greater in the renal disease group than in the group without renal disease (59.4% [38/64] *vs* 20.0% [4/20], P = 0.002). Hemorrhagic bullous lesions and/or erosions were observed in 20.3% (13/64) of the patients with renal manifestations, whereas no such lesions were observed in those without renal manifestations (P = 0.028). Gastrointestinal symptoms were more common in adult patients with renal disease than those without renal disease (48.4% [31/64] *vs* 30.0% [6/20]), but the difference was statistically insignificant (P = 0.147). Arthralgia was seen in approximately 40% of patients in both groups. Adult patients with IgA vasculitis and renal involvement had higher rates of hospitalization than those without renal disease (76.6% [49/64] *vs* 45.0% [9/20], P = 0.008). Disease recurrence was similar in both groups, while occurrence of recalcitrant disease was higher in the renal disease group compared with the group without renal disease (45.3% [29/64] *vs* 20.0% [4/20], P = 0.043).

Serum Immunoglobulin Levels and Clinical Manifestations in Adult IgA Vasculitis

Table **5** shows that serum IgA levels in adult patients exceeded the normal range (140.0–240.0 mg/dl) but no significant difference was observed between those with renal disease and those without renal disease (410.1 ± 124.0 mg/dl *vs* 385.3 ± 150.3 mg/dl, P = 0.531). Immunoglobulin levels were also compared between groups of adult patients with

Table 5. Renal manifestations in adult cases of IgA vasculitis.

	Renal Manifestations[1] +		Renal Manifestations −		P
	(n = 64)		(n = 20)		
	n	(%)	n	(%)	
Sex					
Male:Female	34:30 (1.13:1)		13:7 (1.86:1)		0.350
Age (years)					
Mean ± SD	52.4 ± 16.4		48.9 ± 21.0		0.495
Range	21–83		24–91		
Recent signs of infection	33/64	(51.6)	14/20	(70.0)	0.147
Serum IgA level (mg/dl)[2]	410.1 ± 124.0		385.3 ± 150.3		0.531
Clinical manifestations					
Purpura					
Distributed on the trunk and/or upper extremities	38/64	(59.4)	4/20	(20.0)	0.002**
Hemorrhagic bullous lesions/erosions	13/64	(20.3)	0/20	(0.0)	0.028*
Gastrointestinal symptoms[3]	31/64	(48.4)	6/20	(30.0)	0.147
Arthralgia	24/64	(37.5)	8/20	(40.0)	0.841
Admission rate	49/64	(76.6)	9/20	(45.0)	0.008**
Medical therapy					
Prednisolone	31/64	(48.4)	10/20	(50.0)	0.903
Antibiotics	18/64	(28.1)	8/20	(40.0)	0.316
Dapsone	28/64	(43.8)	6/20	(30.0)	0.274
Outcome					
Recurrence	10/64	(15.6)	5/20	(25.0)	0.339
Recalcitrance	29/64	(45.3)	4/20	(20.0)	0.043*

[1]Proteinuria, hematuria and/or urinary casts.
[2]Normal range of IgA (140.0–240.0 mg/dl).
[3]Abdominal pain, hematochezia and/or fecal occult blood.
*$P < 0.05$, **$P < 0.02$.

and without gastrointestinal and joint involvement (Fig. **2**). It was noted that IgG and IgA levels were significantly lower in patients with gastrointestinal involvement than those without gastrointestinal symptoms ($P < 0.05$), and a similar tendency was observed in patients with joint manifestations for all immunoglobulin levels. Furthermore, as shown in Table **6**, we compared the incidence of renal, gastrointestinal and joint manifestations in patients with elevated levels of immunoglobulins, and found that the 32 patients with a sole increase in IgA level had a higher incidence of renal (87.5% [28/32]) and gastrointestinal (59.4% [19/32]) involvement. This was in contrast to the net incidence of renal (65.1% [28/43], $P = 0.027$) and gastrointestinal (34.9% [15/43], $P = 0.035$) manifestations in the other groups. However, a lower proportion of patients with concurrent elevation of IgA and IgG, or IgA, IgG and IgM had gastrointestinal manifestations (11.9% [3/14], $P = 0.046$; and 0% [0/8], $P = 0.006$; respectively).

DISCUSSION

The present study showed that adult-type IgA vasculitis is different from pediatric-type IgA vasculitis. Preceding upper respiratory infections were relatively less common in

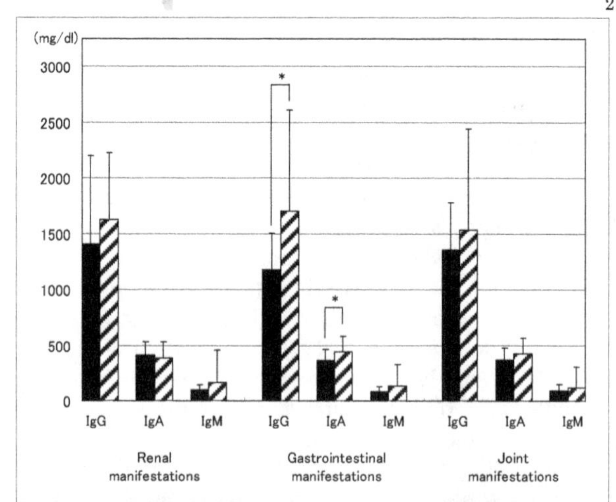

Fig. (2). Comparison of serum IgG, IgA and IgM levels in adult patients with and without renal, gastrointestinal and joint manifestations. Solid bars represent patients with the clinical manifestation and hatched bars represent those without the manifestation. Immunoglobulin levels are expressed as mean ± SD. *$P < 0.05$.

Table 6. Patients with increased serum immunoglobulin levels and clinical manifestations in adult IgA vasculitis.

Ig Increase[1]	No. of Adult Cases		Renal Manifestations			Gastrointestinal Manifestations			Joint Manifestations		
	n	(%)	n	(%)	P^2	n	(%)	P	n	(%)	P
IgG only	1/75[3]	(1.3)	0/1[4]	(0)	0.084	0/1[5]	(0)	0.359	0/1[6]	(0)	0.411
IgA only	32/75	(42.7)	28/32	(87.5)	0.027*	19/32	(59.4)	0.035*	13/32	(40.6)	0.924
IgM only	4/75	(5.3)	2/4	(50.0)	0.244	3/4	(75.0)	0.221	2/4	(50.0)	0.675
IgG and IgA	14/75	(18.7)	8/14	(57.1)	0.095	3/14	(11.9)	0.046*	5/14	(35.7)	0.717
IgA and IgM	14/75	(18.7)	12/14	(85.7)	0.292	7/14	(50.0)	0.697	5/14	(35.7)	0.717
IgG, IgA and IgM	8/75	(10.7)	5/8	(62.5)	0.403	0/8	(0)	0.006**	3/8	(37.5)	0.879
All WNL[7]	2/75	(2.7)	1/2	(50.0)	0.416	2/2	(100)	0.115	2/2	(100)	0.079
Total	75/75	(100)	56/75	(74.7)		34/75	(45.3)		30/75	(40.0)	

[1]Patients with an increase of immunoglobulin (Ig) subtypes were grouped as shown in this column. Normal ranges for IgG, IgA and IgM are 850–1,500 mg/dl, 140–240 mg/dl, and 40.0–100 mg/dl, respectively.
[2]P-value: incidence of renal, gastrointestinal or joint manifestations in specific groups with Ig increase was compared with the incidence of renal, gastrointestinal or joint manifestations in the net number of patients in the other groups i.e., total number of patients minus the number of patients in the specified group.
[3]Number of patients with the specified Ig increase/75 cases who had complete data for all three immunoglobulin levels.
[4]Number of patients with renal manifestations/number of patients with the specified Ig increase.
[5]Number of patients with gastrointestinal manifestations/number of patients with the specified Ig increase.
[6]Number of patients with joint manifestations/number of patients with the specified Ig increase.
[7]WNL, within normal limits.
$^*P < 0.05$, $^{**}P < 0.02$.

adult-type disease (56.5%) than in pediatric disease (89.2%). However, adult cases were associated with a range of infections, and clinicians should be vigilant for infections such as pneumonia, cellulitis and other infectious foci associated with palmoplantar pustulosis [16] and acrodermatitis continua of Hallopeau.

Our findings revealed that adult-type IgA vasculitis might be associated with malignancy. This is consistent with the findings described by Zurada *et al.* [14]. They concluded that lung and prostate carcinomas and hematologic malignancies such as multiple myeloma and non-Hodgkin's lymphoma are the most commonly associated malignancies. In our study, seven cases (8.2%) of adult-type IgA vasculitis were associated with malignancy: four had lung cancers and the other three had hematological disorders. Six of the seven cases were over 56 years of age, and the malignancies were found at the onset of IgA vasculitis in three of seven cases. Mitsui *et al.* compared their 53 cases of adult-type IgA vasculitis and reported that the cases with malignancy were significantly older, with a lesser prevalence of arthralgia and a higher erythrocyte sedimentation rate than those without malignancy [17]. In our study, except for the higher serum IgA levels in the patients with advanced lung carcinoma, other examined features were not different between patients with and without malignancy. Two cases of lung carcinoma only had persistent cough. Therefore, we need to be vigilant for solid and hematologic malignancies in adult-type IgA vasculitis in cases over 60 years of age, especially in recalcitrant cases or those without apparent infectious triggers. We did not investigate the causative antigen(s) complexed with IgA in the present study. The cancer-related antigen(s) in comparison with infection-related antigens in IgA vasculitis have not been studied.

Renal disease was more common in the adult group as evidenced by proteinuria, hematuria and/or urinary casts in approximately three quarters (76.2%) of adult patients, and tended to be more severe. In an analysis of 100 pediatric cases of IgA vasculitis, Saulsbury [7] concluded that 40% of patients showed signs of nephritis but the vast majority resolved within nine weeks, except for one case. Similarly, Roberts *et al.* [8] reported that the majority of renal disease in pediatric patients resolved spontaneously, with 1% progressing to end-stage renal disease. In contrast, Diehl *et al.* [13] described eight cases of elderly-onset, IgA-positive HSP requiring corticosteroid therapy. In their six patients with renal disease, three patients required both corticosteroids and immunosuppressants, and one patient with severe renal disease required hemodialysis. In the present study, 8 of 84 cases with renal manifestations required a renal biopsy, and five of them needed more aggressive therapy, but none resulted in renal failure. We agree with the suggestion by Diehl *et al.* [13] that elderly patients with IgA vasculitis are more vulnerable to severe renal disease compared with pediatric patients.

Gastrointestinal involvement was more common in adult-type IgA vasculitis (45.2%) compared with pediatric disease (33.3%). A study of intestinal biopsies showed IgA deposition and LCV affecting the submucosal vessels of the small intestine [18], similar to that seen in the skin. Abdominal pain may precede cutaneous signs [19]. It was noted that one case was associated with fatal jejunal artery bleeding, peritonitis and decreased factor XIII activity. Matayoshi *et al.* investigated 44 cases of adult-type IgA vasculitis and showed that factor XIII activity reflected the severities of digestive tract and joint disorders, but not renal symptoms [20]. Clinicians should be aware that a similar outcome might occur in severe gastrointestinal disease. We think that the measurement of plasma factor XIII activity, fecal occult blood test and endoscopy would aid the management of patients with abdominal symptoms.

The distribution of skin lesions was different between adult and pediatric IgA vasculitis. Our findings suggest that purpura on the abdomen and/or waist was more frequently observed in adults, and purpura on the trunk and/or upper extremities and change into hemorrhagic bulla may be associated with renal involvement. Thus, close observation of the morphology and distribution pattern of the skin lesions may lead to better management of adult IgA vasculitis, since renal involvement in adult and elderly patients should be carefully managed. On the other hand, proteinuria and hematuria should be monitored and routine administration of steroids is not beneficial in pediatric patients [21]. In the present study, dapsone was often used for IgA vasculitis, especially in adult patients with extensive skin lesions. Dapsone decreases neutrophil chemotaxis and their activity, suppresses the oxidative pathway, and has an anti-inflammatory effect in IgA vasculitis [22, 23]. We believe that dapsone is useful for adult patients, but care must be taken to avoid possible side effects.

The serum level of IgA was increased in the majority of adult patients with IgA vasculitis, but the increase in serum IgA level did not correlate with renal involvement (P = 0.531). Calvo-Río V *et al.* reported that increased levels of serum IgA were more commonly observed in the subgroup of patients with nephropathy than in those without renal involvement among HSP patients including children and adults (41.8% *vs* 10%, respectively; P = 0.027) [24]. Our analysis was limited to adult patients because of the relatively low number of cases of children with common IgA vasculitis and the significant difference in serum IgA levels between the adult and pediatric group (405.1 ± 129.6 mg/dl *vs* 232.5 ± 89.1 mg/dl, respectively; $P < 0.001$). Further examination of adult patients in our study revealed that a high proportion of patients with sole elevation of IgA had renal involvement compared with the other groups (87.5% *vs* 65.1%, P = 0.027). Similarly, gastrointestinal involvement was more common in patients with a sole increase in IgA level (59.4% *vs* 34.9%, P = 0.035), whereas this association was not seen in patients with increased IgA and IgG, or concurrent IgA, IgG and IgM elevation. In children, it has been reported that renal involvement is seen in 32% of patients with increased IgA, and raised IgA in association with reduced IgM levels is predictive of severe complications [25]. This suggests that an unknown interaction exists between circulating IgA and other immunoglobulins in IgA vasculitis, and may be related to its complications. Lau *et al.* [5] suggested that anti-glycan IgG and IgA1 interact to form a complex that reacts to glomerular and mesangial cells in nephritis associated with IgA vasculitis, but the roles of IgG and IgM in the pathogenesis of IgA vasculitis-associated complications remain unknown. Further study of the role of immunoglobulin subtypes in IgA vasculitis is required.

Byun *et al.* [26] recently suggested that relapse is common in adult IgA vasculitis, and predictive factors for relapse include onset at an older age, persistent rash, abdominal pain, hematuria, and the presence of underlying disease. Poterucha *et al.* [27] reported that histopathologic markers might predict renal and gastrointestinal involvement, stating that absence of eosinophils and age > 40 years might be important predictors of renal involvement. Our results showed that recalcitrant disease should be carefully monitored because it was significantly more common in the adult group than in the pediatric group (38.8% *vs* 18.9%, P = 0.031); specifically, it was more common in adults with renal manifestations than in those without (45.3% *vs* 20.0%, P = 0.043). Approximately half of the adult patients were treated with corticosteroids, together with immunosuppressants in some cases.

In summary, we analyzed patients with IgA vasculitis comprising 35 pediatric and 87 adult patients, and suggest that adult IgA vasculitis should be managed carefully because of the greater risk of complications, especially renal damage. Furthermore, we should pay attention to the possible association with malignancy. Although statistical analysis did not show significance, and the IgA vasculitis guidelines of the Japanese Dermatological Association [28] and Japanese Circulation Society [29] did not suggest this possibility, we should consider the possible association of malignancy when we see adult IgA vasculitis. Although the retrospective nature of the study is a limitation, this study provides additional insight into adult-type IgA vasculitis and the information is useful for the management of this condition.

CONFLICT OF INTEREST

The authors confirm that they have no conflicts of interest.

ACKNOWLEDGEMENTS

Declared none.

REFERENCES

[1] Jennette JC, Falk RJ, Bacon PA, *et al.* 2012 revised International Chapel Hill Consensus Conference Nomenclature of Vasculitides. Arthritis Rheum 2013; 65: 1-11.

[2] Linskey KR, Kroshinsky D, Mihm MC Jr, Hoang MP. Immunoglobulin-A-associated small-vessel vasculitis: a 10-year experience at the Massachusetts General Hospital. J Am Acad Dermatol 2012; 66: 813-22.

[3] Kawana S, Shen GH, Kobayashi Y, Nishiyama S. Membrane attack complex of complement in Henoch-Schönlein purpura skin and nephritis. Arch Dermatol Res 1990; 282: 183-7.

[4] Yamamoto T, Kaburagi Y, Izaki S, Tanaka T, Kitamura K. Leukocytoclasis: ultrastructural in situ nick end labeling study in anaphylactoid purpura. J Dermatol Sci 2000; 24: 158-65.

[5] Lau KK, Suzuki H, Novak J, Wyatt RJ. Pathogenesis of Henoch-Schönlein purpura nephritis. Pediatr Nephrol 2012; 25: 19-26.

[6] Kato S, Ebina K, Naganuma H, Sato S, Maisawa S, Nakagawa H. Intestinal IgA deposition in Henoch-Schönlein purpura with severe gastro-intestinal manifestations. Eur J Pediatr 1996; 155: 91-5.

[7] Saulsbury FK. Henoch-Schönlein purpura in children. Reports of 100 patients and review of the literature. Medicine 1999; 78: 395-409.

[8] Roberts PF, Waller TA, Brinker TM, Riffe IZ, Sayre JW, Bratton RL. Henoch-Schönlein purpura: a review article. South Med J 2007; 100: 821-4.

[9] Mills JA, Michel BA, Bloch DA, *et al.* The American College of Rheumatology 1990 criteria for the classification of Henoch-Schönlein purpura. Arthritis Rheum 1990; 33: 1114-21.

[10] Blanco R, Martínez-Taboada VM, Rodríguez-Valverde V, García-Fuentes M, González-Gay MA. Henoch-Schönlein purpura in adulthood and childhood: two different expressions of the same syndrome. Arthritis Rheum 1997; 40: 859-64.

[11] Tancrede-Bohin E, Ochonisky S, Vignon-Pennamen MD, Flaguel B, Morel P, Rybojad M. Schönlein-Henoch purpura in adult patients. Predictive factors for IgA glomerulonephritis in a retrospective study of 57 cases. Arch Dermatol 1997; 133: 438-42.

[12] García-Porrúa C, Calviño MC, Llorca J, Couselo JM, González-Gay MA. Henoch-Schönlein purpura in children and adults: clinical differences in a defined population. Semin Arthritis Rheum 2002; 32: 149-56.

[13] Diehl MP, Harrington T, Olenginski T. Elderly-onset Henoch-Schönlein purpura: a case series and review of the literature. J Am Geriatr Soc 2008; 56: 2157-9.

[14] Zurada JM, Ward KM, Grossman ME. Henoch-Schönlein purpura associated with malignancy in adults. J Am Acad Dermatol 2006; 55: S65-70.

[15] Ozen S, Pistorio A, Iusan SM, *et al.* EULAR/PRINTO/PRES criteria for Henoch-Schönlein purpura, childhood polyarteritis nodosa, childhood Wegener granulomatosis and childhood Takayasu arteritis: Ankara 2008. Part II: Final classification criteria. Ann Rheum Dis 2010; 69: 798-806.

[16] Izaki S, Goto Y, Kaburagi Y, Kitamura K, Nomaguchi H. Antibody production to heat shock protein with Mr 65 kD (HSP65) in cutaneous inflammation: a possible relation to focal infection. Acta Otolaryngol (Stockh) 1996; Suppl 523: 197-200.

[17] Mitsui H, Shibagaki N, Kawamura T, Matsue H, Shimada S. A clinical study of Henoch-Schönlein Purpura associated with malignancy. J Eur Acad Dermatol Venereol. 2009; 23: 394-401.

[18] Elbert EC. Gastrointestinal manifestations of Henoch-Schonlein purpura. Dig Dis Sci 2008; 53: 2011-9.

[19] Chen XL, Tian H, Li JZ, *et al.* Paroxysmal drastic abdominal pain with tardive cutaneous lesions presenting in Henoch-Schönlein purpura. World J Gastroenterol 2012; 18: 1991-5.

[20] Matayoshi T, Omi T, Sakai N, Kawana S. Clinical significance of blood coagulation factor XIII activity in adult Henoch-Schönlein purpura. J Nippon Med Sch 2013; 80: 268-78.

[21] Smith G. Management of Henoch-Schönlein purpura. Pediatr Child Health 2008; 18: 358-63.

[22] Chen KR, Carlson JA. Clinical approach to cutaneous vasculitis. Am J Clin Dermatol 2008; 9: 71-92.

[23] Bech AP, Reichert LJ, Cohen-Tervaert JW. Dapsone for the treatment of chronic IgA vasculitis (Henoch-Schonlein). Neth J Med 2013; 71; 220-1.

[24] Calvo-Río V, Loricera J, Mata C, *et al.* Henoch-Schönlein purpura in northern Spain: clinical spectrum of the disease in 417 patients from a single center. Medicine (Baltimore) 2014; 93: 106-13.

[25] Fretzayas A, Sionti I, Moustaki M, Nicolaidou P. Clinical impact of altered immunoglobulin levels in Henoch-Schönlein purpura. Pediatr Int 2009; 51: 381-4.

[26] Byun JW, Song HJ, Kim L, Shin JH, Choi GS. Predictive factors of relapse in adult with Henoch-Schönlein purpura. Am J Dermatopathol 2012; 34: 139-44.

[27] Poterucha TJ, Wetter DA, Gibson LE Camilleri MJ, Lohse CM. Histopathology and correlates of sysytemic disease in adult Henoch-Schönlein purpura: A retrospective study of microscopic and clinical findings in 68 patients at Mayo Clinic. J Am Acad Dermatol 2013; 68: 420-4.

[28] Katsuoka K, Kawakami T, Ishiguro N, *et al.* Guidelines for management of vasculitis and vasculopathy (in Japanese). Nippikaishi 2008; 118: 2095-187.

[29] Ozaki S, Ando M, Isobe M, *et al.* Guideline for management of vasculitis syndrome (JCS 2008). Japanese Circulation Society. Circ J 2011; 75: 474-503.

Parental and Child Attitudes Towards Pediculosis are a Major Cause of Reinfection

Deon V. Canyon*, Chauncey Canyon and Sami Milani

Office of Public Health Studies, University of Hawaii at Manoa, 1960 East-West Rd, Biomed Building #T103, Honolulu, HI 96822, USA

Abstract: Pediculosis can elicit considerable emotional distress in the infected and their carers, but the role of attitude in head lice reinfection has not been explored. Failure of head lice control is often attributed to insecticide resistance because human aspects of reinfestation are unknown. This study collected data from 128 teenagers with a history of pediculosis to retrospectively explore attitudes towards head lice. One third of female and two thirds of male teenagers were unconcerned about having head lice. One fifth of parents did nothing about their child's head lice infections, while a few male students did not inform their parents when they had pediculosis. This is the first study on the prevalence of human lice carriers who are a primary cause of head lice reinfection. Medical and public health professions need to understand the social reasons for the failure of insecticide-based head lice control.

Keywords: Apathy, pediculosis, reinfection, reservoir, teenager.

INTRODUCTION

Head lice are a six-legged insect known by the scientific name of *Pediculus humanus capitis* (De Geer) and infection in humans is called pediculosis. Head lice are very common in all countries around the world and they are spreading because of increased travel and resistance to insecticides [1,2].

Pediculosis elicits great alarm among adults that is out of proportion to their medical significance [3,4]. They can be a source of amusement or stigma for the uninfected and an embarrassing nuisance to the infected [5]. Head lice and human beings have evolved together partly because head lice depend totally on humans for their existence. This is a very old relationship since preserved head lice have even been found in the hair of mummies from Egypt buried 9000 years ago [6]. This pest has evolved closely with humans over time and now cannot survive on the blood of any other animal host.

Parison and Canyon (2010) collected data on pediculosis knowledge and attitudes [7]. They found that parents and carers focused on experiences while head lice treaters focused on control issues. The dominant themes that emerged from this study included concerns about treatment products, issues with treating children, blaming others for reinfection, stigma and social issues. The latter two mental health themes represent difficult aspects of pediculosis management, but have largely been ignored by researchers [8].

The stigma 'inherited' from older generations concerned with fatal louse-borne infections appears to be diminishing in younger generations. The concern is that this will lead to diminishing concern for lice presence and will lead to greatly enhanced transmission rates. In fact, the prevalence we have already observed all over Australia of 10-40% and globally in all schools may already be a result of this emerging attitude [1,9]. Prevalence of pediculosis significantly varies by country, region, school and classroom. One large and well-conducted study on 135 classrooms throughout the state of Victoria in Australia reported an average infection rate of 13% [10]. It found that commonly assumed risk factors, such as long hair, living in a rural area and age, were not associated with active infection.

Two issues remain fundamental to controlling head lice – resistance and reinfection. Resistance can be addressed by modifying treatment protocols, but reinfection is a behavioral and a social problem that requires more research. We already know that certain key individuals (school students) serve as potent carriers who continually reinfect associates [11]. They maintain lice infections due to greater susceptibility, apathy, lack of treatment or lack of awareness due to lack of symptoms.

However, when children are infected, there are always two sides to the infection equation – parents and children. While the behavior of an infected child is often considered primarily responsible for transmission, parental or career behaviors can also have a large impact. Therefore, this study aimed to gain insight into the experiences and attitudes of teenagers who recalled having lice infections to learn what they thought about their infections and their parent's attitudes towards pediculosis.

METHODS

A multicultural school in Perth, Western Australia with approx. 1700 students from grades 8 to 12 agreed to allow this study to take place on 480 middle-school students in grades 8 and 9. Grade 7 is the last primary school grade in

*Address correspondence to this author at the Office of Public Health Studies, University of Hawaii at Manoa, 1960 East-West Rd, Biomed Building #T103, Honolulu, HI 96822, USA;
E-mail: dcanyon@hawaii.edu

Australia and head lice infections predominantly occur in primary school grades 1 through 6 [1,2]. Ethics approval H2954 was obtained from James Cook University. Consent letters and information sheets were sent home to parents along with a hard copy of the survey. Parents were asked to complete the consent form and return it to the school. Eligible teenagers with parental consent were asked by their parents to complete an anonymous survey and return it to the school. Completed consent forms and surveys were collected from the school for storage and analysis. Participation was thus based on voluntary self-selection. This sampling strategy combines criterion based and convenience approaches, since the targeted participants are those who have direct experience coping with a head lice infestation (criterion) and they are accessible (convenience) [12].

The questionnaire requested basic non-identifying demographic information (grade, gender and hair details) followed by four open-ended questions:

1. When you think about the last time you had head lice, how did you feel?
2. Why do you think you felt that way?
3. How did your parents feel and behave when they found out you had head lice?
4. Why do you think they felt and behaved that way?

Only students who could recall being infected with head lice were included in the study. The anonymous responses were analyzed for salient themes that addressed the questionnaire focus using the computer software package SPSS 21. Cross-tabulations with Chi-square Tests were employed but since 20% of the frequencies were usually less than 5, this test was not applicable. Thus Goodman and Krustal tau/Uncertainty Coefficient Tests were performed.

RESULTS

The response rate was good with 133 students out of 480 (27.7%) participating in the study and 128 surveys that were sufficiently complete to enable analysis. These students had a history of head lice infection and were willing to volunteer to be in the study. The temporal proximity of participants to the infection event and the nature of the event being recalled indicate that recall would have been reasonably accurate. While adult retrospective reports of adverse childhood experiences involve a substantial rate of false negatives, false positive reports are rare [13]. Only 9th graders reported on 8th Grade infections (Fig. **1**).

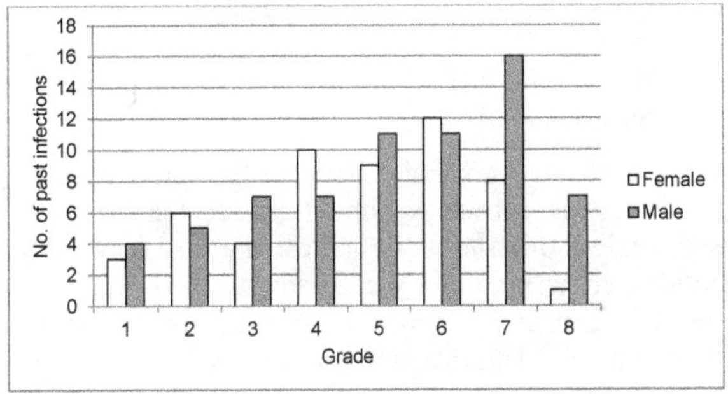

Fig. (1). Number of students who recalled having a head lice infection and the grade in which that infection occurred.

Overall there were 45.3% females and 53.1% males while 3% did not indicate gender (Table **1**). There were two Aboriginal females and one African male, but these were omitted from the analysis because there were too few to represent an ethnic background. This left a total of 128 valid questionnaires for Caucasians and Asians.

Table 1. Study Participants by Gender and Race

Gender	Ethnicity		Total
	Caucasian	Asian	
Female	50	7	57
Male	57	10	67
Missing	-	-	4
Total			128

In response to the question, 'What grade are you in now?' there were 66 responders in Grade 8, 59 in Grade 9 and 3 did not respond. Thus the dataset was well distributed between the two grades. In response to the questions about hair thickness, 17.2% had thin hair, 50.0% had medium and 32.8% had thick hair. Blonds made up 16.4% of the data while 67.2% had brown hair and 16.4% had black hair. Shorthaired participants made up 46.4% of the survey population, 28.0% had medium hair and 25.6% had long hair. Short brown medium thickness hair was the most common hair type. This data was unbalanced with only one female and 57 males having short hair, while 28 females and eight males had shoulder length hair, and 29 females and two males had long hair.

Question 1. When You Think About the Last Time You had Head Lice, How Did You Feel at the Time?

More than half of the total respondents (53.6%) did not care that they had head lice and most of these were males. A quarter said that they were disgusted or angry about having head lice (26.4%). Females made up most of the 7.2% who were embarrassed and the 12.8% who were scared or worried about being infected (Fig. **2**). When these data were statistically tested using Pearson chi-square and uncertainty coefficient analyses, a significant relationship between the responses to the question and the gender was observed

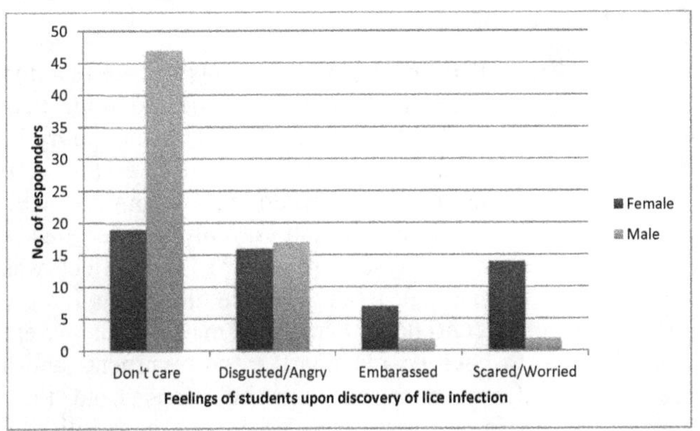

Fig. (2). The range of feelings students had when they found out they had head lice.

(24.62, p<0.001). This relationship was moderately strong (u=0.118) and more gender dependent (u=0.156). Female responses were fairly evenly distributed, but most males did not care at all. When the responses to this question were statistically tested against ethnicity (Caucasian *vs* Asian), there was no significant difference.

Question 2. Why Do You Think You Felt that Way?

A quarter of the students gave answers that indicated that they did not know or did not care about why they did not know or did not care at all (24.8%), and most of these were males. Very few stated concerns about treatment and these focused on avoidance of painful or smelly treatments (6.4%). One third of responders cited pain or itch (36.8%) and another third cited social issues (32.0%) (Table **2**). When these data were statistically tested using Pearson chi-square and uncertainty coefficient analyses, a significant relationship between the responses to the question and the gender was observed (12.764, p<0.01). This relationship was weak (u=0.056) and more dependent on gender rather than the question (u=0.079). There were no significant differences when the responses to this question were statistically tested against race, hair thickness and hair color. However, hair length was significantly associated with attitude (15.051, p<0.05). This relationship was weak (u=0.053) and slightly more hair-length dependent (u=0.058) (Table **2**). Shorthaired students were less inclined to care, treatment issues were more common in longhaired students, itch was greater in shorter haired students, and social issues elevated in shorthaired students.

Table 2. Number of Students Expressing Reasons for their Attitudes About Head Lice Infection Compared with Gender and Hair Length

Reasons for Attitudes	Student Gender		Student Hair Length		
	Female	Male	Short	Shoulder	Long
Don't know/care	7	24	21	6	3
Treatment issues	6	2	1	2	5
Painful/ Itchy	21	25	18	15	11
Social Issues	23	15	16	12	12

Question 3. How did Your Parents React When They Found Out You had Head Lice?

Students indicated that 15.1% of parents had no reaction upon finding out that their child was infected with lice, 61.1% of parents treated the infection, 21.4% were angry or horrified and 2.4% did not find out about the infection. When the responses to this question were compared with gender, ethnicity, and hair variables, only gender had a statistical effect on the results (Table **3**). This effect was significant (8.867, p<0.05) but weak (u=0.049) and more gender dependent (u=0.060). Parents of male students were more inclined to have no reaction (i.e. no treatment) and a few male students concealed their infections from their parents. If it is conservatively assumed that all the angry/horrified parents treated their children, then 83.1% of parents treated their children with some head lice control method and 16.9% of infected students remained untreated.

Table 3. Number of Students Indicating Parental Reactions on Discovering Head Lice Infections in their Children

Parental Reactions	Student Gender		Student Hair Length		
	Female	Male	Short	Shoulder	Long
Did not do anything	4	14	12	3	3
Treated hair	42	35	30	24	22
Angry/Horrified	12	14	13	6	7
Did not find out	0	3	3	0	0

4. Why Do You Think Parents Felt that Way?

The answers to this question mostly repeated the answers to the last question. Students did not know why their parents had no reaction. They stated that their parents treated because treatment was needed. They stated that parents were angry and horrified because they were concerned about transmission. None of these answers were statistically significant.

DISCUSSION

The aim of this study was to determine if there were any social factors that played an important role in the transmission and control of head lice and the results provided good evidence to show that social factors are involved and that attitude modification should play an essential role in head lice management.

Question 1. When You Think About the Last Time You had Head Lice, How Did You Feel at the Time?

The female answers were fairly evenly distributed between the response types, but the male answers were mostly 'don't care' or 'angry'. From the results we see that one third of the females and two thirds of the males answered that they were not concerned about having head lice. This may be because they consider head lice to be a normal part of life and they are confident of being able to eliminate them. However, "Success breeds complacency [and] complacency breeds failure" [14], which translates to increased opportunities for head lice to spread. If these students do not care about being infected then there is a good chance that they will delay informing their parents which will delay treatment and increase transmission. Maunder's (1985) comment that embarrassment and secrecy support the continued survival of head lice is not supported by the results in this study since there was little evidence of stigma driven human behavior [15]. It may be that attitudes have changed over time or that they differ between populations rather than that Maunder was incorrect.

Having a strong personal reaction of disgust was quite common and was shown by one third of females and a quarter of males. But almost no males said that they reacted by becoming embarrassed or scared and worried. Males may thus be less concerned about the social implications of having pediculosis. This reaction was a very female reaction in response to finding out that they had head lice. The lack of significant difference between Caucasians and Asians, does not support the speculation that there is a strong cultural basis for the origin of the feelings about lice [7]. However, these two populations resided in the same geographic area and may have not been culturally distinct.

These results indicate that female and male children and teenagers often assume the role of head lice carriers since they apathetically allow their parasites to breed, multiply and spread to other heads. It is important to understand the nature of carriers because they increase the number of head lice in a group of socially linked people, they continuously reinfect the people around them, and they infect new people who come into the social group. Males are twice as likely to act as carriers than females and both genders should be targeted with educational material.

Question 2. Why Do You Think You Felt that Way?

The information gathered to answer this question showed that gender and hair length were the most important variables. Table **2** shows that a quarter of the students did not care to explain why they felt the way that they did, while half the males who previously said that they did not care, now attributed this feeling to a mixture of treatment issues, pain and itch or social concerns. It may be that this half of the initial 'don't care' group are more important carriers and transmitters of head lice. While male and female attitudes were equally motivated by pain/itch, female feelings were more motivated by social issues. This shows that some teenagers are very self-conscious about having pediculosis because of the way their peers think about head lice. Thus even though these teens might not have negative emotions towards head lice, they will try to control their head lice infection to conform with the values of their peer group. Thus strategies to control head lice, especially in females, need to have a strong component of social motivation to be effective.

Hair length was the other variable that was significantly related to this question. A fairly equal number of students with different hair lengths was concerned about pain/itch and social issues, so hair length was only of interest with regard to the 'don't know/care' and 'treatment' groups. Students in the 'don't know/care' group were more likely to have short hair and students in the 'treatment' group were more likely to have long hair. Since the data already shows a large percentage of males in the 'don't know/care' group, it is clear that they comprise most of the shorthair group. Thus the relationship between shorthair and 'don't know/care' is probably not very important. The treatment reason for attitudes was more interesting because it was clear that longhaired students were more concerned about getting treated and this affected how they felt about their last head lice infection. This was most likely due to painful treatment methods such as fine-toothed combing.

Question 3. How Did Your Parents React (How Did They Behave) when They Found Out You had Head Lice?

There was a large difference in parental reactions depending on the gender of their child, especially in the 'Did not do anything' category. Parents did not do anything (e.g. treat) to a fifth of their male offspring, whereas almost all of their female offspring experienced a more concerned reaction. This group of head lice infected males is left to fend for themselves so it is also possible that parental reactions have trained some male children not to care and not to be concerned about getting head lice. It is possible that this cycles since a lack of embarrassment and worry in male offspring acts to calm the parents who feel okay about doing nothing.

The lower male score for treatment indicates that less infected males are treated. This result, in combination with other results for males, indicates that they may become important carriers and transmitters of head lice. The last interesting result was that some male students actively concealed their infections from their parents. This behavior may be driven by apathy or a desire to avoid a bad parental reaction or an uncaring parental reaction or unpleasant treatment options. These students are prime carrier candidates because they actively avoid revealing that they have pediculosis.

It has been argued that negative social effects and stigma associated with pediculosis create more problems than the infection itself [8,16,17]. This study shows that stigma is a parental and societal issue rather than a child or teen issue since only a quarter of teenagers showed negative emotions towards head lice. Thus head lice control strategies and programs that focus on stigma and negative emotional reactions in teenagers will not be effective. Rather, control strategies should focus on identifying and treating potent apathetic human carriers of head lice who are largely responsible for the perpetual reintroduction of head lice into society.

CONFLICT OF INTEREST

The authors confirm that this article content has no conflict of interest.

ACKNOWLEDGEMENTS

Declared none.

REFERENCES

[1] Gratz NG. Human lice: their prevalence, control and resistance to insecticides: a review 1985-1997. Geneva: World Health Organization, Division of Control of Tropical Diseases, WHO Pesticide Evaluation Scheme, 1997.

[2] Speare R, Buettner PG. Head lice in pupils of a primary school in Australia and implications for control. Int J Dermatol 1999; 38: 285-90.

[3] Counahan M. Scratching for answers? Public health aspects of head lice control. PhD thesis. Townsville, Qld: James Cook University, 2006.

[4] Falagas M, Matthaiou DK, Petros IP, Panos G, Pappas G. Worldwide prevalence of head lice. Emerg Infect Dis. 2008; 14: 1493-4.

[5] Hochman D. One louse, ick. two lice, call for help! New York Times. 9 April 2010.

[6] Mumcuoglu KY, Zias J. Head lice, *Pediculus humanus capitis* (Anoplura: Pediculidae), from hair combs excavated in Israel and dated from the first century B.C. to the eighth century A.D. J Med Entomol 1988; 25: 545–7.

[7] Parison J, Canyon DV. Head lice and the impact of knowledge, attitudes and practices - a social science overview. In: Management and control of head lice infestations. Bremen: UNI-MED Verlag AG, 2010; 103-9.

[8] Parison J, Speare R, Canyon DV. Head lice: The feelings people have. Int J Dermatol 2013; 52(2): 169-71.

[9] Canyon DV, Speare R. Clinical decision support: Dermatology: Pediculosis. Wilmington, DE: Decision Support in Medicine LLC, 2012.

[10] Counahan M, Andrews R, Büttner P, Byrnes G, Speare R. Head lice prevalence in primary schools in Victoria, Australia. J Paediatr Child Health 2004; 40(11): 616-9.

[11] Canyon DV, Speare R. Head lice transmission and risk factors. In: Heukelbach J, Ed. Management and control of head lice infestations. Bremen: UNI-MED Verlag AG, 2010; 34-40.
[12] Patton MQ. Qualitative research & evaluation methods, 3rd Ed. Thousand Oaks, CA: Sage, 2002.
[13] Grove A. Untitled. Brainy Quote. Retrieved 30 Jan 2014 from http://www.brainyquote.com/quotes/quotes/a/andygrove471638.html.
[14] Hardt J, Rutter M. Validity of adult retrospective reports of adverse childhood experiences: Review of the evidence. J Child Psychol Psych 2004; 45(2): 260-73.
[15] Maunder B. Attitude to head lice--a more powerful force than insecticides. J R Soc Health 1985; 105(2): 61-4.
[16] Counahan M. A conditioned response to head lice. Melbourne Vic: Department of Human Services; 2002; May 1-4.
[17] Parison J, Speare, R, Canyon, DV. Uncovering family experiences with head lice: The difficulties of eradication. Open Dermatol J 2008; 2: 9-17.

Single-Pedicled Myocutaneous Flap of the Nose: A Case Study with Scar Quality Assessment

Christine Schopper[§], Eva Maria Valesky[§], Roland Kaufmann and Markus Meissner[*]

Department of Dermatology, Venereology und Allergology, Johann Wolfgang Goethe-University, Frankfurt am Main, Germany

Abstract: The plastic reconstruction of the nose after microscopically controlled tumor surgery poses a particular challenge. The single pedicled nasalis myocutaneous flap is suited for the repair of defects of the distal nose. The flap is characterized by great tissue mobility and ensured vascular supply. Below a case study is presented that involves 4 patients who were treated with this special flap in our hospital after excision of a basal cell carcinoma. The scar quality was measured after one year with the scar assessment tool POSAS (The Patient and Observer Scar Assessment Scale). The single pedicled nasalis myocutaneous flap healed without any complication in all 4 patients. The nose shape could be preserved by the almost tension-free shift of the flap on the myocutaneous pedicle. The evaluation with the POSAS showed good results for all individual parameters and in the overall assessment. The single pedicled nasalis myocutaneous flap offers a good alternative to repair defects on the distal nasal bridge, nasal ala and the nasal tip. The pedicle provides a maximum on mobility combined with a good perfusion of the flap. As the flap is built out of nose tissue the color and texture can be kept which leads to an excellent cosmetic result. The good results are also reflected by the evaluation of the POSAS data.

Keywords: Myocutaneous, pedicled flap, POSAS, scar, skin flap.

INTRODUCTION

The closure of nasal defects is a particular challenge due to the special anatomical conditions of the nose, which limits the ability to shift tissue. Cosmetic considerations also play a decisive role in this process, due to the central position and visibility of the nose. In principle, such defects can be closed by full-thickness skin grafts or local skin flaps. Full-thickness skin grafts may be distinguishable from surrounding tissue, due to primarily differences in surface structure and color, and they also tend to shrink. Skin flaps thus produce superior cosmetic results and are preferred to free transplants.

Frequently used local flap techniques that are particularly suitable for the coverage of defects on the ala and lateral tip of the nose include the nasolabial transposition or bilobed flap. As an alternative, subcutaneous island pedicle flaps are suitable for the closure of defects at the distal bridge, ala nasi, or tip of the nose, but they are characterized by limited mobilization capability in most cases. The single-pedicled myocutaneous flap is a nasal flap variant with good mobilization ability that provides a safe blood supply through the arteria angularis nasi. Rybka [1] first described the use of a myocutaneous island pedicle flap to cover nasal defects in 1983, and several authors have subsequently described the application of a modified form of this flap [1-4]. In this article, we describe the use of the single-pedicled nasalis myocutaneous flap in a case series of four patients. We also report the first evaluation of flap and scar quality using the Patient and Observer Scar Assessment Scale (POSAS) [5-7].

METHODS

Patients

Between August 2011 and August 2012, four patients (two women, two men; age, 77–91 years) with sclerodermiforme basal cell carcinoma at the distal bridge of the nose were treated with this flap in our ward. Tumor excision was controlled by micrographic surgery in all cases. Defect size ranged from 1.3 cm to 1.8 cm.

Technique

To create the single-pedicled nasalis myocutaneous flap, the triangular flap is first defined above the defect (Fig. **1a**). An incision is made to the depth of adipose tissue to define the lateral side of the triangle, which is then mobilized laterally and subcutaneously above the musculus transversalis to the sulcus nasofaciale (Fig. **1b**). On this side, the muscle remains intact and serves as a subcutaneous flap pedicle. At the medial flap margin, an incision is then made to the depth of the nasal cartilage or bone, through the musculus transversalis nasi. The flap is then released from the nasal cartilage below the musculature (Fig.**1c**). This bilayer (above and below the muscle) subcutaneous mobilization, which Papadopoulos *et al.* referred to as

*Address correspondence to this author at the Department of Dermatology, Venereology und Allergology, Johann Wolfgang Goethe-University, Theodor-Stern-Kai 7, D-60590 Frankfurt/Main, Germany;
E-mail: markus.meissner@kgu.de

[§]Both authors contributed equally.

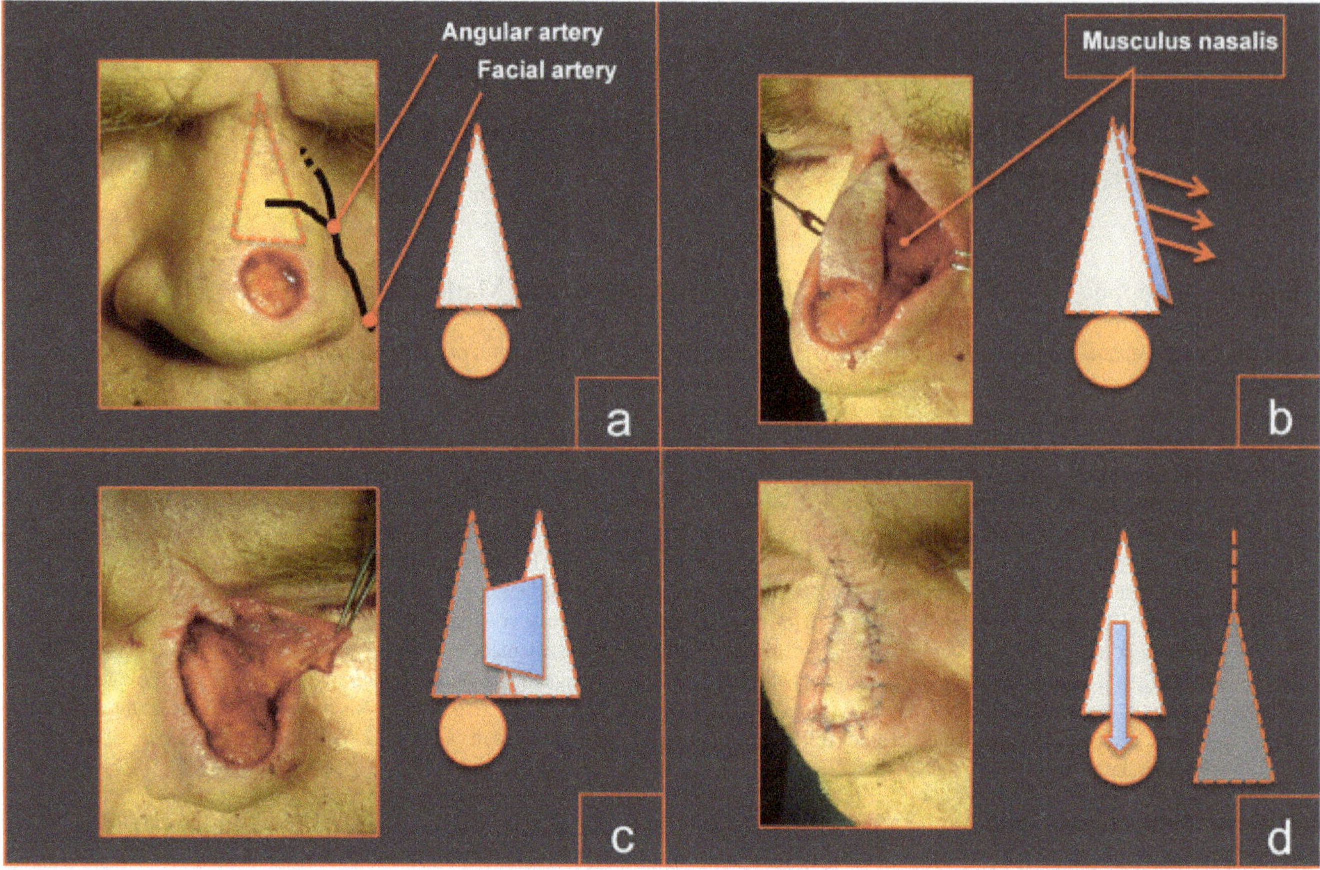

Fig. (1). (**a**) Triangular incision above the defect; (**b**) Mobilization lateral and subcutaneously above the musculus transversalis; (**c**) Release of the muscle from the nasal cartilage below the musculature; (**d**) Transfer to the defect without tension using its pedicle, and closure of the donor area in a V-Y shape.

"bilevel undermining" of the "nasalis myocutaneous island pedicle flap" generates great flap mobility [3].

The flap is then transferred to the defect without tension using its pedicle, and the donor area is closed in a V-Y shape (Fig. **1d**). Blood supply to the flap is guaranteed by the circulation of the musculus transversalis nasi through the arteria angularis nasi.

RESULTS

Flaps were vital after 24 h and subsequently healed with no complication and good cosmetic results in all patients. Fig. (**2**) shows the initial defects and postoperative results after 1 year.

After 1 year, scar quality was evaluated as part of regular follow-up care using the POSAS, which consists of two parts: the patient and observer scales. Each scale is used to evaluate six parameters (e.g., scar color) using a 10-point scale (1:best result; 10: worst result) and obtain a summarizing judgment (Tables **1** and **2**). The observer scale also allows the description of deviations, such as whether the scar is thinner or thicker than normal skin. Several survey studies have determined that the POSAS is a suitable means of evaluating scars [5-7]. Summary patient and observer scale scores (summarizers: C.S., E.V., M.M.) for the four patients in this case series are presented in Tables **1** and **2**, respectively. Scores for all patient scale parameters were very good (1–2), indicating that patients were satisfied with scar quality. In contrast, observer scale scores ranged from 2 to 5, indicating that surgeons classified scar quality as satisfactory to good. In particular, differences in relief and pigmentation were regarded as problematic.

DISCUSSION

The single-pedicled nasalis myocutaneous flap offers an alternative for the closure of defects of the lower bridge, ala nasi, and tip of the nose. The myocutaneous pedicle of the flap provides maximum mobility and a good blood supply *via* the arteria angularis nasi. Thus, lifting of the tip of the nose can be prevented. As the flap is generated from nose tissue, color and texture are preserved, producing a good cosmetic result. The disadvantages of this flap include its geometric shape, which results in a more conspicuous contour than that of a bilobed flap. This disadvantage is partially compensated by the excellent vascularization and great mobilization capability. The perfect vascularisation is assured by the arteria angularis nasi which originates not only from the facial arteria but also from the opthalmic arteria, infraorbital or transverse facial arteria [8]. In addition, the complex network between branches of the angular arteria and the dorsonasal artria might contribute to the good vascularisation of the musculus nasalis.

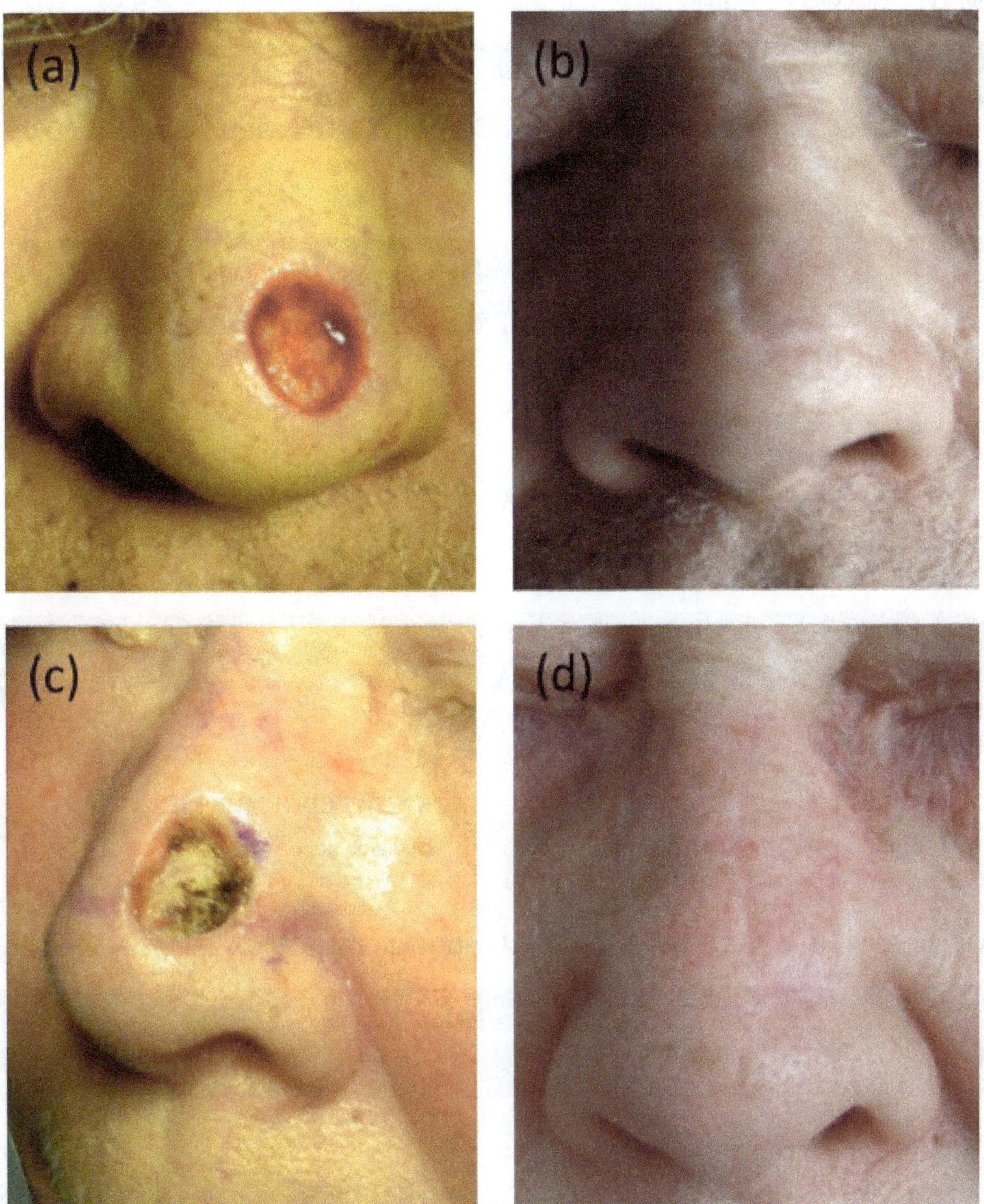

Fig. (2). Two examples of the single-pedicled nasalis myocutaneous flap. Primary defect (a, c) and postoperative results (b, d) after one year.

POSAS patient scale scores reflected great satisfaction in this small case series. The patient's evaluation indicated that scars were thinner than normal skin, with slight hypopigmentation compared with the surrounding skin. No hypertrophic scar or scar contraction was perceived. Overall patient scale scores ranged from 1 to 2, indicating that patients perceived the flap as almost completely resembling normal skin.

Observer scale scores were generally lower than patient scale scores, indicating that surgeons had more critical appraisals of the cosmetic results of the surgery. Evaluators noted essential differences in relief and pigmentation.

Of course, comparison of the results of several different skin closure techniques using the POSAS would enable more objective assessment of the flap technique described here. This instrument is suitable for the assessment of flap and scar quality because it takes patients' perceptions into account, unlike other scales. This small case series provides only limited evidence, but it reveals some divergence in patients' and surgeons' evaluations of postoperative scar conditions following the use of the single-pedicled nasalis myocutaneous flap. Hence, the POSAS is also suitable for detecting differences between observers' and patients' perceptions. In summary, the described flap is nevertheless a very good option for the closure of nasal defects with good cosmetic outcome and high patient satisfaction. In the future, larger prospective studies should be performed to investigate whether this myocutaneous flap is superior or not to other ways of skin closure.

Table 1. Results of the patient POSAS scale.

N=4	1=no, not at all									Yes, very much=10
	1	2	3	4	5	6	7	8	9	10
Has the scar been painful the last few weeks?	4									
Has the scar been itching the past few weeks?	4									
	1=no, as normal skin									Yes, very different=10
	1	2	3	4	5	6	7	8	9	10
Is the scar color different from the color of your normal skin at present?	4									
Is the stiffness of the scar differentfrom your normal skin at present?	3	1								
Is the thickness of the scar different from your normal skin at present?	4									
Is the scar more irregular than your normal skin at present?	2	2								
	1=as normal skin									Very different=10
	1	2	3	4	5	6	7	8	9	10
What is your overall opinion of the scar compared to normal skin?	2	2								

CONFLICT OF INTEREST

The authors confirm that this article content has no conflict of interest.

ACKNOWLEDGEMENTS

Declared none.

Table 2. Results of the observer POSAS scale as the mean value of the results of three different observers (dermatologic surgeons).

N=4	1=normal skin									Worst scar imaginable=10					
Parameter	1	2	3	4	5	6	7	8	9	10	Category				
Vascularity		2	1	1							pale	pink	red	purple	mix
											3				1
Pigmentation			2	2							hypo	hyper	mix		
											4				
Thickness		1	3								thicker	thinner			
												4			
Relief			2	1	1						more	less	mix		
												2	2		
Pliability		3		1							supple	stiff	mix		
												1			
Surface area		1	1	2							expansion		contraction		mix
													2		2
Overall opinion		1	1	2											

REFERENCES

[1] Rybka FJ. Reconstruction of the nasal tip using nasalis myocutaneous sliding flaps. Plast Reconstr Surg 1983; 71: 40-4.

[2] Constantine VS. Nasalis myocutaneous sliding flap: repair of nasal supratip defects. J Dermatol Surg Oncol 1991; 17(5): 439-44.

[3] Papadopoulos DJ, Trinei FA. Superiorly based nasalis myocutaneous island pedicle flap with bilevel undermining for nasal tip and supratip reconstruction. Dermatol Surg 1999; 25(7): 530-6.

[4] Wee SS, Hruza GJ, Mustoe TA. Refinements of nasalis myocutaneous flap. Ann Plast Surg 1990; 25(4): 271-8.

[5] Falder S, Browne A, Edgar D, *et al.* Core outcomes for adult burn survivors: a clinical overview. Burns 2009; 35(5): 618-41.

[6] Idriss N, Maibach H. Scar assessment scales: a dermatologic overview. Skin Res Technol 2009; 15(1): 1-5.

[7] Vercelli S, Ferriero G, Sartorio F, Stissi V, Franchignoni F. How to assess postsurgical scars: a review of outcome measures. Disabil Rehabil 2009; 31(25): 2055-63.

[8] Hou D, Fang L, Zhao Z, Zhou C, Yang M. Angular vessels as a new vascular pedicle of an island nasal chondromucosal flap: Anatomical study and clinical application. Exp Ther Med 2013; 5(3): 751-6.

Characterizing the Nature of Human Carriers of Head Lice

Deon V. Canyon*, Chauncey Canyon and Sami Milani

Office of Public Health Studies, University of Hawaii at Manoa, 1960 East-West Rd, Biomed Building #T103, Honolulu HI 96822, USA

Abstract: Pediculosis is a ubiquitous disease common throughout the globe and managed entirely through the application of insecticides and natural therapies with varying success. Resistance and reinfection are known to be responsible for increases in prevalence reported in many countries since the 1900s. This study investigated reinfection, which has been neglected by researchers, by attempting to learn more about the role of reservoir hosts. Open-ended questions were asked from 126 students of Grades 8 and 9 to explore this issue from the perspective of the infected population. A majority of females (60%) and 40% of males had no idea that they had pediculosis until it was discovered by themselves, a friend or a carer. Some female (12.1%) and male (14.5%) students did not tell their parents when they became aware that they had pediculosis. Hair thickness was significantly related to this question with 23.3% of thick-haired students concealing their infections. The results from this study suggest that brown- and short-haired White boys should be a primary target in lice awareness and control programs, because they are much more likely to harbor lice than long-haired girls. Health professionals should be aware of the social reasons for why this pest is so difficult to control.

Keywords: Carrier, head lice, pediculosis, reservoir, transmission.

INTRODUCTION

Pediculosis is a classic global health disease since it affects all people in all nations, crosses national boundaries and most countries have experienced increases in the detection of *Pediculus humanus* var. *capitis* (De Geer) since the 1900s [1]. Head lice are obligate human parasites that have coexisted with humans for at least 9000 years [2]. Physical, botanical and chemical methods have been used to control head lice since earliest recorded history with limited success.

While reducing transmission is fundamental to control the spread of any infection, pediculosis often eludes management efforts and the way forward is not clear when treatment fails. The persistence of head lice in modern society has often been attributed to lack of hygiene, a mobile population and insecticide resistance while the underlying social aspects of head lice transmission have received far less attention. Despite multiple treatments with effective pediculicides, lice may continually return to cause great alarm to parents that exceeds their medical significance [3,4]. Reinfection is a highly problematic and understudied social issue that merits further consideration and study [5,6]. Is it due to an unfortunate chance meeting of an uninfected child with an infected child or are there patterns of social behavior that enable head lice populations to persist in a population? Do these behaviors have something to do with the newfound role of feelings and emotions related to head lice infection [7-9]? These questions have remained unexplored by researchers, so this study sought to shed light on the nature of human head lice carriers.

*Address correspondence to this author at the Office of Public Health Studies, University of Hawaii at Manoa, 1960 East-West Rd, Biomed Building #T103, Honolulu HI 96822, USA; Tel: (808) 956-6263; E-mail: dcanyon@hawaii.edu

METHODS

The site for this study was a multicultural, middle-class, public school in Perth, Western Australia, which was one of the top performing schools in the state. The student body totaled around 1700 students in Grades 8 to 12 with 480 middle-school students in Grades 8 and 9. Participants for this study were sought from the middle school and information on the study was provided to parents who completed the consent form. Teenagers with parental consent were asked to complete an anonymous survey, which they deposited in a box in the school front office. This retrospective study requested information on pediculosis incidence based on student recall. In Australia, primary schools, in which head lice infections predominantly occur, run from Grades 1 to 7. Completed consent forms and surveys were collected from the school for analysis. Participation was thus voluntary and self-selecting. Only students who could recall being infected with head lice were included in the study. This sampling strategy combines criterion based and convenience approaches, since the targeted participants are those who have direct experience coping with a head lice infestation (criterion) and they are accessible (convenience) [10].

The questionnaire requested basic non-identifying demographic information (grade, gender and hair details) followed by three open-ended questions:

1. Have you ever been surprised to find out that you had head lice when you did not know that you had them?
2. Have you ever known you had head lice and didn't tell your parents?
3. If you had lice and you did not tell your parents, why didn't you tell them?

The anonymous responses were analyzed using the computer software package SPSS 21. Cross-tabulations with Chi-Square tests were employed, but since frequencies were occasionally less than five per cell, this test was replaced with the Uncertainty Coefficient analysis. Ethics approval H2954 was obtained from James Cook University.

RESULTS

Out of 480 students contacted, 133 confirmed a history of head lice infection, volunteered to participate and submitted study surveys with a response rate 27.7%. Six surveys were discarded due to being too incomplete for analysis, leaving 127 participant surveys for the study (Table **1**). The temporal proximity of participants to the infection event and the nature of the event being recalled indicate that recall would have been reasonably accurate. While adult retrospective reports of adverse childhood experiences involve a substantial rate of false negatives, false positive reports are rare [11].

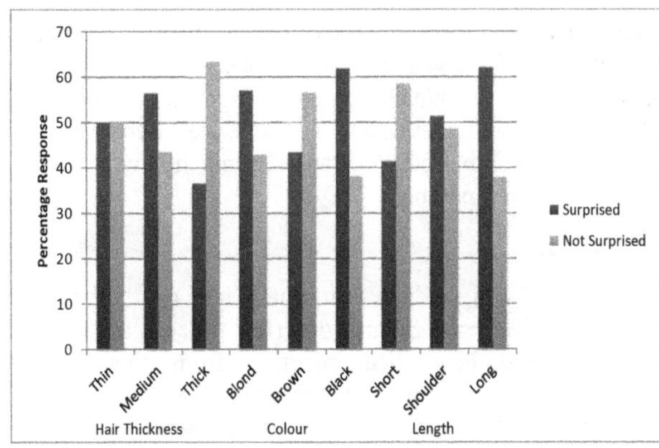

Fig. (2). The relationship between hair thickness, colour and length in participants who were unsurprised and surprised to find out they were infected with head lice.

Six female and ten male students concealed their infection from their parents and there was no significant gender effect. All those who concealed their infection were Caucasian. Uncertainty coefficient analysis showed that the relationship between the responses to the question and ethnicity was significant ($p<0.05$), although the relationship was weak ($u=0.052$). This was reflected in the hair color result which showed that all black-haired students told their parents and 17.9% of brown-haired students did not tell their parents (Chi square 6.264, $p<0.05$). Only one blond haired student concealed an infection. Uncertainty coefficient analysis also showed a trend in the relationship between the responses to the question and hair thickness (Chi square 5.475, $p=0.066$), with thick-haired students being twice as likely as medium-haired students to conceal an infection from their parents (Fig. **3**).

Table 1. Demographic data for the sample.

Grade	Females (%)	Males (%)	Missing	Caucasians (%)	Asians (%)	Missing (%)
8	28 (41.2)	38 (55.9)	2 (2.9)	59 (86.8)	8 (11.9)	1 (1.5)
9	30 (50.8)	29 (49.2)	0 (0)	49 (83.1)	9 (15.3)	1 (1.7)

In response to the question, "Have you ever been surprised to find out that you had head lice when you did not know that you had them?" males were less likely than females to be surprised that they had a head lice infection. Pearson's Chi-Square analysis showed that the relationship between the responses to the question and gender was significant (4.310, $p<0.05$), but that ethnicity was not. Nevertheless, there were distinct ethnic differences observable in Fig. (**1**).

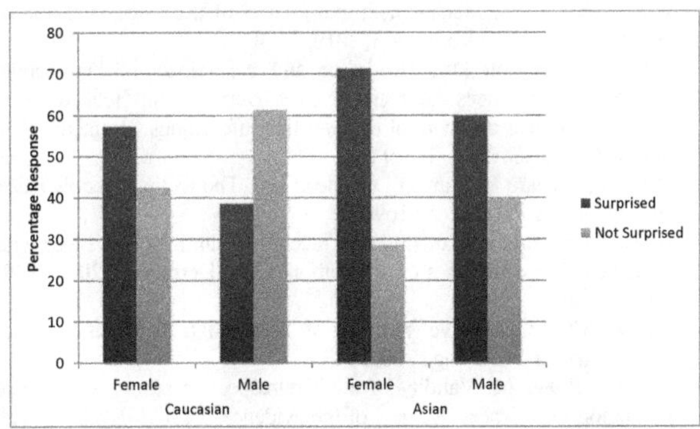

Fig. (1). The percentage of Caucasian and Asian females and males that were surprised or not surprised to find out they were infected with head lice.

Hair thickness, color and length were not significantly associated with surprise in this analysis ($p>0.05$). However, Fig. (**2**) shows that respondents with short brown thick hair were more often not surprised to find that they had pediculosis. The most surprised were those with medium thickness blond or black long hair.

Participants were then asked if they had ever known they had head lice and had concealed the infection from their parents.

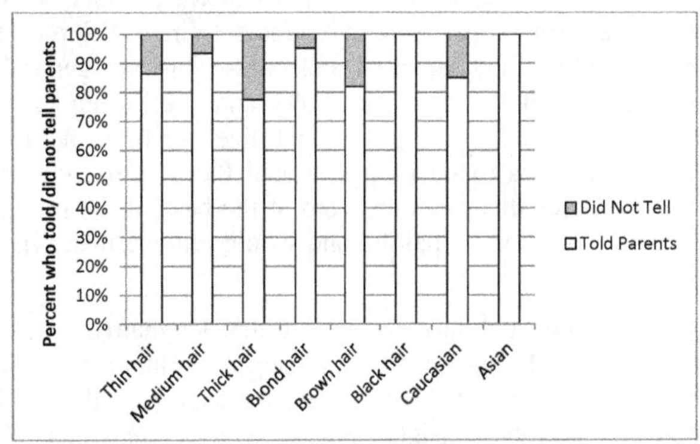

Fig. (3). Percentage of students who concealed a head lice infection from their parents compared with hair thickness and color.

When asked the third question, "If you had lice and you did not tell your parents, why didn't you tell them?" twelve males and nine females stated reasons. Five answered that they did not want their parents to get annoyed, angry or have problems; three were embarrassed or ashamed; five did not want to be treated; and eight did not know the reason. None of the study factors were significantly related to this question. Uncertainty coefficient analysis revealed a moderate trend (p=0.77, u=0.111) for thick-haired students who did not want to have problems with their parents.

DISCUSSION

The aim of this study was to shed light on the nature of human head lice carriers and describe the extent to which children conceal head lice infection from their parents. Concealment is an important prevalence and transmission variable because it results in individuals becoming carriers, which invariably increases the availability of head lice in a community. Concealment is thought to derive mainly from social and emotional feelings that influence the behavior of infected individuals and their carers [7-9]. The results from this study provided evidence to suggest that brown-haired, shorthaired boys should be a primary target in lice awareness and control programs, but that other people should not be overlooked.

Results from the question, "Have you ever been surprised to find out that you had head lice when you did not know that you had them?" indicated that females were more likely to be surprised than males upon discovering that they have pediculosis. The important point here is that 60% of females and 40% of males had no idea that they had pediculosis until it was discovered. This means that they may act as head lice carriers and transmitters for a considerable amount of time until the infection becomes noticed by themselves or someone else. Hair length is a likely explanation because head lice infections are harder to detect on people with longer hair.

In response to the very direct question, "Have you ever known you had head lice and didn't tell your parents?" 10.7% of female and 14.7% of male students admitted to not telling their parents when they became aware that they had pediculosis. Hair thickness was significantly related to this question with 22.0% of thick-haired students concealing their infections. It may be that combing with a fine-toothed comb would be more painful for thick-haired people, which gives them a practical reason for concealing infection. The diameter of hairs on the human head varies between individuals from 0.017 mm to 0.181 mm [12]. Fine, medium and coarse hair are generally classified as <0.05, 0.06 to 0.09, and >0.1 mm wide, respectively. The most popular head lice comb is the Lice Meister which has metal prongs spaced 0.094 mm wide and splaying reduces this to almost zero at the base of the prongs. The comb would prove painful and would remove many hairs upon use.

The common public perception is that longhaired females who do a lot of head-to-head socializing are primary head lice carriers and transmitters. By questioning teenagers, this study gained considerable insight which demonstrated that this perception is incorrect. Of those teenagers who were aware of their head lice infections, 64.5% were males and 35.5% were females; of those who did not inform their parents when they knew that they had lice, 53.7% were males and 46.3% were females; of those who did not tell their parents because they did not want to be treated, 80% were males and 20% were females; and of those who could not explain why they did not tell their parents or thought the infection was not important, 57.1% were males and 42.9% were females. Maunder (1985) had a healthy suspicion when he stated that attitude to head lice is a more powerful force than insecticides [13]. If there is to be any generalized perception of who carries head lice in a western multicultural setting, it is that boys with short brown hair should be suspected well before longhaired girls.

CONFLICT OF INTEREST

The authors confirm that this article content has no conflict of interest.

ACKNOWLEDGEMENTS

Declared none.

REFERENCES

[1] Gratz NG. Human lice: their prevalence, control and resistance to insecticides: a review 1985-1997. Geneva: World Health Organization, Division of Control of Tropical Diseases, WHO Pesticide Evaluation Scheme, 1997.

[2] Mumcuoglu KY, Zias J. Head lice, *Pediculus humanus capitis* (Anoplura: Pediculidae), from hair combs excavated in Israel and dated from the first century B.C. to the eighth century A.D. J Med Entomol 1988; 25: 545–7.

[3] Counahan M. Scratching for answers? Public health aspects of head lice control. PhD thesis, Townsville, Qld: James Cook University 2006.

[4] Falagas M, Matthaiou DK, Petros IP, Panos G, Pappas G. Worldwide prevalence of head lice. Emerg Infect Dis 2008; 14: 1493-4.

[5] Canyon DV, Speare R. Clinical decision support: Dermatology: Pediculosis. Wilmington, DE: Decision Support in Medicine LLC, 2012.

[6] Canyon DV, Speare R. Head lice transmission and risk factors. In: Heukelbach J, Ed. Management and control of head lice infestations. Bremen: UNI-MED Verlag AG, 2010; 34-40.

[7] Parison J, Canyon DV. Head lice and the impact of knowledge, attitudes and practices - a social science overview. In: Heukelbach J, Ed. Management and control of head lice infestations. Bremen: UNI-MED Verlag AG, 2010; 103-9.

[8] Parison J, Speare R, Canyon DV. Head lice: The feelings people have. Int J Dermatol 2013; 52(2): 169-71.

[9] Parison J, Speare, R, Canyon DV. Uncovering family experiences with head lice: The difficulties of eradication. Open Dermatol J 2008; 2: 9-17.

[10] Patton MQ. Qualitative research & evaluation methods, 3rd ed. Thousand Oaks, CA: Sage 2002.

[11] Hardt J, Rutter M. Validity of adult retrospective reports of adverse childhood experiences: Review of the evidence. J Child Psychol Psych 2004; 45(2): 260-73.

[12] Ley B. Diameter of a human hair; 1999; http://hypertextbook.com/facts/1999/BrianLey.shtml [Accessed: Apr 2014].

[13] Maunder B. Attitude to head lice--a more powerful force than insecticides. J R Soc Health 1985; 105(2): 61-4.

Chronic Cutaneous Hyalohyphomycosis by Paecilomyces

N. Boufflette[1], J.E. Arrese[2], P. Leonard[3] and A.F. Nikkels[*,1]

Departments of [1]Dermatology, [2]Dermatopathology and [3]Infections Diseases, University Hospital of Liège, Liège, Belgium

Abstract: *Paecilomyces lilacinus* is a ubiquitous saprophytic fungus that rarely causes infections in humans, frequently affecting the eyes and the skin. Cutaneous and subcutaneous infections mainly occur in immunocompromised hosts but have occasionally been reported in immunocompetent patients. The clinical spectrum is highly heterogeneous and diagnosis is often delayed.

A 60-year-old woman with idiopathic chronic necrotizing vasculitis treated since 10 years with a series of immunosuppressive therapies presented since three years various clinical presentations of chronic hyalohyphomycosis caused by *P. lilacinus*. Diagnosis was only obtained three years after the first clinical signs, following the histologic analysis of the surgical excision of a cutaneous abscess. Treatment with oral voriconazole was successful.

This case report illustrates the highly heterogeneous clinical aspects of hyalohyphomycosis by *P. lilacinus* leading to a delay in diagnosis and treatment, particularly in the immunosuppressed patient.

Keywords: Hyalohyphomycosis, immunosuppression, *paecilomyces lilacinus*, voriconazole, skin infection.

INTRODUCTION

Hyalohyphomycosis is a rare infection caused by fungi that produce hyaline septate hyphae in tissues [1]. Etiological agents include, among others, species of *Acremonium*, *Fusarium*, *Scopulariopsis*, *Paecilomyces* and *Beauveria*. The genus *Paecilomyces* was identified for the first time in 1907 [2]. *P. lilacinus* has only been assigned since 1974 to the genus *Paecilomyces* [3]. The lilac-colored colony and the production of a deep purplish-red pigment on Czapek solution agar are characteristic. *P. lilacinus* and *P. variotii* are the two major species, which are most frequently associated with infections in human. Most of these occur in immunocompromised hosts, while the incidence in immunocompetent hosts is also increasing [4]. *Paecilomyces* species are rare but emerging causes of hyalohyphomycosis. These fungi are regularly isolated from soil and air, decaying plants and food products [1]. Their potential resistance to sterilization techniques increases their clinical significance. *Paecilomyces* infections usually concern oculomycosis as well as cutaneous and subcutaneous infections [1], and occasionally sinusitis, fungaemia, onychomycosis, lung abscess, pleural effusion, osteomyelitis, peritonitis and endocarditis.

Cutaneous and subcutaneous infections have been reported to be highly heterogeneous and may be notoriously difficult to diagnose. Herein, the polymorphous clinical and histologic features of chronic cutaneous hyalohyphomycosis related to *P. lilacinus* are illustrated in a patient with longstanding immunosuppressive therapies for idiopathic necrotizing vasculitis.

*Address correspondence to this author at the Department of Dermatology, University Hospital of Liège, Liège, Belgium;
E-mail: af.nikkels@chu.ulg.ac.be

CASE REPORT

A 60-year-old woman presented a tender and asymptomatic swelling, 5 cm in diameter, at the posterior aspect of her left arm (Fig. **1**). According to the patient, she had this swelling for over 12 months. The lesion appeared progressively and increased in size over time. The lesion was mistaken clinically as a lipoma and echographically as a hematic collection and no treatment was initiated. The patient also noticed the development of three subcutaneous nodular and pustular lesions in the immediate vicinity of the swelling during the last few weeks (Fig. **2**). Furthermore, she complained of an erythematous-violaceous irregularly shaped infiltrated large plaque of the entire anterolateral aspect of her left thigh (Fig. **3**). This lesion was also present since more than three years and several punch and excisional biopsies were performed without however evidencing the presence of fungal agents despite periodic acid-Schiff (PAS) and Gomori-Grocott histochemical stainings. She denied any trauma related to these areas and had no systemic complaints. She was a febrile and without palpable regional lymph nodes.

The patient had been followed for over 10 years in the rheumatology department for anecrotizing vasculitis. Extensive and repetitive workups remained negative (antinuclear antibodies, p and cANCA's cryoglobulines, anti-phospholipids, etc) and the vasculitis was classified as idiopathic. Over time, she received several lines of immunosuppressive therapies: cyclophosphamide, rituximab IV (anti-CD20 monoclonal antibodies), azathioprine and systemic corticosteroids. The cutaneous lesions of her idiopathic necrotizing vasculitis occurred most of the times on her legs. Every time noticing a new lesion in the lower extremities, the rheumatologist suspected a recurrence of vasculitis and treated the patient with systemic corticosteroids. Current medication included methylprednisolone 12 mg daily, azathioprine 50mg tid, esomeprazol 40 mg daily, calcium carbonate 1250mg daily and vitamin D 100.000UI weekly. On physical examination, blood pressure was 140/90mmHg, respiratory rate was 18 breaths/min and pulse rate 100/min with a regular rhythm. All laboratory work including a complete blood count, chemistry and liver panel was in normal range.

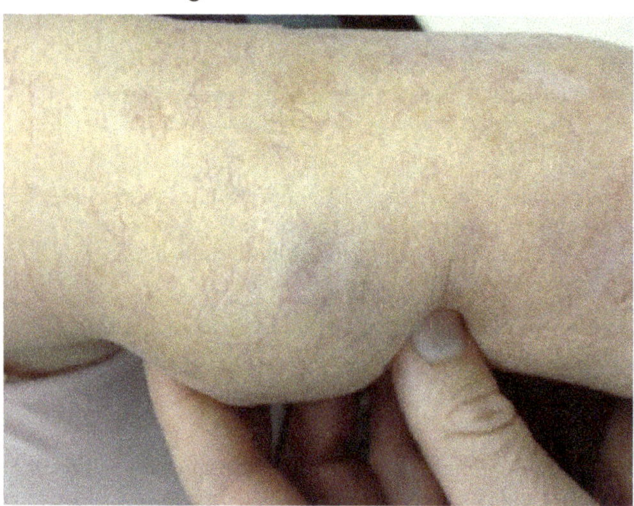

Fig. (1). Cutaneous *Paecilomyces lilacinus* infection onthe left arm characterized bya large and tender swelling.

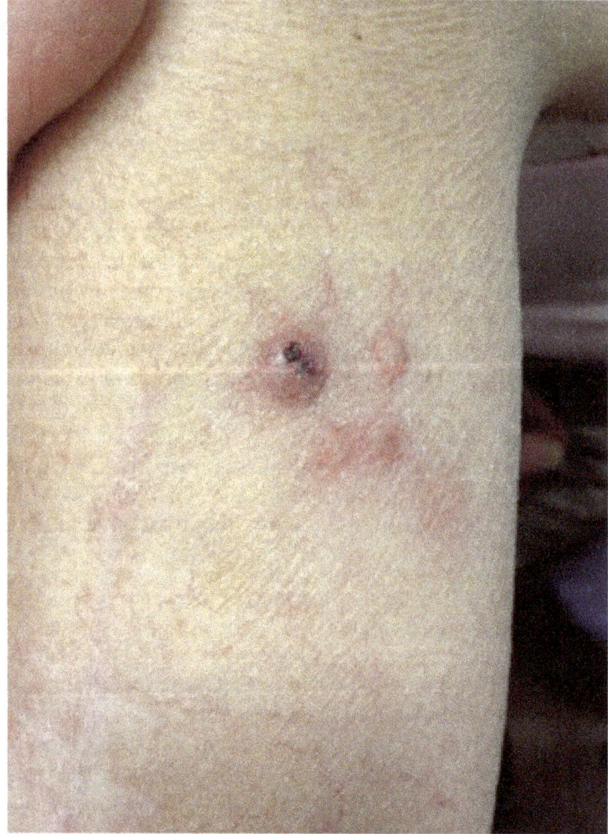

Fig. (2). Cutaneous nodular lesions by *Paecilomyces lilacinus* on the left arm.

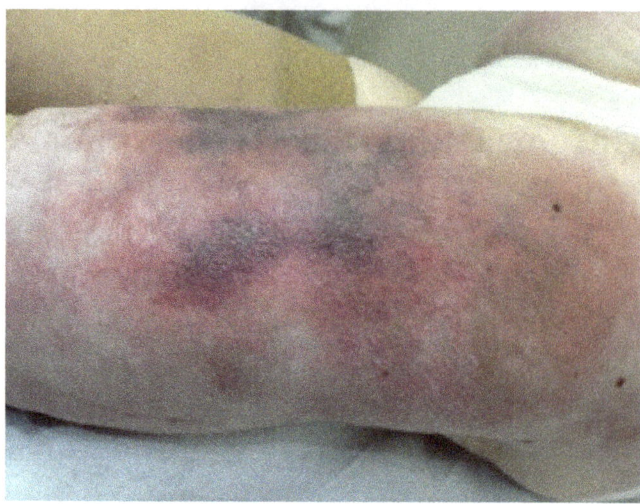

Fig. (3). Chronic cutaneous *Paecilomyces lilacinus* infection on left thigh characterized byan erythematous-violaceous, partially necrotic and infiltrated plaque.

Due to the longstanding administration of azathioprine and her fair phototype, the patient had already presented several squamous cell carcinomas (SCC). She presented with a clinical suspicion of three new SCC's on her left upper arm. Surgical excision was decided and simultaneously she requested the excision of the large swelling on the anterior aspect of her left upper arm. On excision, a large amount of pustular secretions was evidenced requiring the insertion of a drain. Histology of the biopsy specimens revealed a heavily necrotic and granulomatous reaction with giant cells and few inflammatory cells in the dermis on haematoxylin/eosin staining (Fig. **4**). PAS (Fig. **5**) and Gomori-Grocott methenamine-silver (Fig. **6**) histochemical stainings noted the presence of hyaline hyphae within the dermal necrotic tissue with numerous septate hyphae associated with the presence of spores. Giemsa staining was negative. The final histologic result was a hyalohyphomycosis. Bacterial cultures of the fluid were negative. Fungal culture, however, grew a mold, which was subsequently identified as *P. lilacinus* after a subculture on an enriched medium. Fungal cultures of blood presented no growth. Although no

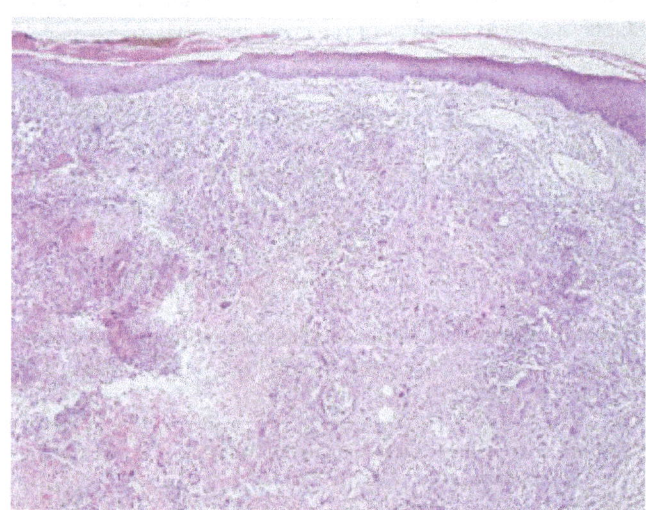

Fig. (4). Granulomatous and necrotic infiltration of the entire reticular dermis (H/E, x 4).

breakpoints have been established for molds, antifungal susceptibility showed an elevated minimum inhibitory concentration (MIC) for amphotericin B (MIC >32µg/ml) and itraconazole (MIC >32µg/ml). However, a low MIC for voriconazole (MIC =0,094µg/ml) was noted. Therefore, a treatment with oral voriconazole was initiated. The loading dose was 300mg bid on the first day, followed by 200mg bid, prescribed for a period of 3 months. During the first 4 weeks of treatment, clinical resolution progressed nicely in the left thigh and the scar of the surgery performed in the left arm was healthy. The patient suffered no major side effects related to the treatment except for a slight elevation of liver enzymes. Unfortunately, the patient died during the fifth week of treatment from a bacterial pneumonia.

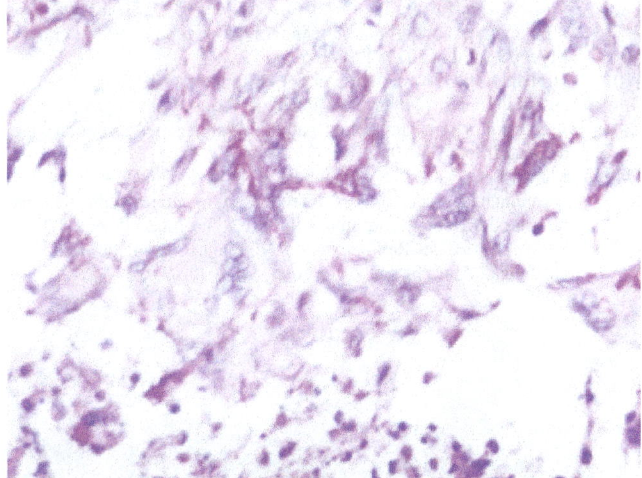

Fig. (5). Demonstration of septate hyphae in red (PAS, x40).

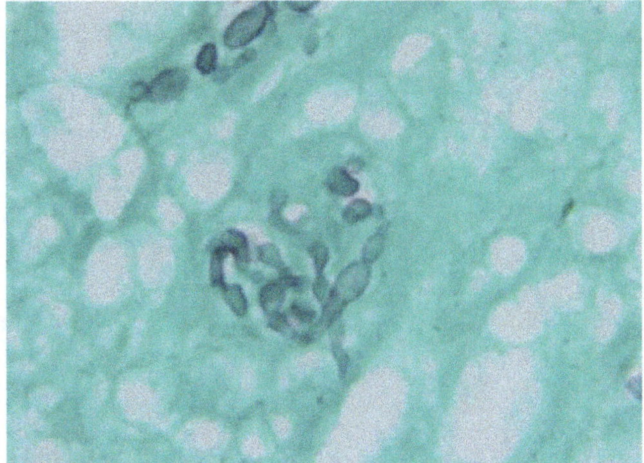

Fig. (6). Grocott-Gomori methenamine-silver staining of a biopsy specimen showing regular filamentous fungi and spores.

DISCUSSION

In most of the infections caused by these environmental fungi, some predisposing factors were found. As to cutaneous and subcutaneous *P. lilacinus* infections, risk factors were mainly solid organ and bone marrow transplantation, malignancies, corticosteroid therapy, primary immunodeficiency, diabetes mellitus and AIDS [1]. Our patient presented a chronic and severe iatrogenic immunosuppression following several immunosuppressive regimens used for over 10 years to treat her necrotizing vasculitis. The portal of entry attributed to this fungus usually involves a breakdown of the skin barrier, in dwelling catheters or inhalation. There was no evidence of hematogenous spread in our patient and fungal blood cultures were negative. We hypothesized that our patient was contaminated by direct inoculation through an unnoticed, minor skin abrasion, facilitated by a highly atrophic skin induced by chronic systemic corticosteroids [5].

Cutaneous and subcutaneous infections present numerous clinical manifestations such as solitary or disseminated skin eruptions with erythematous macules, papules, vesicles, or nodules with a necrotic center [1]. Our patient presented several clinical presentations such as nodular lesions and a swelling of the arm, as well as a large, irregular, infiltrated and indurated plaque on the thigh. As illustrated in our case, these highly polymorphous clinical images frequently lead to a delay in diagnosis subsequently interfering with adequate treatment.

Fungal culture and histology of the lesions are required to diagnose a *P. lilacinus* infection. Even if histological examination can identify fungal structures, the fungal culture remains the gold standard for fungal identification. *Paecilomyces* molds grow fast on Sabouraud dextrose agar and the pathogen can be identified within one to two weeks [6].

Because of their different antifungal susceptibilities, the differentiation between *Paecilomyces* species is mandatory to treat the disease correctly. *P. lilacinus* has a high resistnce to conventional antifungal drugs unlike *P. variotii*, which has a greater susceptibility to these agents [7]. Given *P. lilacinus'* broad resistance, it is always useful to realize a susceptibility test in order to define the most appropriate treatment. *In vitro* studies of *P. lilacinus* antifungal susceptibility have shown poor activity of older antifungal drugs (amphotericin B, flucytosine and fluconazole) and contradiction exists concerning data regarding the activity of the first-generation azoles, such as ketoconazole, miconazole, clotrimazole and itraconazole [7]. The second-generation triazoles, such as voriconazole, posaconazole and ravuconazole present a good antifungal effect [8]. More specifically, the last two drugs show very low MICs although no data have been published concerning their clinical use. Currently, there is no standard treatment regimen for *P. lilacinus* infections. Although the clinical experience with voriconazole is limited, it is recommended as first-line therapy [9]. Up to date, only seven published cases of skin infection treated with voriconazole, which were all successful. Although we were unable to follow the entire evolution of the lesions, a spectacular regression was observed during the first 4 weeks with voriconazole treatment.

Treatment duration with voriconazole remains undetermined, ranging from 3 weeks to 10 months [10,11]. The treatment duration should rely on the clinical resolution of the infection and/or the presence of adverse effects linked to the medication. The most common adverse effects of voriconazole included visual disturbances, increased levels of hepatic enzymes and skin rash through photosensitization [12]. Surgical excision should also be considered on a case-by-case basis.

In conclusion, this case illustrates the highly polymorphous spectrum of *P. lilacinus* skin infection. Performing susceptibility tests is mandatory as resistance is not uncommon. Surgery should not be overlooked as treatment option.

AUTHORS' CONTRIBUTIONS

All authors provided substantial contributions to the conception and design, acquisition of data, or analysis and interpretation of data, to the drafting of the article or revising it critically for important intellectual content. All authors provided final approval of the version to be published.

CONFLICT OF INTEREST

The authors confirm that this article content has no conflict of interest.

ACKNOWLEDGEMENTS

Declared none.

REFERENCES

[1] Pastor FJ, Guarro J. Clinical manifestations, treatment and outcome of *Paecilomyces lilacinus* infections. Clin Microbiol Infect. 2006; 12: 948-60.

[2] Bainer G. Mycothèque de l'école de pharmacie XI. *Paecilomyces*, genre nouveau de mucédinées. Bull Soc Mycol Fr 1907; 23: 26-7.

[3] Samson RA. *Paecilomyces* and some allied hyphomycetes. Stud Mycol 1974; 6: 58-62.

[4] Carey J, D'Amico R, Sutton DA, Rinaldi MG: *Paecilomyces lilacinus* vaginitis in an immunocompetent patient. Emerg Infect Dis 2003; 9: 1155-8.

[5] Itin PH, Frei R, Lautenschlager S, *et al.* Cutaneous manifestations of *Paecilomyces lilacinus*infection induced by a contaminated skin lotion in patients who are severely immunosuppressed. J Am AcadDermatol1998; 39: 401-9.

[6] Hall VC, Goyal S, Davis MD, Walsh JS. Cutaneous hyalohyphomycosis caused by *Paecilomyces lilacinus*: report of three cases and review of the literature. Int J Dermatol 2004; 43: 648-53.

[7] Aguilar C, Pujol I, Sala J, Guarro J. Antifungal susceptibilities of *Paecilomyces* species. Antimicrob Agents Chemother 1998; 42: 1601-4.

[8] Castelli MV, Alastruey-Izquierdo A, Cuesta I, *et al.* Susceptibility testing and molecular classification of *Paecilomyces* spp. Antimicrob Agents Chemother 2008; 52: 2926-8.

[9] Rimawi RH, Carter Y, Ware T, Christie J, Siraj D. Use of voriconazole for the treatment of *Paecilomyces lilacinus*cutaneous infections: case presentation and review of published literature. Mycopathologia 2013; 175: 345-9.

[10] Hilmarsdottir I, Thorsteinsson SB, Asmundsson P, Bodvarsson M, Arnadottir M: Cutaneous infection caused by *Paecilomyces lilacinus*in a renal transplant patient: treatment with voriconazole. Scand J Infect Dis 2000; 32: 331-2.

[11] Martin CA, Roberts S, Greenberg RN. Voriconazole treatment of disseminated *Paecilomyces* infection in a patient with acquired immunodeficiency syndrome. Clin Infect Dis 2002; 35: e78-81.

[12] Sabo JA, Abdel-Rahman SM: Voriconazole: a new triazole antifungal. Ann Pharmacother 2000; 34: 1032-43.

18

CEA (Carcinoembryonic Antigen) and CEACAM6 (CEA-Related Cell Adhesion Molecule 6) are Expressed in Psoriasis Vulgaris

Akihiko Fujisawa[1], Kiyofumi Egawa[2,3], Yumi Honda[4], Masahide Kuroki[5], Masatoshi Jinnin[1] and Hironobu Ihn[*,1]

[1]*Department of Dermatology and Plastic Surgery, Faculty of Life Sciences, Kumamoto University, Japan*

[2]*Department of Dermatology, The Jikei University School of Medicine, Tokyo, Japan*

[3]*Department of Microbiology, Kitasato University School of Allied Health Science, Sagamihara, Japan*

[4]*Department of Surgical Pathology, Kumamoto University Hospital, Kumamoto, Japan*

[5]*Department of Biochemistry, Faculty of Medicine, Fukuoka University, Fukuoka, Japan*

Abstract: Carcinoembryonic antigen-related cell adhesion molecules (CEACAMs) belong to a group of mammalian immunoglobulin-related glycoproteins. The CEACAM family of proteins has been implicated in intracellular-signaling-mediated effects that govern the growth and differentiation of normal and cancer cells.

In this study, the expression of CEACAMs was studied immunohistochemically in the skin of patients with psoriasis, using a panel of polyclonal (PoAb) and monoclonal (F34-187, F33-104, and F106-88) antibodies that recognize different epitopes of CEA and related molecules (CEACAMs), in comparison with the expression of cell differentiation and proliferation markers, such as involucrin, PCNA, Ki-67 and CK16. The expression of these molecules in adjacent parts without eruptions was also investigated for comparison.

The three CEACAMs, CEACAM1, CEA and CEACAM6, were expressed, limited to the upper part of the proliferated epidermal cells which expressed involucrin in the psoriatic lesions. Only the upper epidermal cell layers of the psoriatic lesions expressed these markers more highly than the adjacent normal skin. These results suggested that the expression of CEACAMs is related to epidermal cell de-differentiation in the diseased skin of psoriasis vulgaris.

Keywords: Psoriasis, CEA, CEACAM5, CEACAM6, CD66.

INTRODUCTION

The carcinoembryonic antigen (CEA) family consists of two subfamilies, the CEACAM subgroup and the pregnancy specific glycoprotein (PSG) subgroup [1, 2]. Recent studies have shown that CEACAMs are members of the immunoglobulin superfamily, and that they are composed of an N-terminal domain (N) and six very homologous immunoglobulin constant region-like domains (A1, B1, A2, B2, A3 and B3) [3, 4]. The CEACAMs in the human being consist of 18 genes and 11 pseudogenes on chromosome 19q13.2.

CEACAMs are now recognized as being important not only as tumor markers but also as cell adhesion molecules [5,6]. Furthermore CEACAMs are considered to be capable of transmitting the signals that result in a variety of effects depending on the tissue, including tumor suppression, tumor promotion, angiogenesis, neutrophil activation, lymphocyte activation and the cell cycle regulation [1].

CEACAMs expression has been reported not only in normal and malignant mucosa of the gastrointestinal tract, but also in some inflammatory diseases [3] and epithelial neoplasms [7] of the skin, gall bladder and extrahepatic biliary tract [8]. CEACAMs are also expressed in follicular keratinocytes [3,9] and sweat gland apparatus [10,11] in normal skin.

Concerning the psoriatic skin, CEACAM1 has been reported to be expressed in outer epidermal cell layers of the psoriatic skin [12]. Over expression of CEA was also demonstrated immunohistochemically [3, 13]. However, it remains unclear whether other CEACAMs are expressed in psoriatic skin.

In the present study, we aimed to evaluate the expression of CEACAMs by immunoblotting as well as immunohistochemical staining analysis. In the present study, we also developed an antigen retrieval method suitable for in situ CEACAMs expression in formalin-fixed materials.

MATERIAL AND METHODS

Materials

Totally 37 tissue samples of psoriasis vulgaris (28 formalin-fixed and 9 frozen specimens) were obtained from 28 patients who received biopsy in the Department of Dermatology and Plastic Surgery at Kumamoto University

*Address correspondence to this author at the 1-1-1 Honjo, Kumamoto 860-8556, Kumamoto, Japan;
E-mail: ihn-der@kumamoto-u.ac.jp

Hospital. Written informed consent to participate in the study was obtained from all the patients, which was approved by the institutional review board.

For histological and immunohistochemical analyses, 28 specimens were fixed in 10% formalin and embedded in paraffin. Nine of 28 specimens were divided into two pieces, one of which was frozen in liquid nitrogen and kept at -80°C for further analysis.

Antibodies Used

Three mouse monoclonal antibodies (F34-187, F33-104 and F106-88; developed by Kuroki *et al.*) and one rabbit polyclonal antibody raised against human CEACAMs (Dako-PoAb) were used as primary antibodies. Epitope mapping analysis, using CEA and related antigens and various CEA and related recombinant proteins, has revealed the specificity of the monoclonal antibodies used here [14, 15].

F34-187, which recognizes an epitope on domain N of CEA, reacts with CEA, CEACAM1 and CEACAM6 [14, 15]. F33-104, which recognizes an epitope on the B3 domain of CEA, seems to be specific for CEA [14, 15]. F106-88 reacts only with CEACAM6 [14, 15]. Dako-PoAb reacts with CEA and other CEACAM members.

A well-characterized PoAb against involucrin (Paesel), MoAbs against PCNA (Dako), Ki-67 (MIB-1, SANTA CRUZ BIOTECHNOLOGY, INC.) andCK16 (Novocastra) were also used as proliferation and/or differentiation markers to investigate the histological localization of the CEACAMs in comparison with the molecules.

Immunoblotting Analysis

Four frozen samples of psoriasis vulgaris and 3 of normal skin were used for immunoblotting analysis. The samples were frozen in liquid nitrogen and kept at -80°C. One frozen sample of rectal carcinoma was also used for positive control and human fibroblasts cultured in modified Eagle's medium supplemented with 10% fetal calf serum (FCS) and 50 μg/ml amphotericin for negative control.

The specimens were homogenized and added phosphatidylinositol-specific phospholipase C (PI-PLC; Sigma) to cleave off the GPI-anchored proteins, such as CEA and CEACAM6, from the extracellular membrane. Then 20μl of the supernatant of the sample were exposed to 7.5% SDS-polyacrylamide gel electrophoresis before transferring to a nitrocellulose membrane. Blocking was achieved by incubating the membrane in 3% skimmed milk/Tris buffered saline with 0.2% Twin-20 (TBST) overnight at 4°C.

Dako-PoAb was applied at the dilution of 1:1000 and incubated overnight at 4°C, after which the membrane was incubated with goat anti-rabbit IgG-HRP for 60 min. Likewise, F33-104 (specific for CEA) and F106-88 (specific for CEACAM6) were applied at the dilution of 1:1000 and incubated overnight at 4°C, after which the membranes were incubated with goat anti-mouse IgG-HRP for 60 min. Membranes were washed with TBST and signals detected using the enhanced chemiluminescence system (Amersham Biosciences). β-actin was used as a loading control.

Immunohistochemical Staining Analysis

Immunohistochemical staining for the expression of CEACAMs and the proliferation/differentiation markers was performed with Vectastain ABC kit (Vector Laboratories) on serial sections of frozen and/or formalin-fixed specimens.

In regard to the frozen material, 4μm cryostat sections were air-dried and fixed in acetone at 4°C for 10 min, whereas in regard to formalin-fixed material, after the sections were deparaffinized and rehydrated, antigen retrieval of CEACAMs was achieved by microwave treatment for 10 min in EDTA (1mmol/l, pH6.0), followed by cooling at room temperature for 60 min. After being washed in phosphate-buffered saline (PBS), the sections were treated with 3% hydrogen peroxide solution to reduce endogenous peroxidase activity. Those slides were incubated with the respective primary antibodies at 4°C overnight, washed in phosphate-buffered saline, treated with biotinylated anti-mouse (for MoAbs) or anti-rabbit (for Dako-PoAb) IgG (Vector Laboratories) for 30 min at room temperature, and rewashed. After 60 min of incubation with the avidin-biotin peroxidase complex (ABC, Vector Laboratories), the sections were washed in phosphate-buffered saline, developed in 0.05% diaminobenzidine diluted in phosphate-buffered saline with 0.01% hydrogen peroxide, dehydrated, and mounted.

11C2A4 (hybridoma protein; for F34-187, F33-104 and F106-88), normal mouse (Cappel Division, Organon Teknika Co.; for MoAbs), or rabbit serum (Cappel Division, Organon Teknika Co.; for PoAbs) were used as the negative controls. For positive controls, we examined normal eccrine glands and ducts in each section.

Double Immunoenzymatic Staining Analysis

Since the expression of CEACAMs was restricted to the upper epidermal cell layers, we performed the double immunoenzymatic staining analysis to compare the expression of the CEACAMs with that of involucrin, a well-characterized differentiation marker for the epidermal keratinocytes.

In brief, the sequential immunostaining procedure was carried out by first performing immunoperoxidase staining against F34-187, the monoclonal antibody attaining the clearest staining in our protocol, using the ABC method with a Vectastain ABC Kit (Vector Laboratories), and then the immunoalkaline phosphatase–antialkaline phosphatase (APAAP) method against involucrin (PoAb) was conducted with an APAAP Kit (Zymed Laboratories.). The sections were stained for peroxidase with diaminobenzidine and then stained with second primary antibody. As substrate solution for the alkaline phosphatase reaction, naphthol-AS-phosphatase (Sigma) and Fast Blue BB (Sigma) were dissolved in dimethylformamide and diluted with 0.1 mol/l Tris buffer, pH 8.2. To inhibit endogenous alkaline phosphatase activity, the incubation medium was supplemented with 0.25 mmol/l levamisole (Sigma).

RESULTS

Immunoblotting Analysis

Immunoblotting analysis revealed that the expression of both CEA and CEACAM6was up-regulated in psoriatic skin compared to normal skin, in which CEACAM6 expression was detected, but not CEA (Fig. **1**).

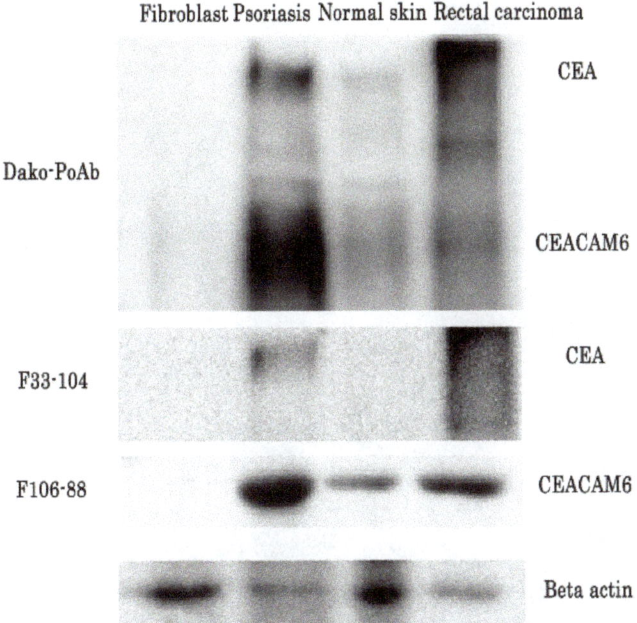

Fig. (1). Immunoblotting analysis of CEA and CEACAM6 expression in dermal fibroblasts, psoriasis skin, normal skin and rectal carcinoma. With F33-106 (specific for CEA), positive signal was seen only in psoriatic skin, whereas positive signal was seen in both psoriasis and normal skin with F106-88 (specific for CEACAM6), with much stronger signal in psoriatic skin than in normal skin. The β-actin was used as a loading control.

Immunohistochemical Staining Analysis

Using a Dako-PoAb against CEACAMs, the histological distribution of all the CEACAM-expressing cells was visible in the psoriatic skin. The expression was obtained in the epidermal keratinocytes only in the upper epidermal cell layers, while no expression was seen in the basal and lower prickle cell layers and in perilesional normal skin (Fig. **2**). Positive signal was also seen on neutrophils in Munro's microabscess and some dermal and epidermal inflammatory infiltrating cells; the infiltration of the CEACAM-expressing inflammatory cells was restricted to the dermis just beneath the epidermis expressing the CEACAM, and was the denser infiltration of the CEACAM-expressing inflammatory cells seen in the dermis where the stronger expression of the CEACAM was seen in the overlying epidermis (Fig. **2**). Eccrine sweat glands and ducts were also positive for the antibody.

Heamatoxylin and eosin stain shows hyperkeratosis, parakeratosis, acanthosis and Munro's microabcess (Fig **3a**). In higher magnification, both membranous and cytoplasmic expression of the CEACAMs was seen in the epidermal keratinocytes (Fig. **3b**). Similar expression pattern was also seen with the F34-187 and F33-104 (Fig. **3c**) in the epidermal keratinocytes, suggesting that CEA was expressed in the psoriatic keratinocytes and this was confirmed by the result of immunoblotting analysis. Neither neutrophils in Munro's microabscess nor inflammatory infiltrating cells showed positive signals with the F33-104, suggesting that CEA was not expressed in these cells (Fig. **3c**).

Using F106-88 (specific for CEACAM6), negative (Fig. **3d**) to weak (Fig. **4**) signal was obtained in the epidermal keratinocytes, depending on the samples studied, in contrast to that strong expression was seen by immunoblotting analysis using the same antibody as mentioned above. Neutophils in Munro's microabscess and inflammatory infiltrating cells were positive for F106-88, suggesting that CEACAM6 was expressed in the cells.

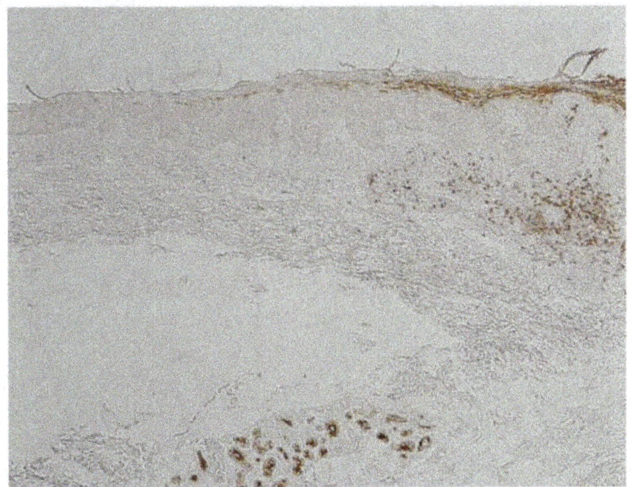

Fig. (2). Immunohistochemistry with Dako-PoAb shows strong CEACAM expression in the epidermal keratinocytes restricted to the upper epidermal cell layers, inflammatory infiltrating cells, and eccrine glands (x 20).

Up-regulated expression of PCNA, Ki-67, CK16 and involucrin was also shown in the epidermal keratinocytes of the psoriatic skin: PCNA and Ki-67 were expressed in the keratinocytes of basal and lower prickle cell layers, while CK16 and involucrin were expressed in middle to upper epidermal cell layers (Fig. **5**).

The expression of the CEACAM was restricted to more de-differentiated. This finding was well demonstrated by double immunoenzymatic staining analysis (Fig. **6**).

DISCUSSION

Using a panel of antibodies that recognize different epitopes of CEACAMs, we clearly demonstrated that CEA and CEACAM6 were overexpressed in inflamed psoriasis skin. The expression was detected in membrane and cytoplasm of the epidermal keratinocytes whose distribution was restricted to the upper cell layers of the acanthotic epidermis.

While, even though our immunoblotting analysis showed strong expression of CEACAM6 with F106-88 (MoAb specific for CEACAM6), our immunohistochemical analysis showed only a week positive signal (some lesions were even negative) with the same antibody in the epidermal keratinocytes. The reason for this weak staining could be because F106-88 antibody is not suitable for detecting naive protein, in contrast to its high immunoreactivity in immunoblotting.

Infiltrating inflammatory cells showed strong positive signal for not only Dako-PoAb and F34-187 but also F106-88, suggesting that CEACAM6 was strongly expressed in the inflammatory cells.

Immunohistochemical and double immunoenzymatic revealed that the CEACAMs expression correlated with the overexpression of involucrin, PCNA, Ki-67 and CK16.

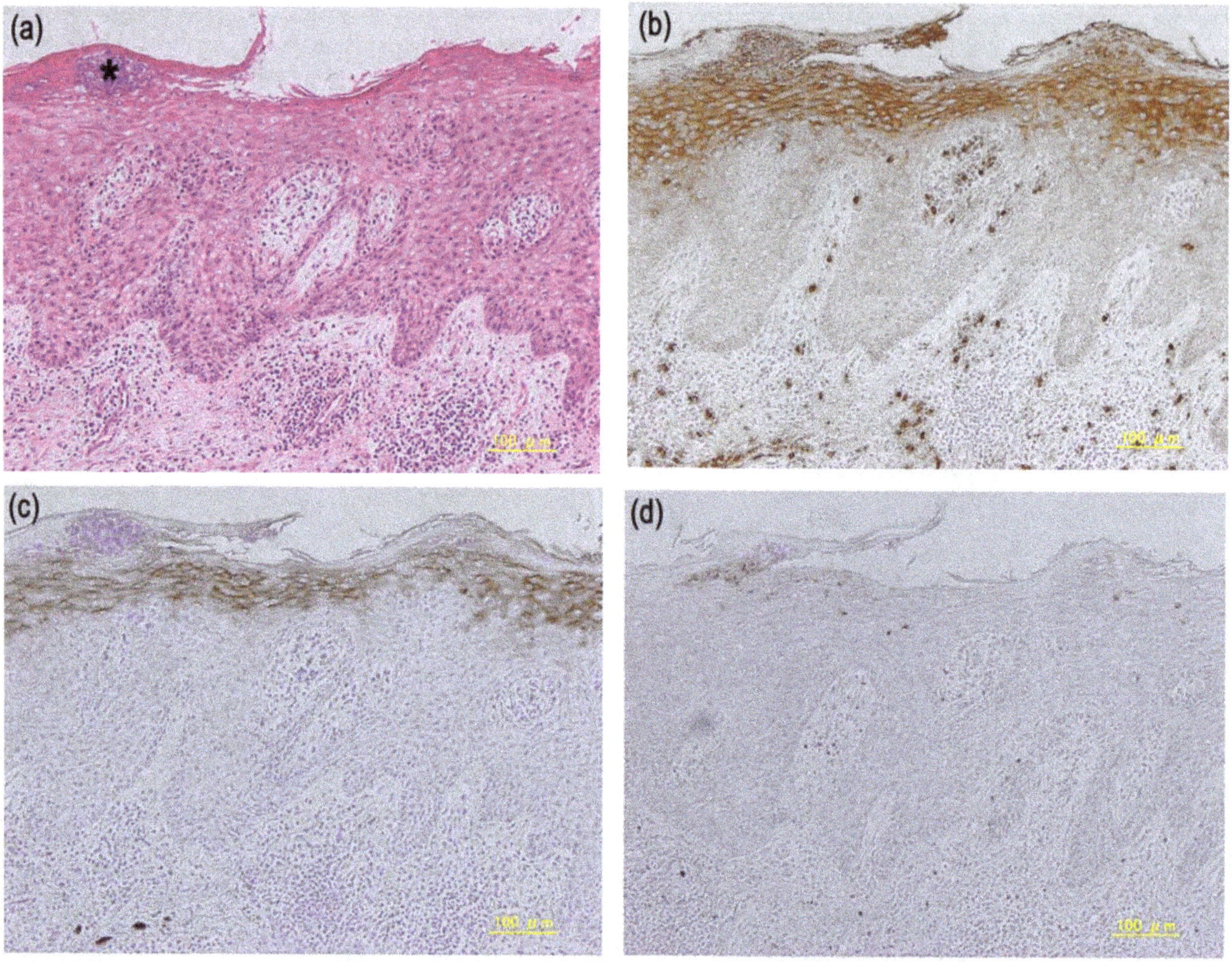

Fig. (3). Representative staining for CEACAMs in psoriasis skin. Haematoxylin and eosin stain (**a**) shows hyperkeratosis, parakeratosis, acanthosis and Munro's microabscess (*). Lymphocytes and a few neutrophils are present in the perivascular infiltrates. In immunohistochemical analysis, Dako-PoAb (**b**) shows positive signal in keratinocytes restricted to the upper epidermal cell layers and inflammatory infiltrating cells, including those in Munro's microabscess (*); F33-104 (**c**) shows positive signal in the epidermal keratinocytes and eccrine ducts, but not in the inflammatory infiltrating cells;F106-88 (**d**) shows positive signal only a few inflammatory infiltrating cells. Bar 100µm.

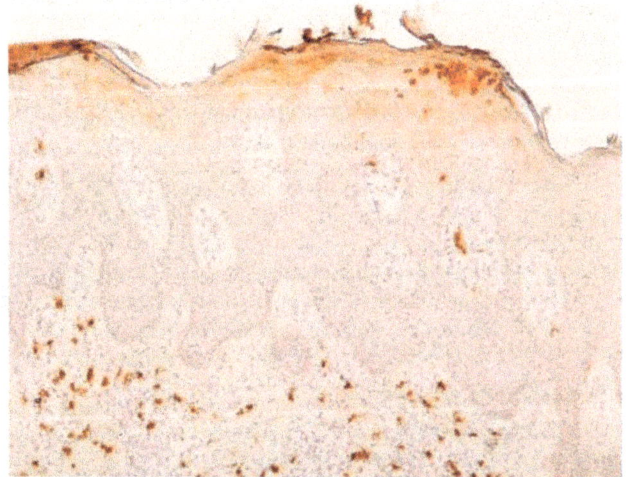

Fig. (4). Immunohistochamical staining with F106-88 showed week to moderate positive signal in keratinocytes of upper epidermal cell layers, in addition to the strong signal in inflammatory infiltrating cells (x 40).

These results suggest that both CEA and CEACAM6 are induced on epidermal keratinocytes in psoriasis lesions, and that the expression may be associated with the state of de-differentiation of the actively proliferating keratinocytes of the disease. Up-regulated expression of CEA and other CEACAM members only in the upper epidermal cell layers was also demonstrated in keratinocytic neoplasma [7] and verruca vulgarisin in our previous studies [7,16], suggesting the differentiation-related expression of these molecules also exists in the proliferatively active keratinocytes in the neoplastic skin conditions.

It is currently well known that CEA and CEACAM6 are up-regulated in a wide variety of human cancers, including colon, breast, pancreatic, and lung cancer [17]. Functional analyses have indicated that CEA and CEACAM6 can inhibit differentiation [18] and anoikis [19] of a number of different cell lines. An inverse correlation between the cell surface levels of CEA and CEACAM6 and the degree of differentiation of the tumors has also been shown [20].

CEACAM1 was reported to be expressed only in outer epidermal cell layers in association with Munro's

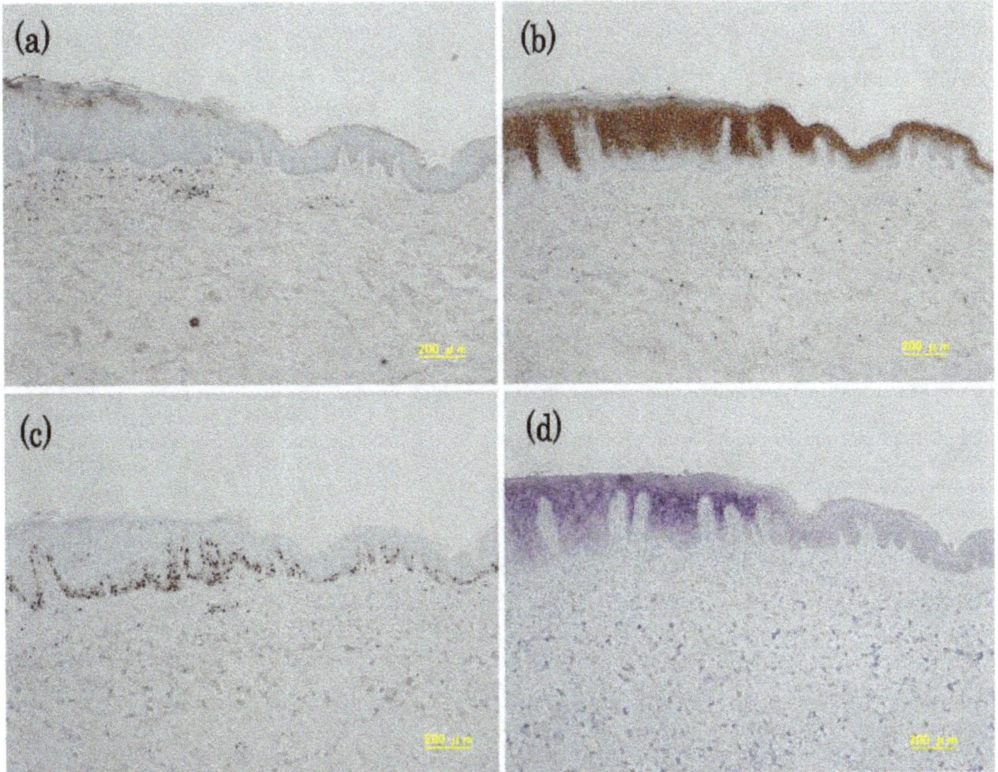

Fig. (5). Immunohistochemical staining for CEACAMs (**a**), involucrin (**b**), Ki-67 (**c**) and CK16 (d). (**a**) Membranous and cytoplasmic expression of CEACAMs is seen on keratinocytes only in the upper part of the epidermis. (**b**) Expression of involucrin existed at the lower epidermal cell layers. (**c**) In psoriasis lesions, overexpression of Ki-67 is seen in the nuclei in the basal and lower epidermal cell layers. (**d**) Expression of CK16 was seen only in the psoriasis lesions. Bar 200μm.

microabscess [12]. However, in the present study, CEA was expressed diffusely in the upper epidermal cell layers, not only in association with the Munro's microabscess.

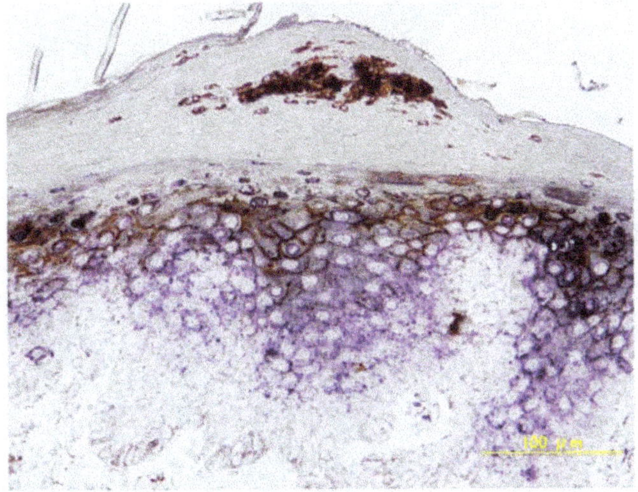

Fig. (6). Double immunoenzymatic staining with F34-187 (avidin-biotin peroxidasecomplex) and involucrin (alkaline phosphatase-antialkaline phosphatase) shows the CEACAM expression (brown) exists at the epidermal cell layers above that of involucrin (blue) in psoriasis lesion. Neutrophils in Munro's microabcess also express the CEACAM (brown). Bar 100μm.

Indeed these limited data are insufficient to elucidate true roles of CEACAMs in the pathogenesis of psoriasis vulgaris. Interstingly, immunohistological studies have failed to show CEACAMs expression in atopic dermatitis [12], suggesting the difference of underlying pathogenesis of these skin disorders. In fact, it is generally accepted that the immune response in atopic dermatitis is mediated by Th2 lymphocytes, whereas Th1 cells are important in the pathogenesis of psoriasis [21]; it has recently been revealed that both CEA and CEACAM6 are major target for Smad3-mediated TGF-β signaling [22]; and that IFN-γ or oncostatin M induces the expression of CEACAM1 [12].

ABBREVIATIONS

CEA	=	Carcinoembryonic antigen
CEACAM	=	CEA-related cell adhesion molecule
MoAb	=	Monoclonal antibody
PoAb	=	Polyclonal antibody

CONFLICT OF INTEREST

The authors confirm that this article content has no conflict of interest.

ACKNOWLEDGEMENTS

Declared none.

REFERENCES

[1] Skubitz K, Skubitz A. Interdependency of CEACAM-1, -3, -6, and -8 induced human neutrophil adhesion to endothelial cells. J Transl Med 2008; 6: 78.

[2] Beauchemin N, Draber P, Dveksler G, *et al.* Redefined nomenclature for members of the carcinoembryonic antigen family. Exp Cell Res 1999; 252: 243-9.

[3] Egawa K, Honda Y, Kuroki M, Inaba Y, Ono T. Carcinoembryonic antigen and related antigens expressed on keratinocytes in inflammatory dermatoses. Br J Dermatol 1996; 134: 451-9.

[4] Gray-Owen S, Blumberg R. CEACAM1: contact-dependent control of immunity. Nat Rev Immunol 2006; 6: 433-46.

[5] Gold P, Freedman S. Demonstration oftumor-specific antigens in human colonic carcinoma by immunological tolerance and absorption techniques. J Exp Med 1965; 121: 439-62.

[6] Benchimol S, Fuks A, Jothy S, Beauchemin N, Shirota K, Stanners C. Carcinoembryonic antigen, a human tumor marker, functions as an intercellular adhesion molecule. Cell 1989; 57: 327-34.

[7] Egawa K, Honda Y, Ono T, Kuroki M. Immunohistochemical demonstration of carcinoembryonic antigen and related antigens in various cutaneous keratinous neoplasms and verruca vulgaris. Br J Dermatol 1998; 139: 178-85.

[8] Maxwell P, Davis R, Sloan J. Carcinoembryonic antigen (CEA) in benign and malignant epithelium of the gall bladder, extrahepatic bile ducts, and ampulla of Vater. J Pathol 1993; 170: 73-6.

[9] Honda Y, Egawa K, Kuroki M, Ono T. Hair cycle-dependent expression of a nonspecific cross reacting antigen (NCA)-50/90-like molecule on follicular keratinocytes. Arch Dermatol Res 1997; 289: 457-65.

[10] Metze D, Grunert F, Neumaier M, *et al.* Neoplasms with sweat gland differentiation express various glycoproteins of the carcinoembryonic antigen (CEA) family. J Cutan Pathol. 1996; 23: 1-11.

[11] Metze D, Soyer H, Zelger B, *et al.* Expression of a glycoprotein of the carcinoembryonic antigen family in normal and neoplastic sebaceous glands. Limited role of carcinoembryonic antigen as a sweat gland marker. J Am Acad Dermatol 1996; 34: 735-44.

[12] Rahmoun M, Molès J, Pedretti N, *et al.* Cytokine-induced CEACAM1 expression on keratinocytes is characteristic for psoriatic skin and contributes to a prolonged lifespan of neutrophils. J Invest Dermatol 2009; 129: 671-81.

[13] Hagemeier H, Bhardwaj R, Grunert F, *et al.* Carcinoembryonic antigen and related glycoproteins in psoriasis. Pathobiology 1993; 61: 19-24.

[14] Kuroki M, Arakawa F, Higuchi H, Haruno M, Wakisaka M, Matsuoka Y. Immunological and biochemical characterization of the nonspecific cross-reacting antigen epitopes using twenty-three monoclonal antibodies. Hybridoma 1991; 10: 557-74.

[15] Kuroki M, Arakawa F, Haruno M, *et al.* Biochemical characterization of 25 distinct carcinoembryonic antigen (CEA) epitopes recognized by 57 monoclonal antibodies and categorized into seven groups in terms of domain structure of the CEA molecule. Hybridoma 1992; 11: 391-407.

[16] Egawa K, Honda Y, Ono T, Kitasato H, Kuroki M. The glycoprotein of the carcinoembryonic antigen (CEA) gene family expressed on epithelial keratinocytes in viral warts. Arch Dermatol Res 1998; 290: 453-7.

[17] Ordonez C, Zhai A, Camacho-Leal P, Demarte L, Fan M, Stanners C. GPI-anchored CEA family glycoproteins CEA and CEACAM6 mediate their biological effects through enhanced integrin $\alpha5\beta1$-fibronectin interaction. J Cell Physiol 2007; 210: 757-65.

[18] Eidelman F, Fuks A, DeMarte L, Taheri M, Stanners C. Human carcinoembryonic antigen, an intercellular adhesion molecule, blocks fusion and differentiation of rat myoblasts. J Cell Biol 1993; 123: 467-75.

[19] Ordoñez C, Screaton R, Ilantzis C, Stanners C. Human carcinoembryonic antigen functions as a general inhibitor of anoikis. Cancer Res 2000; 60: 3419-24.

[20] Ilantzis C, Jothy S, Alpert L, Draber P, Stanners C. Cell-surface levels of human carcinoembryonic antigen are inversely correlated with colonocyte differentiation in colon carcinogenesis. Lab Invest 1997; 76: 703-16.

[21] Bowcock A, Krueger J. Getting under the skin: the immunogenetics of psoriasis. Nat Rev Immunol 2005; 5: 699-711.

[22] Han S, Kwak T, Her K, *et al.* CEACAM5 and CEACAM6 are major target genes for Smad3-mediated TGF-β signaling. Oncogene 2008; 27: 675-83.

19

Attitudes Towards Pediculosis Treatments in Teenagers

Deon V. Canyon*, Chauncey Canyon, Sami Milani and Rick Speare

Office of Public Health Studies, University of Hawaii at Manoa, 1960 East-West Rd, Biomed Building #T103, Honolulu, HI 96822, USA

Abstract: Research on pediculosis has focused on treatment strategies and social aspects have been largely ignored. Pediculosis and its treatment in are associated with negative emotional responses while in developing countries pediculosis and its treatment may provide more an opportunity for positive social bonding. Attitudes to pediculosis have been proposed as important to successful control. Previous studies in Australia found that parents of primary school children say they treat pediculosis once it has been detected.

This study retrospectively investigated attitudes towards treatment in teenage high school students in an attempt to collect information from those afflicted rather than from parents. Only participants with a history of pediculosis were recruited from a high school in Western Australia and they were asked to complete an anonymous questionnaire. The sample contained 128 Grade 8 and 9 students, aged 13-15 years old with an even gender split. Negative feelings towards being treated for head lice were observed in 41.5% of males and 54.7% of females and 49.5% of Caucasians and 40% of Asians. Anti-treatment sentiment was expressed by 19.7% of males and 10.9% of females. Shampooing with and without combing were the most preferred treatments overall.

The results showed that 63.6% male and 52.7% female high school students were in favour of head lice treatments. This low percentage indicates that current treatments for head lice require improvement to be made more acceptable and that alternative treatments that are less unpleasant need to be developed. Strategies need to be explored to make treatment of pediculosis a more positive emotional experience.

Keywords: Combing, feelings, hair thickness, head lice, treatment,

INTRODUCTION

Pediculus humanus capitis De Geer, the insect ectoparasite that causes pediculosis, has evolved in close association with human hosts with archeological evidence extending back 9000 years [1]. Pediculosis in developed countries is mainly treated by application of liquid compounds to the hair. These typically have an insecticidal action and are often combined with use of a fine-toothed "nit" comb to physically remove lice and lice eggs [2]. Other less commonly used treatments include specialised combs that electrocute lice and equipment to kill lice using hot air [3, 4]. Head lice repellents, although lacking studies to demonstrate efficacy, are being increasingly sought to prevent transmission [5]. Research on pediculosis has focused on treatment strategies and social aspects have been largely ignored.

A study of adults (91% female) on issues associated with treatment of pediculosis found a broad range of technological, biological and social issues [6]. Many respondents in this survey found commercial products and methods ineffective and difficult and had concerns about their safety. Trying several treatments was commonly reported. Pain associated with use of nit combs was also reported. Decades ago a society's attitude to pediculosis was proposed as important to successful control [7]. Previous studies indicated that most parents of primary school children in Australia say they treat pediculosis once detected [8, 9]. This was also the case in Norway [10].

Some researchers propose that perhaps a more important role is played by certain social factors and individual behavior [6, 7, 11, 12]. While chemical or natural treatments may succeed in eliminating lice, the lice-free period may often be short-lived. Reinfection from other infected people is almost guaranteed if associates of the treated person (and their associates) are not treated concurrently. The root cause of reinfection traces back to behavior and attitudes. Product concerns, treating children, blaming others for reinfection, stigma and social issues are major concerns of parents and carers [11, 12] that remain to be adequately investigated in the infected population. Work by Canyon and Speare showed that a significant degree of apathy was present in infected students and their parents [13, 14]. Certain key individuals (school students) who remained apathetic due to a lack of awareness or lack of symptoms or desire to avoid treatment were observed to serve as potent head lice carriers. In fact, the growing global prevalence of pediculosis may be partly a result of this attitude [13]. This study thus aimed to investigate the attitudes of secondary school children to head lice treatments that largely occurred during primary/ elementary school, with a view to providing more informat-

*Address correspondence to this author at the Office of Public Health Studies, University of Hawaii at Manoa, 1960 East-West Rd, Biomed Building #T103, Honolulu, HI 96822, USA;
E-mail: dcanyon@hawaii.edu

ion on teenage attitudes to pediculosis that serve to diminish head lice control efforts.

METHODS

The site of this study was a multicultural school in Perth, Western Australia with around 1700 students from Grades 8 to 12. Consent letters and information sheets were sent home to the parents of 480 middle-school students from Grades 8 and 9. Eligible teenagers with parental consent were asked to complete an anonymous survey that they returned to the school for collection. Participation was thus based on voluntary self-selection and diagnosis of pediculosis was not confirmed. Only students who could recall being infected with head lice were included in the study. It is possible that this sampling strategy introduced non-participation/non-response bias which may have lead to differing results. This sampling strategy combined criterion based and convenience approaches, since the targeted participants are those who have direct experience coping with a head lice infestation (criterion) and they are accessible (convenience) [15]. The questionnaire requested basic non-identifying demographic information (grade, gender and hair details) followed by two open-ended questions:

How do you feel about getting treated for head lice with combs, shampoos and other treatments?

What do you feel are the worst and best treatments for head lice?

"Shampoos" referred to topical liquid treatments, including both shampoos and lotions. The computer software package SPSS 20 was used to analyze responses for salient themes that addressed the questionnaire focus. Cross-tabulations with Chi-Square tests were employed where possible, but low cell frequencies meant that Uncertainty Coefficient Tests were often employed. Ethics approval H2954 was obtained from James Cook University Human Ethics Committee.

RESULTS

The response rate was 27.7% with 133 students out of 480 participating in the study and 128 surveys that were sufficiently complete to enable analysis (Table **1**). However, since only students who had experienced pediculosis were eligible to participate, the true response rate cannot be determined.

Table 1. Frequencies of personal factors in children with pediculosis.

Personal Factors	Frequency (%)
Gender	*2 missing*
Male	68 (53.1)
Female	58 (45.3)
Current Grade ♂/♀	*3 missing*
8	38/28 (30.4/22.4)
9	29/30 (23.2/24.0)
Grade during infection ♂/♀	*10 missing*
1	4/2 (3.4/1.7)
2	5/6 (4.2/5.1)
3	7/4 (5.9/3.4)
4	7/9 (5.9/7.6)
5	11/9 (9.3/7.6)
6	11/12 (9.3/10.2)
7	15/8 (12.7/6.8)
8	7/1 (5.9/0.8)
Ethnicity ♂/♀	*4 missing*
Caucasian	57/50 (46.0/40.3)
Asian	10/7 (8.1/5.6)
Hair Thickness ♂/♀	*2 missing*
Thin	10/12 (7.9/9.5)
Medium	35/27 (27.8/21.4)
Thick	23/19 (18.3/15.1)
Hair Color ♂/♀	*2 missing*
Blond	12/9 (9.5/7.1)
Brown	41/43 (32.5/34.1)
Black	15/6 (11.9/4.8)
Hair Length ♂/♀	*5 missing*
Short	57/1 (46.3/0.8)
Shoulder	8/26 (6.5/21.1)
Long	2/29 (1.6/23.6)

In response to the question, "How do you feel about getting treated for head lice with combs, shampoos and other treatments?" negative experiences included: smell, disgust, phobia, annoyance, inconvenience, wasted time, 'I prefer having lice', and pain. Non-negative experiences included: 'good', 'I like it', and 'I don't mind'. Responses were divided into five categories: anti-process, anti-shampoo, anti-comb, anti-treatment and pro-treatment, which included neutral responses.

Anti-Process: 20.3% of all participants had a problem with the process of lice treatment. Gender was significant with 12.1% of males and 32.7% of females being annoyed or disgusted with the treatment (Chi-Square $p<0.01$). Caucasian females were significantly more anti-process than males ($p<0.05$). Race and hair-related variables were not significant.

Anti-Shampoo: 11.7% of all participants had a problem with lice treatment shampoos. Gender was moderately significant with 4.5% of males and 20.0% of females disliking the smell (Chi-Square $p<0.01$). When gender was broken down by ethnicity, females remained significantly more likely to be anti-shampoo than males (Uncertainty coefficient: Caucasians $p<0.01$, $u=0.062$; Asians $p<0.05$, $u=0.259$). Hair length significantly affected anti-shampoo sentiment among Caucasians with fewer shorthaired people (2.2%) and more longhaired people (22.2%) being anti-shampoo (Chi-square $p<0.05$). Ethnicity, hair thickness and hair color were not significant.

Anti-Combing: 10.9% of all participants had a problem with fine-toothed lice combs. Hair thickness was significant with 17.9% of thick-haired, 11.3% of medium-haired, and 0.0% of thin-haired people disliking the pain ($p<0.05$, u=0.40). Gender, ethnicity, hair color and length were not significant.

Anti-Treatment: 16.3% of participants explicitly expressed anti-treatment sentiment, but the only significant association was that people with thick hair were significantly less likely to be anti treatment ($p<0.05$, u=0.034).

Pro-Treatment: 57.7% of participants explicitly stated that they were in favor of head lice treatments, but all study factors were not significant.

Participant responses to the question "What do you feel are the worst and best treatments for head lice?" are presented in Table **2**.

With regard to the worst treatments for head lice, several significant associations were identified. Hair thickness was moderately significant ($p<0.05$, u=0.071) with more medium-haired people saying 'doing nothing' (adjusted residual [AR] = 1.9), no thick-haired person saying that manual removal or cutting is worst (AR -1.8, -1.9), more medium-haired people saying cutting is worst (AR=2.0), and more thick haired people having no particular distaste for any treatments (AR=2.0) (Figs. **1**, **2**). Hair length was more significant ($p<0.01$, u=0.082) with, more longhaired people saying 'doing nothing' is worse (AR=2.2), more shorthaired people disliking combs (AR=1.6), more shoulder-length-haired people saying they had no preference (AR=4.1). Hair color was not significantly related to worst treatment.

DISCUSSION

Some children are known to under-report infections to parents and some parents are known to avoid treating their children [13, 14]. The aim of this study was to take this further and retrospectively investigate how teenage students felt about getting treated for head lice with combs, shampoos and other methods in primary/elementary school, and which treatments they considered worst and best.

How Do you Feel About Getting Treated for Head Lice?

Negative feelings towards being treated for head lice were observed in almost half of males, females, Caucasians and Asians with specific anti-treatment sentiment expressed by a fifth of males and a tenth of females and pro-treatment sentiment was expressed by over half of females and half of males. These feelings were displayed for the entire treatment experience and particular methods, such as application of topical liquids and combing. These results have implications, primarily for the industries providing these goods and the parents and guardians attempting to use them to treat their children. For manufacturers, smelly liquid treatments can be modified to have a more appealing odor to females and fine-toothed lice combs can be made available in different widths to suit different hair thickness to reduce pain.

Few thick-haired students were anti-treatment compared to a fifth of thin and medium hair types. This may be due to thick-haired individuals being less sensitive or more used to painful treatments or more cognizant of the need for treatment. Hair length was not associated with being more or less anti-treatment. Hair thickness was not strongly associated with being more or less pro-treatment. Shorter

Table 2. Head lice treatments considered worst and best by female and male Caucasians and Asians.

		Caucasian (%)		Asian (%)	
		Female	**Male**	**Female**	**Male**
Worst Treatments	Doing Nothing	9.6	9.6	23.1	7.7
	Combing	11.7	18.1	7.7	30.8
	Shampoo/Herbal	12.8	14.9	0.0	0.0
	Manual Removal	3.2	2.1	0.0	7.7
	Cutting Hair	1.1	3.2	0.0	7.7
	No Preference	9.6	4.3	7.7	7.7
	Totals	48	52	38	62
Best Treatments	Doing nothing	0.0	1.0	0.0	0.0
	Combing	5.1	8.2	0.0	8.3
	Combing + Shampoo/Conditioner	14.3	11.2	8.3	8.3
	Shampoo/Conditioner	10.2	15.3	0.0	16.7
	Chemical/Herbal Treatment + Others	9.2	8.2	16.7	16.7
	Manual Removal	0.0	2.0	0.0	0.0
	Cutting Hair	2.0	2.0	0.0	8.3
	Electro Combing	1.0	3.1	0.0	0.0
	No Preference	6.1	1.0	8.3	8.3
	Totals	48	52	33	67

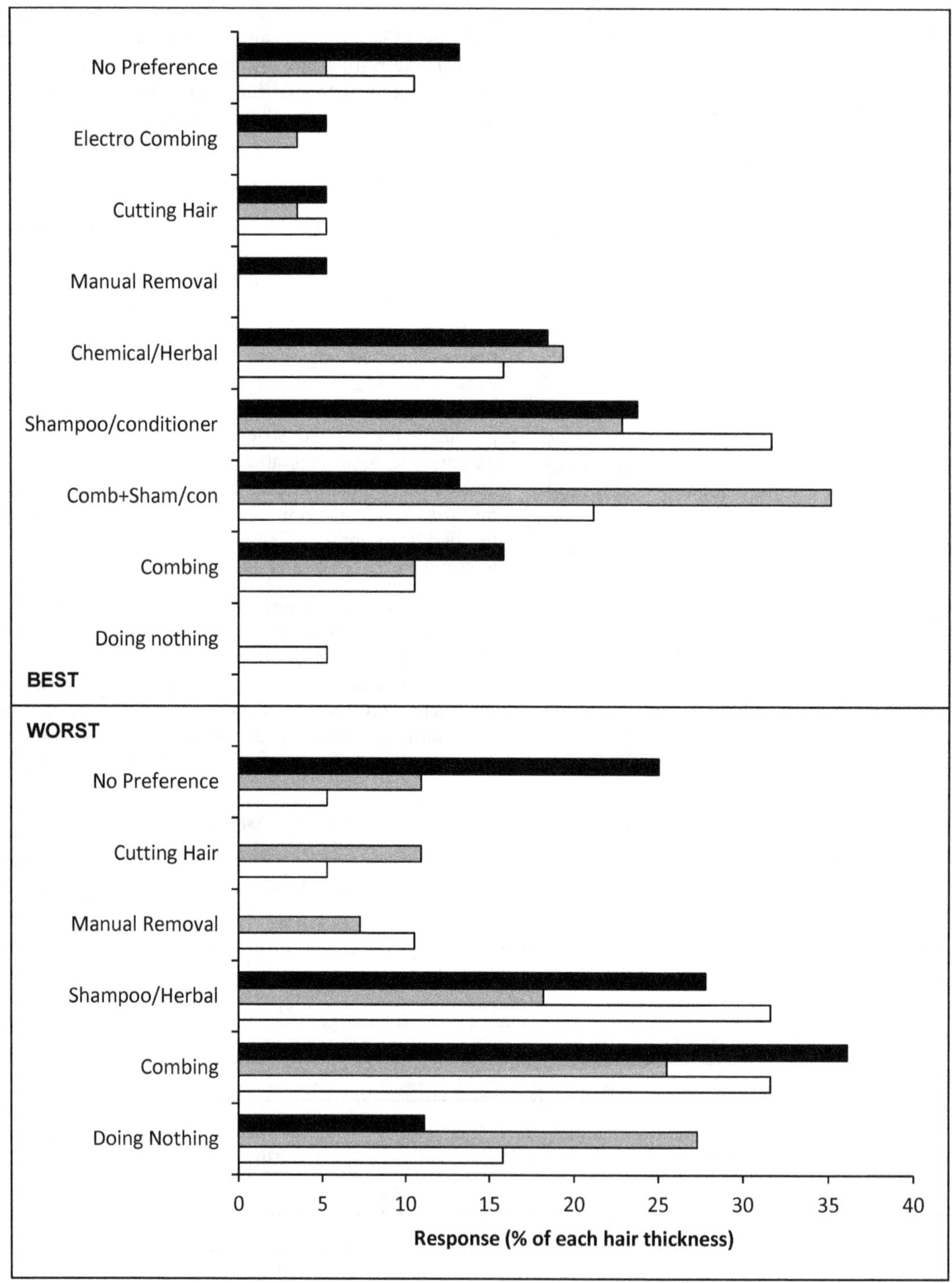

Fig. (1). Treatments considered to be the Best and Worst by participants with thin, medium and thick hair.

hair lengths were associated with being more pro-treatment, but not significantly so.

A small proportion of thin haired people (5.3%) and shorthaired people (2%) indicated that doing nothing was the best treatment. These children are at risk of becoming sources of head lice by concealing infection and avoiding treatment.

What Do you Feel are the Worst and Best Treatments for Head Lice?

Caucasian students thought combing and topical liquids were the worst treatments while Asian students thought doing nothing and combing were the worst. This response revealed more of the social environment in which head lice infections exist. For example, a fifth of Caucasian and a third

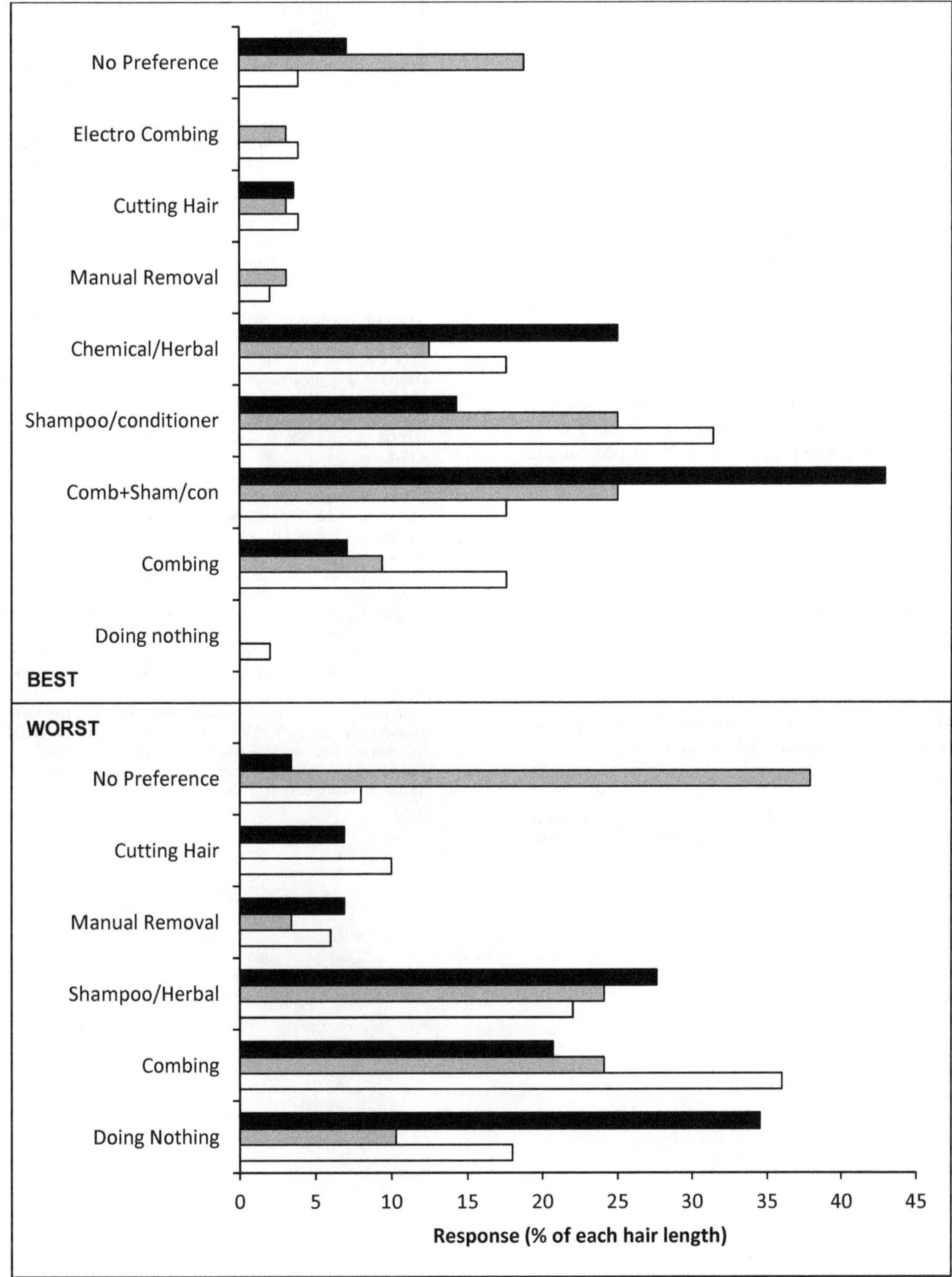

Fig. (2). Treatments considered to be the Best and Worst by participants with short , shoulder and long length hair.

of Asians said that doing nothing was the worst possible treatment. Given that there are a number of treatment options available, this was not expected. It may be that some students are aware of other infected students who chose to do nothing about their head lice infections or it may be that these students were often left untreated by their parents.

Hair thickness and length were significantly related to the stated worst treatments. It was confirmed that thick-haired students had a higher dislike than other hair types for combing. This supports the idea that this more painful method may be responsible for them concealing head lice infections. A higher proportion of shorthaired students disliked combing, so it may be the case that shorthaired students are combed more frequently or more roughly than longhaired students.

A higher proportion of longhaired students were against doing nothing. This may be because head lice eggs are difficult to remove and they stay on long hair for many months. As the hair grows out, the empty eggs from old infections become more visible. Thus long-term head lice infections in longhaired students are more likely to be detected visually by casual observers, which would result in social discomfort. Overall, the application of topical liquid treatments with and without combing were the most preferred treatments, which indicates a certain degree of tolerance in most teenagers to standard methods.

LIMITATIONS

Since most respondents wrote about pediculosis they had experienced in Grades 4 to 7, their recall would have been reasonable. A minority, who recalled episodes of pediculosis more than 3 years previously, may have been less accurate.

CONFLICT OF INTEREST

The authors confirm that this article content has no conflict of interest.

ACKNOWLEDGEMENTS

Declared none.

PATIENTS CONSENT

Informed Consent was given to the Author by the patients in respect of the clinical trials conducted.

REFERENCES

[1] Mumcuoglu KY, Zias J. Head lice, *Pediculus humanus capitis* (Anoplura: Pediculidae), from hair combs excavated in Israel and dated from the first century B.C. to the eighth century A.D. J Med Entomol 1988; 25: 545–7.

[2] Speare R, Canyon DV, Cahill C, Thomas G. Comparative efficacy of two nit combs in removing head lice (*Pediculus humanus* var. *capitis*) and their eggs. Int J Dermatol 2007; 46(12): 1275-8.

[3] O'Brien E. Detection and removal of head lice with an electronic comb: zapping the louse. J Pediatr Nurs 1998; 13(4): 265-6.

[4] Goates BM, Atkin JS, Wilding KG, *et al.* An effective nonchemical treatment for head lice: a lot of hot air. Pediatrics 2006; 118(5): 1962-70.

[5] Canyon DV, Speare R. A comparison of botanical and synthetic substances commonly used to prevent head lice (*Pediculus humanus* var. *capitis*) infestation. Int J Dermatol 2007; 46: 422–26.

[6] Parison J, Speare R, Canyon DV. Uncovering family experiences with head lice: the difficulties of eradication. Open Dermatol J 2008; 2: 9-17.

[7] Maunder B. Attitude to head lice--a more powerful force than insecticides. J R Soc Health 1985; 105(2): 61-4.

[8] Speare R, Buttner P. Prevalence of head lice in a primary school in Australia and implications for control. Int J Dermatol 1999; 38: 285-90.

[9] Counahan M, Andrews R, Speare R. Reliability of written parental reports of head lice in their children. Med J Aust 2005; 182(3): 137-8.

[10] Rukke BA, Birkemoe T, Soleng A, Lindstedt HH, Ottesen P. Head lice in Norwegian households: actions taken, costs and knowledge. PLoS One 2012; 7(2): e32686.

[11] Parison J, Canyon DV. Head lice and the impact of knowledge, attitudes and practices - a social science overview. In: Management and control of head lice infestations. Bremen: UNI-MED Verlag AG, 2010; 103-9.

[12] Parison J, Speare R, Canyon DV. Head lice: the feelings people have. Int J Dermatol 2013; 52(2): 169-71.

[13] Canyon DV, Speare R. Clinical decision support: Dermatology: Pediculosis. Wilmington, DE: Decision Support in Medicine LLC, 2012.

[14] Canyon DV, Speare R. Head lice transmission and risk factors. In: Heukelbach J, Ed. Management and control of head lice infestations. Bremen: UNI-MED Verlag AG, 2010; 34-40.

[15] Patton MQ. Qualitative research & evaluation methods, 3rd Ed. Thousand Oaks, CA: Sage, 2002.

20

Persistent Effects of Adapalene Gel After Chemical Peeling with Glycolic Acid in Patients with Acne Vulgaris

Mikiko Uede*[,1], Chikako Kaminaka[1,2], Nozomi Yonei[3], Fukumi Furukawa[1] and Yuki Yamamoto[1,2]

[1]*Department of Dermatology, Wakayama Medical University, Japan*

[2]*Department of Cosmetic Dermatology and Photomedicine, Wakayama Medical University, Japan*

[3]*Department of Dermatology, Public Naga Hospital, Japan*

Abstract: We investigated the usefulness of adapalene gel as maintenance therapy following chemical peeling with glycolic acid in patients with acne vulgaris. The study period was 14 weeks. The subjects were 23 patients with mild to moderate acne vulgaris (1 male, 22 females). After chemical peeling (CP) of the face was performed 3 times at 2-week intervals, adapalene was applied for 6 weeks using a randomized, double-blind half-side method. On the day of observation, dermatologists examined dermal findings, and measurement was conducted using instruments to analyze the physiological skin function. After the third session of CP was completed, both the inflammatory and non-inflammatory lesion counts significantly decreased. Subsequently, on the adapalene-treated side there were no change in the inflammatory and non-inflammatory lesion counts after the CP 3 times, but on placebo-treated side, there significant increase in the inflammatory and non inflammatory lesion counts. Concerning the results of measurement with instruments, the sebum capacity significantly decreased after the third session of CP. Subsequently, there were no changes after the 6-week application of adapalene or a placebo. These results suggest that post-CP adapalene application is an effective acne treatment method to improve efficacy and treatment adherence.

Keywords: Acne vulgaris(AV), chemical peeling(CP), adapalene.

INTRODUCTION

Acne vulgaris is frequent in clinical practice. It is a chronic, inflammatory dermal disease involving sebaceous hair follicles [1]. Its clinical characteristics include seborrhea, comedones, red papules, and pustules [1]. This disease frequently develops on the faces and thoracic/dorsal regions of persons aged 10 to 29 years, and is experienced by more than 90% of Japanese persons [2,3].

Chemical peeling (CP) is a technique to treat dermal symptoms related to acne, pigment anomalies, and photoaging or cosmetically improve the skin (anti-aging, reduction of spots/dullness, and improvement in the skin quality) [4]. In patients with acne, the thickening cornified layer of the hair follicle infundibulais exfoliated, reducing sebum retention in hair follicles. In particular, this procedure is effective for pimples [4]. Glycolic acid belongs to α-hydroxy acids, with the smallest molecular weight. It is appropriate for peeling of the most superficial (level 1) and superficial (level 1,2) layers [5]. Neither systemic toxicity nor serious complications have been reported, and various products are commercially available. In 2008, the Japanese Dermatological Association prepared the "Guidelines for Acne Vulgaris Treatment" for Japanese [6]. Concerning inflammatory/non-inflammatory lesion, glycolic and salicylic acids (macrogol base) were recommended as recommendation grade C1 (recommended as options, although there was little evidence) [5-7]. On the other hand, adapalene (6-[3-(1-adamantyl)-4-methoxyphenyl]-2-naphthoic acid), a naphthoic acid derivative [8], was approved as an external retinoid preparation in Japan in 2008 [9]. In patients with acne, this drug corrects the alteration of the hyperkeratinization process of the hair follicle infundibular, reducing microcomedones, comedones and inflammatory lesions. Furthermore, it was also strongly recommended as maintenance therapy after the reduction of inflammation. In the guidelines, the recommendation grade was established as A (Strongly recommended to perform (there should be at least one level I or II study that supports effectiveness) [5-7]. However, no study has compared CP with adapalene, although CP may exhibit immediate actions on comedones and cosmetic effects such as whitening [4]. In this study, we used an external adapalene preparation (recommendation grade A) after CP, which reduces lesion in the early phase, and examined its usefulness for acne vulgaris treatment.

*Address correspondence to this author at the Department of Dermatology, Wakayama Medical University, Postal code: 641-0012, 811-1, Kimiidera, Wakayama City, Wakayama Prefecture, Japan;
E-mail: kifubi@wakayama-med.ac.jp

SUBJECTS AND METHODS

Subjects

The subjects were 23 patients with mild to moderate acne, aged over 20 years, in whom there was no laterality in the acne count, and from whom written informed consent was obtained in the Department of Dermatology, Wakayama Medical University between 2009 and 2010. Patients were excluded if they had cyst, scar, and keloids, or other dematologic conditions requiring systemic treatment.

Exclusion criteria included males/females aged 19 years or younger and pregnant or lactating women. The purpose and contents of this study were examined and approved by the Ethic Review Board of Wakayama Medical University in accordance with the Helsinki Declaration.

Methods

The study period was 12 weeks. Chemical peeling with 40% glycolic acid (pH3.2) was performed 3 times at 2-week intervals [9]. From 2 weeks after the completion of CP, adapalene or a placebo (supplied by Galderma, Inc.) was applied to the half-face before bedtime every day for 6 weeks. Each drug was randomly assigned using the double-blind method.

EVALUATION

The severity of acne was evaluated according to the guidelines [6]. The exanthema count and skin condition were examined by dermatologists every two weeks (total: 7 times). For physiological skin function analysis, the water content (%) was measured using a CORNEOMETER®, the sebum capacity (μg/cm^2) using a SEBMETER®, and the transepidermal water loss (TEWL) (g/cm^2) using a TEWAMETER® (Multi-probe adaptor, Courage + Khazaka Co., Ltd., Cologne, Germany) at the start of this study, 2 weeks after the completion of the third session of CP, and 6 weeks after the start of adapalene application (total: 3 times) in a room with constant temperature(22 ~ 23℃) and humidity (relative humidity 40 ~ 45%).

STATISTICAL ANALYSIS

Statistical analysis was conducted using Wilcoxon's t-test. A p-value <0.05 was regarded as significant.

RESULTS

The subjects were 23 patients with acne vulgaris (1 male, 22 females), with a mean age of 25.3±5.8 (standard deviation) years.

Changes in the Lesion

Time dependent changes in the inflammatory lesion are shown in Fig. (**1**). After the completion of the third session of CP (6th week), the lesion significantly decreased in comparison with the pre-study value ($p<0.001$). Subsequently, there was a significant decrease after the 6-week (12th week) application of adapalene in comparison with the pre-study value ($p<0.01$). However, 6 weeks (12th week) after the start of application in adapalene group, there was no significant difference in comparison with the value after the third session of CP (6th week), although there was a slight decrease from 2 weeks after the start of application (8th week). In the placebo group, the lesion significantly increased in comparison with that after the third session of CP (12th week) ($p<0.01$).

The changes in the non-inflammatory lesion are shown in Fig. (**2**). After the third session of CP (6th week), the non-inflammatory lesion significantly decreased in comparison with the pre-study value ($p<0.001$). Subsequently, there were significant decreases after the 6-week (12th week) application of adapalene or the placebo in comparison with the pre-study value ($p<0.01$). In the adapalene group, there was no significant difference in comparison with the value after the third session of CP (6th week), although there was a slight decrease. In the placebo group, the exanthema was significantly greater than after the third session of CP (6th week) ($p<0.05$).

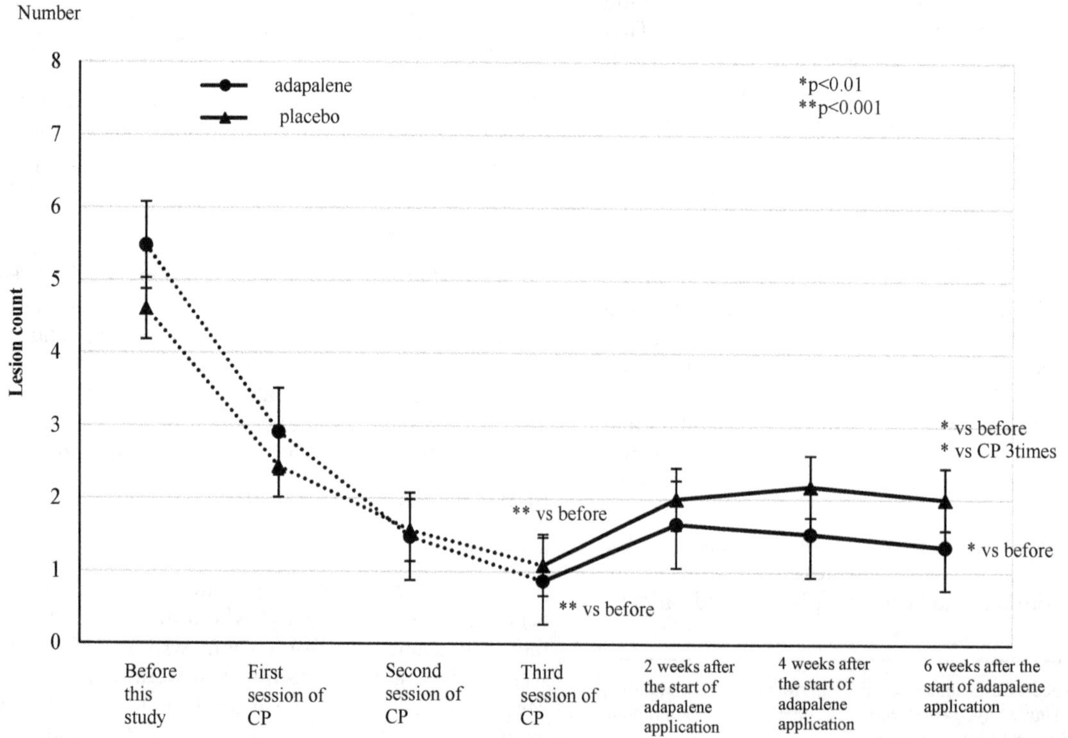

Fig. (1). Changes in the inflammatory lesion count (N=23).

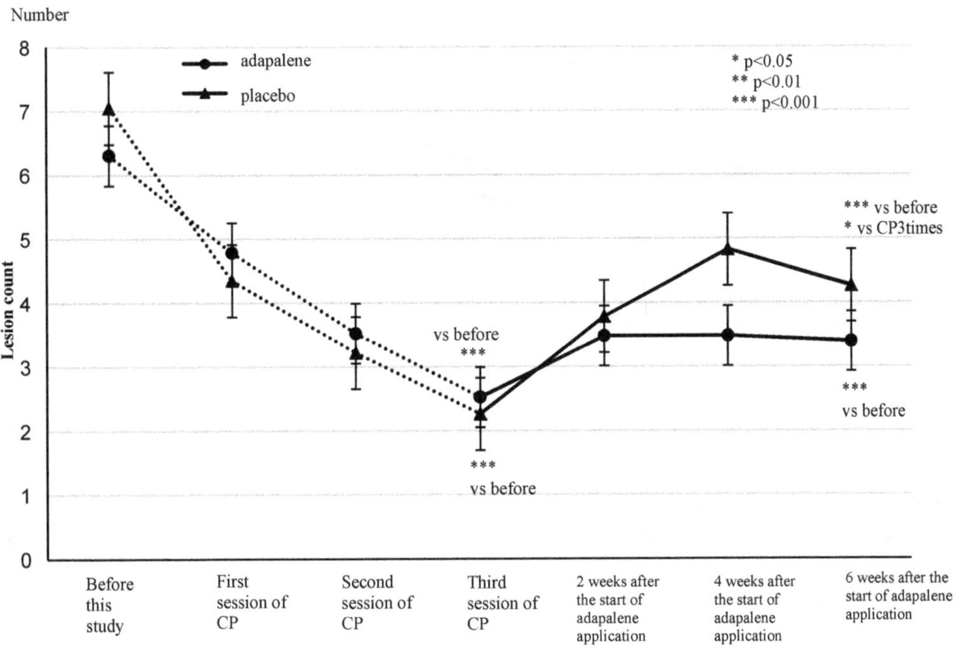

Fig. (2). Changes in the non-inflammatory lesion count (N=23).

Analysis of the Physiological Skin Function

Changes in the Sebum Secretion

After the third session of CP, the sebum secretion significantly decreased in comparison with the pre-study value ($p<0.05$). Subsequently, there were slight increases in both the adapalene and placebo groups, although there were no significant differences (Fig. **3**).

Changes in TEWL

After the third session of CP, the TEWL value significantly decreased in comparison with the pre-study value ($p<0.05$). Subsequently, the values in the adapalene and placebo groups were significantly higher than after the third session of CP (Fig. **4**).

Changes in the Cornified Layer Water Content

There was no significant difference in the cornified layer water content before and after this study.

Safety

During the study period, there were no side effects of CP. In the adapalene group, more than 90% (21/23) of the patients complained of dryness, desquamation, erythema, or

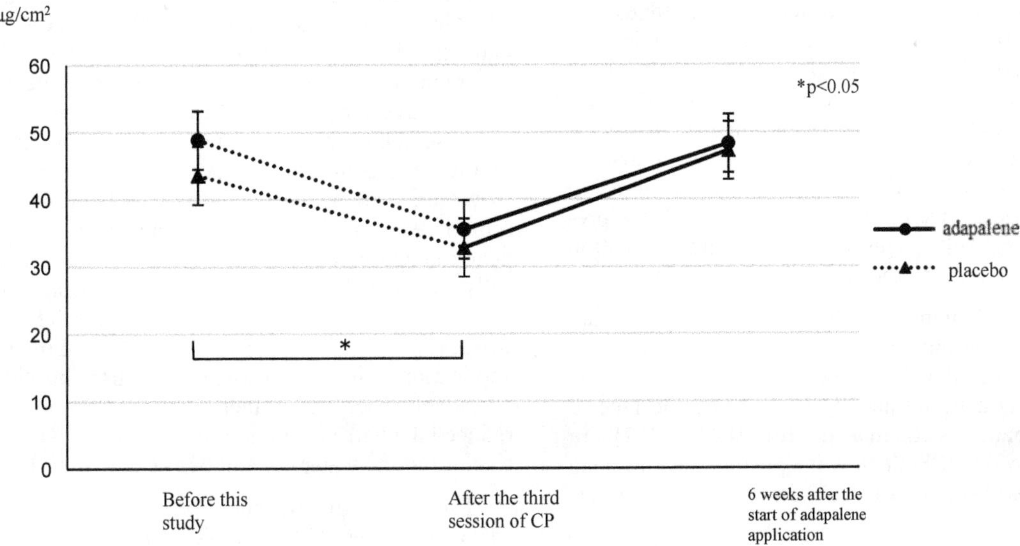

Fig. (3). Changes in the sebum secretion (N=23).

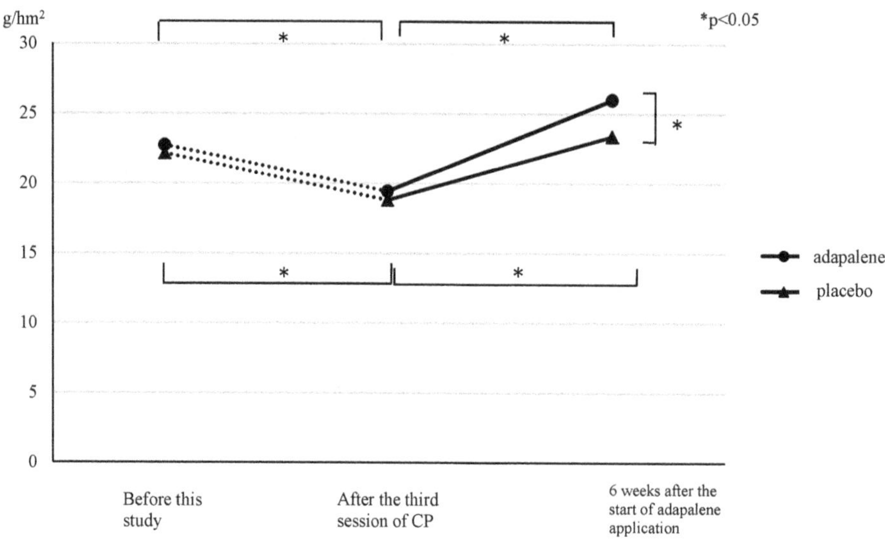

Fig. (4). Changes in the TEWL (N=23).

irritation within 2 weeks. However, in all patients, it was possible to continue treatment until the completion of this study.

DISCUSSION

Recently, patients have been strongly interested in acne treatment, and acne has been reviewed as an important dermal disease. Chemical peeling shows immediate actions on acne vulgaris, and its results are satisfactory for females and young patients, who have a strong esthetic sense. According to several studies, CP with glycolic acid significantly decreases the lesion count 2 weeks after the start of treatment; glycolic acid may exhibit more immediate actions compared to adapalene [10,11]. However, as a limitation of CP, continuous visits are required, which is stressful. In this study, we examined the usefulness of adapalene application as maintenance therapy following CP with glycolic acid. After the third session of CP, both inflammatory and non-inflammatory lesion significantly reduced. Subsequently, adapalene was applied for 6 weeks. The lesion count slightly increased with no statistical significance 2 to 4 weeks after the start of application, but there was a significant decrease in comparison with the pre-study value. These results suggest that adapalene application is useful for maintaining the therapeutic effects of CP.

Acne is often thought to affect the teenaged group. However, a significant number of patients either continue to experience acne or develop new-onset acne after the teenaged years. As acne frequently develops on the face, it influences the patient's quality of life (QOL) [12]. In particular, QOL of most patients with post adolescent acne markedly reduces because of their strong esthetic sense [12,13].

In this study, the mean age of subjects are 25.3±5.8 (standard deviation) years, mostof who have post-adlescent acne [14]. Irregular menstruation, mental stress, and hormones, especially androgen, are closely involved in post-adlescent acne [15]. Androgen acts on the sebaceous gland, promoting sebum production and leading to comedones formation through the excessive cornification of hair follicles. Furthermore, marked mental stress enhances the production of corticotropin-releasing and adrenocorticotropic hormones, increasing the secretion of androgen. As a result, acne exacerbates, reducing the treatment responsiveness [15].

For physiological skin function analysis, the sebum secretion, TEWL, and cornified layer water content were measured before this study, after the third session of CP, and after the completion of this study. The sebum secretion significantly decreased after the third session of CP. Subsequently, it increased after the application of adapalene/a placebo. As the facial secretion of sebum in patients with acne is higher than in healthy adults, sebum secretion is associated with the onset of acne [16]. Several studies have reported that retinoid/hormonal/laser therapies decrease sebum secretion through the destruction/reduction of the sebaceous gland, leading to the remission of acne. However, there are few studies on a CP-related decrease in sebum secretion [17]. A study indicated that glycolic acid penetratedpores of the skin, acting on the sebaceous gland cells and contributing to a decrease in sebum secretion [17]. There was a significant decrease in the TEWL after CP, whereas there was a significant increase following adapalene application. This was possibly because the side effects of adapalene, such as erythema, desquamation, and dryness, reduced the barrier function of the skin [9,18]. There were no changes in the water content before and after this study.

The results of this study suggest that the application of adapalene after CP remission of acne treatment is an effective acne treatment method to maintain and further improve treatment effect and adherence in patients wishing to completely cure acne earlier.

CONFLICT OF INTEREST

Adapalene and placebo were given by Galderma R&D, France.

ACKNOWLEDGEMENTS

Funding for this study was provided by Galderma R&D, Tokyo.

REFERENCES

[1] Arnold Odom J. William LAndrew's Diseases of the skin Clinical Dermatology. 8th ed. Philadelphia: Harcourt Brace Jovanovich, Inc. 1990; pp. 250-7.

[2] Miyachi Y, Hayashi N, Furukawa F, *et al.* Acne management in Japan: study of patient adherence. Dermatology 2011; 223(2): 174-81.

[3] Shimizu H. Shimizu's Textbook of Dermatology. Tokyo: Nakayama Ltd 2007; pp. 316-9.

[4] Harold J. Chemical Peeling and Resurfacing. St.Louis: Mosby Inc 1997; pp. 94-100.

[5] Yamamoto Y, Funasaka Y, Matsunaga K, *et al.* Guidelines for chemical peeling in Japan (3rd edition). J Dermatol 2011; 38: 1-5.

[6] Hayashi N, Akamatsu H, Iwatsuki K, *et al.* The guideline for the treatment of acne vulgaris. Jpn J Dermatol 2004; 14: 195-202.

[7] Hayashi N, Akamatsu H, Kawashima M, *et al.* Establishment of grading criteria for acne severity. J Dermatol 2008; 35(5): 255-60.

[8] Michel S, Jomard A, Demarchez M. Pharamacology of adapalene. Br J Dermatol 1998; 139: 3-7

[9] Kawashima M, Harada S, Christian Loesche, *et al.* Adapalene gel 0.1% is effective and safe for Japanese patients with acne vulgaris: A ranomized, multicenter, investigator-blinded, controlled study. J Dermatol Sci 2008; 49(3): 241-8.

[10] Hayashi N, Kawashima M. The usefulness of chemical peeling with 30% glycolic acid (pH1.5) for acne vulgaris. Jpn J Clinic Dermatol 2003; 57: 1213-6 (in Japanese).

[11] Kishioka A, Yamamoto Y, Miyazaki T, *et al.* Clinical evaluation of chemical peeling with glycolic acid for acne. Aesthet Dermatol 2004; 14: 195-202.

[12] Hayashi N, Higaki Y, Kawamoto K, *et al.* A crosssectional analysis of quality of life in Japanese acne patients using the Japanese version of Skinde-16. J Dermatol 2004; 31(12): 971-6.

[13] Golden V, Clark SM, Cunliffe WJ. Post-adolescent-acne : a review of clinical features. Br J Dermatol 1997; 136(1): 66-70.

[14] Chiristina W, Layton AM. Persistent acne in woman. Am J Clin Dermatol 2006; 7(5): 281-90.

[15] George R, Clarke S, Thompson EB, *et al.* Hormonal therapy for acne. Semin Cutan Med Surg 2008; 27(3): 188-96.

[16] Watanabe R, Ito M. The structure and functional of sebaceous glands Aesthet Dermatol 2009; 19: 155-9 (abstract in English).

[17] Lee SH, Huh CH, Park KC, Youn SW.Effects of repetitive superficial chemical peels on facial sebum secretion in acne patients. J Eur Acad Dermatol Venereol 2006; 20: 964-8.

[18] Yonei N, Yamamoto Y, Kaminaka C, *et al.* Effect of chemical peeling with Keisei jorbi GA gel in treatment of acne vugaris, lichen pilaris, and postinflammatory pigmentation in aopic dermatitis. Aesthet Dermatol 2002; 12: 103-8 (abstract in English).

The Use of Topical Calcineurin Inhibitors in Atopic Dermatitis

Annie Crissinger[1] and Nicholas V. Nguyen[*,2]

[1]*Department of Pharmacy, Cleveland Clinic Foundation, Cleveland, OH, USA*

[2]*Department of Dermatology, University of Colorado, Aurora, CO, USA*

Abstract: In recent years, two topical calcineurin inhibitors have emerged as effective alternatives to corticosteroids for the treatment of atopic dermatitis. Decisions regarding first line therapy between pimecrolimus and tacrolimus are often based on anecdotal evidence. Herein, we review the current evidence supporting the use of pimecrolimus and tacrolimus in atopic dermatitis as well as key differences in safety, tolerability, and cost between the drugs.

Keywords: Atopic dermatitis, calcineurin inhibitors, pimecrolimus, tacrolimus.

BACKGROUND

Atopic dermatitis (AD) is a chronic condition that affects 10-20% of children living in developed nations [1]. Implicated in the multifactorial etiology of AD are genetic, environmental, and immunologic factors [1,2]. In susceptible individuals, external allergens or irritants may trigger an immune response that involves T-cells, dendritic cells, mast cells, and proinflammatory cytokines [3]. The pruritic nature of AD may lead to a vicious "itch-scratch" cycle, further aggravating the flares, and leading to inflammation, infection, and scarring. Recent studies have linked the presence of null mutations of the gene encoding filaggrin, a filament-aggregation protein important to the development of a healthy epidermal barrier, to an increased susceptibility of developing AD [4].

For years, topical corticosteroids have remained the mainstay of pharmacological treatment for AD. When prescribed appropriately, cutaneous and systemic adverse effects are rare. However, chronic use, particularly of high potency topical steroids and particularly on areas such as the face, neck, and intertriginous areas, has been limited by a propensity to cause cutaneous atrophy. Topical steroids may also cause or exacerbate rosacea and perioral dermatitis [1,5,6]. Systemic side effects, such as reduced bone density and growth and hypothalamic-pituitary-adrenal axis suppression are theoretical concerns in children as their higher body surface area-to-weight ratio puts them at increased risk for systemic absorption. Additionally, risk of relapse after discontinuation of treatment and steroid tachyphylaxis must be considered when using a corticosteroid in the treatment of AD. Given the potential for these adverse effects, coupled with the high prevalence of parental "steroid phobia," there remains a need for safe and effective therapeutic alternatives for the treatment of AD.

In recent years, two topical calcineurin inhibitors have emerged as effective alternatives to corticosteroids for the treatment of AD. Decisions regarding first line therapy between pimecrolimus and tacrolimus are often based on anecdotal evidence. Herein, we review the current evidence supporting the use of pimecrolimus and tacrolimus in atopic dermatitis as well as key differences in safety, tolerability, and cost between the drugs.

PHARMACOLOGY

Tacrolimus and pimecrolimus are classified as topical calcineurin inhibitors (TCIs). Topical application reduces inflammation by inhibition of T-cells. Both drugs bind the FK binding protein-12 (FKBP12) to inhibit calcineurin, a protein phosphatase responsible for the dephosphorylation of the nuclear factor of activated T-cells (NF-AT). Without dephosphorylation, NF-AT cannot be translocated into the nucleus, and thus the production of inflammatory interleukins is inhibited [7]. Adjunctive mechanisms of action have been proposed for tacrolimus including binding at cell surface steroid receptors, inhibition of mast cell mediator release, and downregulation of chemoattractant IL-8 receptors, intracellular adhesion molecule-1, E-selectin, and Langerhans cells IgE receptors [8-11]. Pimecrolimus has also been shown to prevent the release of pro-inflammatory mediators from both human cutaneous mast cells and rodent cell lines [7,12,13]. In addition to their effects on T-cells, NF-AT and calcineurin are involved in keratinocyte differentiation. Tacrolimus and pimecrolimus have been shown to produce sustained improvements of epidermal barrier function [14,15].

PHARMACOKINETICS

Topical application of tacrolimus in pediatric and adult patients rarely produces serum tacrolimus levels in excess of 2 ng/mL. In point of fact, the AUC produced by this serum level is 30-fold below the levels seen with oral immunosuppressive doses used in transplant patients [9]. Similar results are seen in pharmocokinetic studies of adult patients on pimecrolimus, where levels above 1.4 ng/mL

*Address correspondence to this author at the Department of Dermatology, University of Colorado, 1655 Aurora Ct, Mail Stop F703, ACP Rm 3233, Aurora, CO 80045-0510, USA; E-mail: nicholas.v.nguyen@ucdenver.edu

were not observed after topical administration [16]. These findings were validated by a study involving 22 infants, where blood levels were below 2 ng/ml in 96% of blood samples, with the highest concentration measured at 2.26 ng/ml [17]. These levels are far below the pimecrolimus levels required for systemic immunomodulation (≥15 ng/ml) [18]. Both drugs are metabolized by the CYP3A-subfamily of metabolizing enzymes and are primarily eliminated through the feces. There are no clinically significant differences in the distribution, metabolism, and elimination of the two drugs [9,16].

INDICATIONS

Topical tacrolimus and pimecrolimus have been developed for use as short-term treatment of atopic dermatitis or intermittently as chronic therapy in adults and children over the age of 2 years. Currently, both are indicated for second-line treatment in patients who have not exhibited an adequate response to topical corticosteroid treatments or in those in which such treatments are contraindicated. The 0.03% tacrolimus ointment is FDA-approved for use in adults and children over the age of 2 years, while the 0.1% formulation is approved for adult use only [9,16].

EFFICACY

Pimecrolimus Versus Vehicle

Pimecrolimus was first shown to be effective in the short-term management of AD in a 3-week trial comparing pimecrolimus 1% cream to vehicle in 34 adults with moderate to severe AD. A twice-daily application proved to be significantly more effective than both the once-daily treatment and treatment with vehicle without any notable side effects [19]. Significant improvements in eczema area and severity index (EASI) scores along with rapid onset of action further established the usefulness of pimecrolimus in the treatment of AD in pediatric patients. In a 20-week, randomized, 3-phase trial, Kaufmann *et al.* studied twice daily pimecrolimus 1% compared to vehicle in 196 patients ages 3 months to 23 months with mild to severe atopic AD [20]. For the first 4 weeks of the trial treatment was double-blinded, followed by 12 weeks of open-label pimecrolimus. The trial concluded with a 4 week follow-up period. Treatment with pimecrolimus 1% reduced the mean EASI by 71.5% compared with an increase of 19.4% with vehicle at 4 weeks ($P < 0.001$). Differences in EASI scores between groups were significant by day four of the trial. Response to pimecrolimus was maintained throughout the 12 week open-label period without any significant difference in side effects between the two groups. After discontinuation, symptoms of atopic dermatitis gradually returned in the 4 week follow-up period.

Eichenfield and colleagues [21] performed two identical phase III, randomized, vehicle-controlled, multi-center 6 week studies evaluating the safety and efficacy of pimecrolimus 1% cream when used to treat mild to moderate AD in children and adolescents. The studies included 403 pediatric patients from 2-17 years old. At baseline, patients' EASI scores were determined, and patients were further evaluated for disease severity based on the Investigator's Global Assessment (IGA) score, pruritis severity, and subjective assessment of disease control. At study entry, 59% of patients were classified with moderate disease according to the IGA score and the mean body surface area (BSA) affected was 26%. After a seven day treatment with a basic, bland emollient cream, patients were randomized to treatment with twice daily 1% pimecrolimus or vehicle for 6 weeks. Patients were evaluated for treatment response at weekly visits, with the primary efficacy endpoint being the IGA score. Successful therapy was defined as a decrease from a score of 2 to 3 (mild to moderate) to 0 to 1 (clear to almost clear). Significant improvements in IGA score were observed at the first follow-up visit on day 8, with 12% of the pimecrolimus group being rated as clear or almost clear compared to only 2.2% of the vehicle group. Ninety-six percent of the pimecrolimus group either maintained their IGA scores or showed improvement compared to only 80% of the vehicle group.

The efficacy of pimecrolimus for long-term management of AD has been demonstrated adults, infants, and children in multiple trials ranging from 6 months to 2 years [22-27]. In a two year study, Papp *et al.* demonstrated a reduction in EASI of more than 80% at 12 months, which was sustained in the 1-year open-label follow up [28].

Additionally, pimecrolimus has been shown to work particularly well for lesions on the face and neck, areas prone to adverse effects of corticosteroids [21,22,29]. Murrell *et al.* [29] compared pimecrolimus to vehicle in a 12-week trial involving 200 patients ages 12 years and older with mild to moderate head and neck AD intolerant of, or dependent on, topical corticosteroids. Compared to vehicle cream a significantly higher percentage of patients treated with pimecrolimus were cleared or almost cleared of facial AD. Notably, pimecrolimus use was associated with a reversal in skin thinning in patients with skin atrophy from prior corticosteroid use.

Tacrolimus Versus Vehicle

Tacrolimus is indicated for use in both adult and pediatric patients with moderate to severe atopic dermatitis based on the results of three randomized, double-blind, vehicle-controlled, multi-center phase III studies [30,31]. In phase III trials, patients were treated for 12 weeks with either tacrolimus ointment 0.03%, tacrolimus ointment 0.1%, or a vehicle ointment applied twice daily. The pediatric study involved 351 patients between the ages of 2 and 15 years old, and the two adult studies totaled 632 patients between the ages of 15 and 79 years old. The primary efficacy endpoint was improvement based on the physician's global evaluation of clinical response. Results were similar in all three trials; a significantly greater percentage of patients in the tacrolimus groups achieved at least 90% improvement ($P<0.001$ in both pediatric and adult studies). While the pediatric study did not provide evidence that tacrolimus 0.1% ointment was more effective than the 0.03% ointment, the adult studies suggested that the higher strength may be more effective in adult patients with more severe disease at baseline and higher BSA.

Tacrolimus has also proved useful in the long-term treatment of AD and as prophylactic treatment to prevent disease flares. Recently, a 52-week trial studied the effects of tacrolimus applied three times a week in 197 adult and pediatric patients (>2 years old) with at least moderate AD as rated on the Physician's Static Global Assessment (PSGA) scale [32]. In phase I of the trial, patients were first randomized to double-blinded, twice-daily treatment of either tacrolimus ointment (0.03% for pediatric patients and 0.1% for adult patients) or a corticosteroid (alclometasone dipropionate ointment 0.05% for pediatric patients or triamcinolone acetonide ointment 0.1% for adult patients) for 4 days. In the next 12 weeks of phase I, patients were treated with open-label tacrolimus ointment twice daily, the strength of the ointment once again dependent on the age of the patient. Patients were eligible to enter the phase II of the trial if a PSGA scale of 0-1 (clear to almost clear) was achieved. Of the 383 patients who participated in phase I, 197 were eligible to participate in phase II. In phase II of the trial, patients were randomized to double-blind treatment of either a continuation of three-times weekly application of tacrolimus ointment or a vehicle ointment (2:1) for 40 weeks. Disease relapse (PSGA score > 2) was treated with open-label tacrolimus ointment twice daily. If a PSGA score of 0-1 was not achieved within 8 weeks of relapse, patients discontinued the trial. A significant difference between the tacrolimus group compared to the vehicle group was found for the primary efficacy endpoint in phase II: The mean number of flare-free treatment days was 177 for tacrolimus and 134 for vehicle (P=0.003). Patients treated with tacrolimus also experienced a longer time to first relapse compared to the vehicle groups (169 *vs* 43 days, respectively, P=0.037).

Topical Calcineurin Inhibitors Versus Topical Corticosteroids

Ashcroft *et al.* [33] in 2005, performed a meta-analysis comparing the efficacy and tolerability of the TCIs to that of vehicle and topical corticosteroids. Twenty-five randomized controlled trials were included in this analysis, involving 6897 adults, infants, and children. As expected, both tacrolimus and pimecrolimus were found to be superior to vehicle. When compared to betamethasone valerate 0.1%, pimecrolimus was found to be significantly less effective after three weeks of treatment (rate ratio 0.22, 0.09-0.54) on the proportion of patients determined to be clear or almost clear. Pimecrolimus was also compared to the use of a combined treatment of triamcinolone acetonide 0.1% to the trunk and hydrocortisone acetate 1% to face, neck, and intertriginous areas. The corticosteroid treatment was found to be significantly more effective after one week, three weeks, and six months, but there was no significant difference between the two groups at the end of the 12 month treatment period.

Tacrolimus was also compared to corticosteroids. Compared to hydrocortisone acetate 1%, both tacrolimus 0.03% and 0.1% were found to be significantly more effective at three weeks of treatment (rate ratios 2.56, 1.95 to 3.36 and 3.05, 2.12-4.40, respectively). When used on the face and neck, tacrolimus 0.1% was more effective than aclometasone dipropionate 0.1% for the proportion of patients achieving at least marked improvement of greater than 75% (rate ratio 3.94, 2.21 to 7.00). Compared to more potent corticosteroids (hydrocortisone butyrate 0.1% and betamethasone valerate 0.1%), tacrolimus 0.1% was found to be equally effective at 3 weeks. Tacrolimus 0.03% was compared only to hydrocortisone butyrate 0.1% and found to be significantly less effective. Based on the results of this study, tacrolimus is more effective than pimecrolimus when compared to topical corticosteroids.

Tacrolimus Versus Pimecrolimus

In their meta-analysis, Ashcroft *et al.* confirmed the findings of previous studies, which indicated both tacrolimus and pimecrolimus are superior to vehicle. When compared to topical corticosteroids, however, tacrolimus appeared to perform better than pimecrolimus. A head-to-head trial between tacrolimus and pimecrolimus and a more recent meta-analysis validate these findings.

In 2005, Paller *et al.* [34] conducted three multicenter, investigator-blinded, 6-week studies, in which 1065 patients were randomized to twice daily treatment with either tacroliumus or pimecrolimus. Two of the studies included pediatric patients added 2 to 15 years, with one study including patients with AD classified as mild in severity by the IGA scale and the other study including patients with moderate to very severe disease. The other study included patients above the age of 16 years with mild to very severe AD. Following a 4-week washout period, patients were randomized to their study medications: Picrolimus 1%, tacrolimus 0.1%, or tacrolimus 0.03% if in the pediatric group with mild AD. Patients were to apply the medication twice daily for up to 6 weeks, or at least one week, until the affected area was completely cleared. At the end of treatment the percentage of improvement, by reduction of the EASI score, was significantly greater for tacrolimus than for pimecrolimus in adults (54.1% *vs* 34.9%, respectively; P<0.0001) in pediatric patients with moderate to very severe AD (67.2% *vs* 56.4%, respectively; P=0.04) and in the combined analysis (52.8% *vs* 39.1%, respectively; P<0.0001). At week 1 of treatment a significant difference was found in the pediatric mild AD study with a greater percentage of improvement from baseline in the tacrolimus group compared to the pimecrolimus group (39.2% *vs* 31.2%, respectively; P=0.04). Tacrolimus also showed significantly greater improvements in patients' itch scores and reductions in %BSA affected. In all three studies the most common adverse events were application site reactions. Overall, adverse event profiles were similar in both tacrolimus and pimecrolimus groups. However, in the adult study, patients treated with tacrolimus experienced more application site burning compared to patients treated with pimecrolimus (11.4% *vs* 4.9%, respectively, P=0.02). The authors concluded that tacrolimus is more effective than pimecrolimus with a similar safety profile.

A recent meta-analysis of 20 randomized clinical trials was performed to evaluate the safety and efficacy of tacrolimus and pimecrolimus for the treatment of AD in pediatric patients [35]. The 20 studies, involving 6288 patients, included 10 trials comparing the use of tacrolimus to vehicle or corticosteroids, 7 trials comparing the use of pimecrolimus to vehicle or corticosteroids, and 3 trials comparing the two calcineurin inhibitors to each other. The results of the analysis showed that, while both pimecrolimus and tacrolimus were effective in the treatment of AD in pediatric patients, tacrolimus was superior pimecrolimus.

SAFETY CONSIDERATIONS

Topical calcineurin inhibitors may be locally irritating producing burning and pruritus. Both events occur more frequently with tacrolimus [9,16,36]; however, in most cases, the burning sensations are mild and resolve within 1 to 8 days of drug use [37]. Systemically, calcineurin inhibitors produce immunosuppression, nephrotoxicity, and hypertension. However, these adverse effects are seen at serum concentration much greater than those produced from topical use.

Controversy exists regarding the use of TCIs in Netherton syndrome (NS), a syndrome in which impaired skin integrity often results in significant absorption of medications applied topically. In a small case series, 2 of 3 Netherton syndrome patients treated with tacrolimus ointment 0.1% showed marked improvement. All 3 patients demonstrated serum tacrolimus levels within the therapeutic range for organ transplant patients, however, none showed signs of tacrolimus toxicity [38]. A more recent study involving 4 patients with NS failed to validate these findings, demonstrating serum levels ranging from undetectable to 2.7 ng/ml [39]. Pimecrolimus 1% cream also proved to be effective and well tolerated in 3 children with NS. Blood levels ranged from 0.625-7.08 ng/ml, much lower than anticipated when applied to 50% of BSA [40]. In small case series, TCIs have been safe and effective treatments for NS. Larger studies are needed before even tentative conclusions regarding safety and efficacy can be made.

In 2006, the FDA approved the addition of a black box warning for the calcineurin inhibitors, tacrolimus and pimecrolimus. The warning was added because of concerns of a potential link between use of these agents and development of malignancy. These concerns were prompted by reports of cutaneous neoplasms and lymphomas in animal studies and postmarketing case reports. When used as long-term treatment as part of an immunosuppressive regimen, calcineurin inhibitors may increase the risk of developing lymphomas and non-melanotic skin cancers [41,42]. Theoretically, topical preparations could carry the same risk if absorbed sufficiently into the system; however, as evidenced by the aforementioned pharmacokinetic data, this is rarely the case. Conceivably cutaneous lymphomas, particularly cutaneous T-cell lymphoma (CTCL), may masquerade as dermatitis resulting in treatment with a TCI. Upon treatment failure, biopsy of the lesion may lead to discovery of a cutaneous lymphoma, but it would be impossible to determine if lymphoma was caused by the medication or if the condition had been initially misdiagnosed [43].

Based on this data, the FDA concluded that a casual relationship between topical calcineurin inhibitors and development of malignancy has not been established, but that continuous long-term use should be avoided, and TCIs should not be used in children under the age of 2. It is recommended by the American Academy of Dermatology Association Task Force, that tacrolimus and pimecrolimus should remain therapeutic options in AD as they are currently indicated. Although an increased risk of lymphoma with topical use is unlikely, there is potential concern if the medications are to be used on larger areas for lengthy periods of time [43].

DRUG INTERACTIONS

In light of topical administration and minimal systemic absorption, the incidence of significant drug-drug interactions is low. No formal studies have been performed on drug interactions with TCIs. Nonetheless, systemic interactions are still possible, so caution should be used when administering them with CYP3A4 inhibitors including, but not limited to, erythromycin, azole-based antifungals, calcium channel blockers and cimetidine [9,16]. It has also been reported that alcohol consumption during topical tacrolimus therapy can result in facial flushing, irritation, pruritis, and periocular edema [44].

CONTRAINDICATIONS AND PRECAUTIONS

Topical calcineurin inhibitors should be used with caution in patients with Netherton syndrome due to the potential for increased systemic absorption. Safety in patients with erythroderma has yet to be determined. Safety studies have also not been performed on either drug in patients with viral or bacterial skin infections, however, in preliminary studies, TCIs were associated with an increased risk of cutaneous bacterial and viral infections including herpetic infections. Thus, the manufacturer recommends resolution of existing infections prior to initiation of therapy. In animal photo-carcinogenicity studies, TCIs shortened the time to skin tumor formation. Thus, patients should be counseled to limit their exposure to UV radiation during treatment [9,16].

PATIENT MONITORING GUIDELINES

Patients should be regularly evaluated for clinical improvement. If there is not adequate improvement after six weeks of therapy, then a reassessment of diagnosis and therapy choice is recommended. Patients that develop lymphadenopathy should be monitored for the resolution of this condition [9,16].

DRUG DOSING AND ADMINISTRATION

Table **1** lists manufacturer recommended drug dosing and administration guidelines. When applying either drug, patients should rub the drug in gently and completely to clean, dry skin. Patients should not use occlusive dressings as they may promote systemic absorption. Tacrolimus and pimecrolimus should be discontinued upon clearance of active disease [9,16].

PRODUCT AVAILABILITY AND AVERAGE WHOLESALE PRICE

Table **2** lists the average wholesale price (AWP) for Protopic (tacrolimus) and Elidel (pimecrolimus). Although daily cost calculations can be complicated by the variability of the size of affected areas and amount applied to those areas, it can be reasonably predicted that a one-gram dose is sufficient for the average patient. Using the FDA-approved twice-daily dosing, a 60 gram tube would constitute a month's supply. Thus, the predicted daily cost of Elidel and Protopic is \$16.52 and \$16.99, respectively. Using the 60 gram

Table 1. Dosing and Administration of TCIs

Tacrolimus [9]	Pimecrolimus [16]
Adults: Apply a minimal amount of 0.03% or 0.1% ointment to the affected area twice daily. Pediatric patients (≥2 yo): Use only the 0.03% ointment twice daily.	Adults and Pediatric (≥ 2 yo) patients: Apply a thin layer of 1% cream to the affected area twice daily.

Table 2. AWP of TCIs

AWP as of April 2010 [45]	Protopic 0.03%	Protopic 0.1%	Elidel 1%
30 g tube	$254.87	$254.87	$247.79
60 g tube	$509.75	$509.75	$495.57
100 g tube	$849.58	$849.58	$825.94

tube as a reference, the Protopic products are 3% more expensive than Elidel.

SUMMARY AND FINAL RECOMMENDATION

Topical corticosteroids are the established gold standard for the treatment of atopic dermatitis. But given an unfavorable side effect profile when used improperly, coupled with the high prevalence of parental "steroid phobia," there remains a need for safe and effective therapeutic alternatives. In recent years, two topical calcineurin inhibitors have emerged as safe and effective alternatives to corticosteroids for the treatment of AD. Topical calcineurin inhibitors are particularly useful for patients intolerant of or dependant on corticosteroids. It is the authors' opinion that given the high cost of therapy compared to corticosteroids, TCIs should not be considered first line therapy for most patients with AD. However, they should be strongly considered when presented with a patient with existing steroid atrophy or a parent with a level of "steroid phobia" likely to result in non-compliance.

In clinical efficacy trials, tacrolimus was found to be more effective than pimecrolimus when compared to vehicle, representative corticosteroids, and pimecrolimus. For both drugs, twice daily treatment was superior to once daily application. Despite greater efficacy with the oil-based tacrolimus, the water-based pimecrolimus was better tolerated by patients. Furthermore, the predicted cost of pimecrolimus is 3% less than that of tacrolimus. To ensure treatment compliance, decisions regarding first line therapy between pimecrolimus and tacrolimus should be made on a case-by-case basis, considering cost and tolerability issues. One might consider using pimecrolimus during the day and tacrolimus at night for those patients who prefer a water-based cream but respond best to tacrolimus.

With regards to safety, the FDA has issued black box warning for a possible increased risk of lymphomas in patients treated with TCIs. It should be noted that lymphomas were seen in animal studies with high serum concentration of drug. Theoretically, topical preparations could carry the same risk with sufficient systemic absorption; however, serum concentrations are very low with topical application. Although an increased risk of lymphoma with topical use is unlikely, there is potential concern if the medications are to be used on larger areas for lengthy periods of time. Thus, the clinician should be vigilant in this setting. While preliminary data regarding safety and efficacy in NS shows promise, long-term data in larger patient populations is necessary before even tentative conclusions can be made.

CONFLICT OF INTEREST

The authors confirm that this article content has no conflict of interest.

ACKNOWLEDGEMENTS

Declared none.

REFERENCES

[1] Levy ML. Atopic dermatitis: Understanding the disease and its management. Curr Med Res Opin 2007; 23(12): 3091-103.

[2] Cork MJ, Robinson DA, Vasilopoulos Y, *et al.* New perspectives on epidermal barrier dysfunction in atopic dermatitis: Gene-environment interactions. J Allergy Clin Immunol 2006; 118: 3-21.

[3] Akidis CA, Akdis M, Bieber T, *et al.* Diagnosis and treatment of atopic dermatitis in children and adults: European Academy of Allergology and Clinical Immunology/American Academy of Allergy, Asthma, and Immunology/PRACTALL consensus report. Allergy 2006; 61(8): 969-87.

[4] McGrath JA. Filaggrin and the great epidermal barrier grief. Australas J Dermatol 2008; 49: 67-73.

[5] Krakowski AC, Dohil MA. Topical therapy in pediatric atopic dermatitis. Semin Cutan Med Surg 2008; 27: 161-7.

[6] Charman C, Williams H. The use of corticosteroids and corticosteroid phobia in atopic dermatitis. Clin Dermatol 2003; 21: 193-200.

[7] Grassberger M, Baumruker T, Enz A, *et al.* A novel anti-inflammatory drug, SDZ ASM 981, for the treatment of skin diseases: *In vitro* pharmacology. Br J Dermatol 1999; 141: 264-73.

[8] Novak N, Bieber T. The role of dendritic cell subtypes in the pathophysiology of atopic dermatitis. J Am Acad Dermatol 2005; 53(S2): 171S-6S.

[9] Protopic [package insert]. Deerfield, IL: Astellas Pharma; 2009.

[10] Panhans-Gross A, Novak N, Kraft S, Bieber T. Human epidermal Langerhans' cells are targets for the immunosuppressive macrolide tacrolimus (FK506). J Allergy Clin Immunol 2001; 107(2): 345-52.

[11] Wollenberg A, Sharma S, von Bubnoff D, Geiger E, Haberstok J, Bieber T. Topical tacrolimus (FK506) leads to profound phenotypic and functional alterations of epidermal antigen-presenting dendritic cells in atopic dermatitis. J Allergy Clin Immunol 2001; 107(3): 519-25.

[12] Hultsch T, Muller KD, Meingassner JG, Grassberger M, Schopf RE, Knop J. Ascomycin macrolactam derivative SDZ ASM 981 inhibits the release of granule-associated mediators and of newly

synthesized cytokines in RBL 2H3 mast cells in an immunophilin-dependent manner. Arch Dermatol Res 1998; 290: 501-7.

[13] Zuberbier T, Chong SU, Grunow K, *et al.* The ascomycin macrolactam pimecrolimus (Elidel, SDZ ASM 981) is a potent inhibitor of mediator release from human dermal mast cells and peripheral blood basophils. J Allergy Clin Immunol 2001; 108: 275-80.

[14] Proksch E, Jensen J, Braeutigam M, *et al.* Pimecrolimus but not corticosteroid improves the skin barrier in atopic dermatitis. J Invest Dermatol 2008; 128: S104.

[15] Xhauflaire-Uhoda E, Thirion L, Pierard-Franchimont C, Pierard GE. Comparative effect of tacrolimus and betamethasone valerate on the passive sustainable hydration of the stratum corneum in atopic dermatitis. Dermatol 2007; 214: 328-32.

[16] Elidel [package insert]. East Hanover, NJ: Novartis Pharmaceuticals Corp.; 2009.

[17] Staab D, Pariser D, Gottlieb AB, *et al.* Low systemic absorption and good tolerability of pimecrolimus, administered as 1% cream (Elidel) in infants with atopic dermatitis—a multicenter, 3-week, open-label study. Pediatr Dermatol 2005; 22: 465-71.

[18] Wolff K, Fleming C, Hanifin J, *et al.* Efficacy and tolerability of three different doses of oral pimecrolimus in the treatment of moderate-to-severe atopic dermatitis: A randomized controlled trial. Br J Dermatol 2005; 152: 1296-303.

[19] Van Leent EJ, Graber M, Thurston M, Wagenaar A, Spuls PI, Bos JD. Effectiveness of the ascomycin macrolactam SDZ ASM 981 in the topical treatment of atopic dermatitis. Arch Dermatol 1998; 134: 805-9.

[20] Kaufmann R, Floster-Holst R, Hoger P, *et al.* Onset of action of pimecrolimus cream 1% in the treatment of atopic eczema in infants. J Allergy Clin Immunol 2004; 114: 1183-8.

[21] Eichenfield LF, Lucky A, Boguniewicz M, *et al.* Safety and efficacy of pimecrolimus (ASM 981) cream 1% in the treatment of mild and moderate atopic dermatitis in children and adolescents. J Am Acad Dermatol 2002; 46: 495-504.

[22] Zuberbier T, Heinzerling L, Bieber T, Schauer U, Klebs S, Brautigam M. Steroid-sparing effect of pimecrolimus cream 1% in children with severe atopic dermatitis. Dermatol 2007; 215: 325-30.

[23] Meurer M, Folster-Holst R, Wozel G, Weidinger G, Junger M, Brautigam M. Pimecrolimus cream in the long-term management of atopic dermatitis in adults: A six-month study. Dermatol 2002; 205: 271-7.

[24] Wahn U, Bos JD, Goodfield M, *et al.* Efficacy and safety of pimecrolimus cream in the long-term management of atopic dermatitis in children. Pediatrics 2002; 110: e2.

[25] Kapp A, Papp K, Bingham A, *et al.* Long-term management of atopic dermatitis in infacts with topical pimecrolimus, a nonsteroid anti-inflammatory drug. J Allergy Clin Immunol 2002; 110: 277-84.

[26] Simon D, Lubbe J, Wuthrich B, *et al.* Benefits from the use of a pimecrolimus-based treatment in the management of atopic dermatitis in clinical practice. Analysis of a Swiss cohort. Dermatol 2006; 213: 313-8.

[27] Ehrchen J, Sunderkotter C, Luger T, Steinhoff M. Calcineurin inhibitors for the treatment of atopic dermatitis. Expert Opin Pharmacother 2008; 9(17): 3009-23.

[28] Papp KA, Werfel T, Folster-Holst R, *et al.* Long-term control of atopic dermatitis with pimecrolimus cream 1% in infants and young children: a two-year study. J Am Acad Dermatol 2005; 52: 240-6.

[29] Murrell DF, Calvieri S, Ortonne JP, *et al.* A randomized controlled trial of pimecrolimus cream 1% in adolescents and adults with head and neck atopic dermatitis and intolerant of, or dependent on, topical corticosteroids. Br J Dematol 2007; 157: 954-59.

[30] Henifin JM, Ling MR, Langley R, Breneman D, Rafal E. Tacrolimus ointment for the treatment of atopic dermatitis in adult patients. J Am Acad Dermatol 2001; 44: S28-S38.

[31] Paller A, Eichenfield LF, Leung DY, Stewart D, Appell M. A 12-week study of tacrolimus ointment for the treatment of atopic dermatitis in pediatric patients. J Am Acad Dermatol 2001; 44: S47-S57.

[32] Breneman D, Fleischer AB Jr, Abramovits W, *et al.* Intermittent therapy for flare prevention and long-term disease control in stabilized atopic dermatitis: A randomized comparison of 3-times-weekly applications of tacrolimus ointment versus vehicle. J Am Acad Dermatol 2008; 58(6): 990-9.

[33] Ashcroft DM, Dimmock P, Garside R, Stein K, Williams HC. Efficacy and tolerability of topical pimecrolimus and tacrolimus in the treatment of atopic dermatitis: Meta-analysis of randomised controlled trials. BMJ 2005; 330: 516.

[34] Paller AS, Lebwohl M, Fleischer AB Jr, *et al.* Tacrolimus ointment is more effective then pimecrolimus cream with a similar safety profile in the treatment of atopic dermatitis: Results from 3 randomized, comparative studies. J Am Acad Dermatol 2005; 52(5): 810-22.

[35] Chen S, Yan J, Wang F. Two topical calcineurin inhibitors for the treatment of atopic dermatitis in pediatric patients: A meta-analysis of randomized clinical trials. J Dermatolog Treat 2010; 21(3): 144-56.

[36] Kempers S, Boguniewicz M, Carter E, *et al.* A randomized investigator-blinded study comparing pimecrolimus cream 1% with tacrolimus ointment 0.03% in the treatment of pediatric patients with moderate atopic dermatitis. J Am Acad Dermatol 2004; 51(4): 515-25.

[37] Reitamo S, Wollenburg A, Schopf E, *et al.* Safety and efficacy of 1 year tacrolimus ointment monotherapy in adults with atopic dermatitis. The European Tacrolimus Ointment Study Group. Arch Dermatol 2000; 136: 999-1006.

[38] Allen A, Siegfried E, Silverman R, *et al.* Significant absorption of topical tacrolimus in 3 patients with Netherton syndrome. Arch Dermatol 2001; 137: 747-50.

[39] Saif GB, Al-Khenaizan S. Netherton syndrome: Successful use of topical tacrolimus and pimecrolimus in four siblings. Int J Dermatol 2007; 46(3): 290-4.

[40] Yan AC, Honig PJ, Ming ME, Weber J, Shah KN. The safety and efficacy of pimecrolimus, 1% for the treatment of Netherton syndrome. Arch Dermatol 2010; 146(1): 57-62.

[41] Jonas S, Rayes N, Neumann U, *et al.* De novo malignancies after liver transplantation using tacrolimus-based protocols or cyclosporine-based quadruple immunosuppression with an interleukin-2 receptor antibody or antithymocyte globulin. Cancer 1997; 80(6): 1141-50.

[42] Callen J, Chamlin S, Eichenfield LF, *et al.* A systemic review of the safety of topical therapies for atopic dermatitis. Br J Dermatol 2007; 156(2): 203-21.

[43] Berger TG, Duvic M, Van Voorhees AS, VanBeek MJ, Frieden IJ. The use of topical calcineurin inhibitors in dermatology: Safety concerns. Report of the American Academy of Dermatology Association Task Force. J Am Acad Dermatol 2006; 54(5): 818-23.

[44] Knight AK, Boxer M, Chandler M. Alcohol-induced rash caused by topical tacrolimus. Ann Allergy Asthma Immunol 2005; 95: 291-2.

[45] Red Book Online: Available from: http://micromedex.com/redbook

Pressure Ulcer Associated with Critical Colonization Successfully Treated by Transient Usage of Cadexomer-Iodine

Shigeki Inui[*,1], Toshiko Harada[2] and Satoshi Itami[1]

[1]*Departments of Regenerative Dermatology Osaka University Graduate School of Medicine and* [2]*Takarazuka University School of Nursing, Japan*

Abstract: A 56-year-old Japanese man hospitalized for schizophrenia and depression developed pressure ulcer on his greater trochanter due to a long-term bed rest. In spite of applying 0.003% alprostadil alfadex ointment for two months, the ulcer was not improved. Because there was some purulent discharge, we examined semi-quantitative swab bacterial culture from the ulcer and subsequently detected quadrant III of bacteria. Then, 0.9% cadexomer-iodine ointment was applied once a day, resulting in decrease of the discharge and only quadrant I of bacteria culture. Thereafter, by application of polyurethane foams for two months, the wound was completely epithelized. The remarkable acceleration of wound healing after using cadexomer-iodine ointment suggested the initial critical colonization, which might have caused delayed healing.

Keywords: Pressure ulcer, critical colonization, cadexomer-iodine ointment.

INTRODUCTION

Chronic wounds are mostly contaminated with bacteria without harmful effect on healing process. However, when bacteria proliferate up to critical threshold of 10^5 bacteria per gram of tissue, increased toxins and inflammatory mediators may cause local tissue damage and consequently delay of wound healing [1]. This condition is referred as critical colonization. The prevalence of pressure ulcers among nursing home residents was reported to be 7% to 23% and the incidence of pressure ulcers is estimated to be 14/1000 patient-days among high-risk patients [2]. Further, one prospective study of 16 patients with pressure ulcers who were followed for 2184 days reported that the incidence of infection was 1.4 cases per 1000 patient-ulcer days [3]. However, the prevalence of critical colonization in pressure ulcers has not been reported possibly because the differential diagnosis is difficult between critical colonization and infection. Here, we report a case of pressure ulcer associated with critical colonization successfully treated by transient usage of cadexomer-iodine.

CASE PRESENTATION

A 56-year-old Japanese man hospitalized for schizophrenia and depression developed pressure ulcer on his greater trochanter due to a long-term bed rest. In spite of applying 0.003% alprostadil alfadex ointment (Prostandin® ointment 0.003%, Ono pharmaceutical Co. Ltd., Osaka, Japan) for two months, the ulcer was not improved (Fig. **1A**). Because there was some purulent discharge, we examined semi-quantitative swab bacterial culture from the ulcer. Briefly, the bacterial swabs were inoculated onto standard media in a Petri dish and serially diluted and streaked into four quadrants. Five days later, bacterial species isolated from the four quadrants were evaluated as scant (I, first quadrant), light (II, second quadrant), moderate (III, third quadrant), or heavy growth (IV, fourth quadrant). Then we detected quadrant III of *Streptococcus* agalactiae and *Bacteroides* fragilis, quadrant II of α-*Streptococcus*, and quadrant I of methicillin-sensitive *Staphylococcus* aureus (*MSSA*) and *Neisseria* species. Although there were no signs of infection but the purulent discharge, 0.9% cadexomer-iodine ointment was applied once a day for a week, resulting in decrease of the discharge (Fig. **1B**). Simultaneous semi-quantitative swab bacterial culture showed only quadrant I of *MSSA* and *Streptococcus agalactiae*. Then, the cadexomer-iodine ointment was withdrawn and polyurethane foams (HydroSite®, Smith & Nephew, London, UK) were applied. One month later the wound size gradually decreased (Fig. **1C**) and one more month later the wound was completely epithelized (Fig. **1D**). The remarkable acceleration of wound healing after using cadexomer-iodine ointment suggested the initial critical colonization, which might have caused delayed healing.

COMMENTS

Very recently, a standardized UPPER and LOWER mnemonic for wound infection checklist was developed to diagnose critical colonization and deep infection in a randomized controlled trial to evaluate an antimicrobial dressing with silver alginate powder [4]. The UPPER, which is associated with critical colonization, refers to the symptoms of unhealthy tissue, pain, poor healing, exudate and reek and at least 2 signs are required for the identification of critical colonization. On the other hand, the LOWER, associated with deep infection, refers to larger in size, osseous tissue, warmth, edema and redness. In our case

*Address correspondence to this author at the Departments of Regenerative Dermatology Osaka University Graduate School of Medicine, 2-2, G2, Yamadaoka, Suita-shi, Osaka 5650871, Japan;
E-mail: inui@r-derma.med.osaka-u.ac.jp

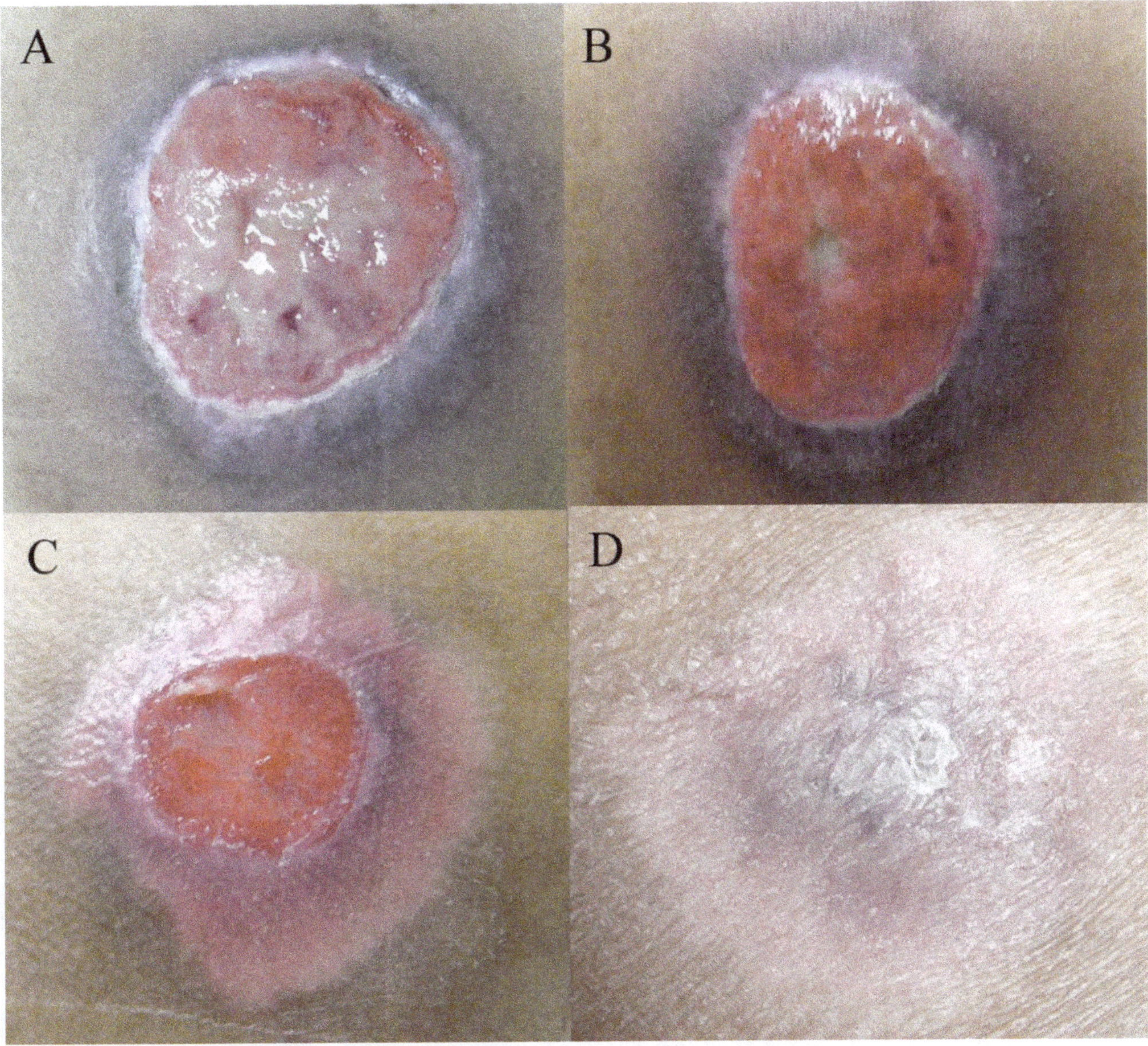

Fig. (1). Clinical course of our patient. A 56-year-old Japanese man developed pressure ulcer on his greater trochanter, which was not improved in spite of applying 0.003% alprostadil alfadex ointment for two months (**A**). The 0.9% cadexomer-iodine ointment was applied once a day for a week. Then, the discharge remarkably decreased (**B**). After using the cadexomer-iodine ointment for a week, the cadexomer-iodine ointment was withdrawn and polyurethane foams were applied. One month later the wound size gradually decreased (**C**). Applying them further for one month, the wound was completely epithelized (**D**).

the two signs such as poor healing and exudate were detected to indicate critical colonization but none of the signs for deep infection were shown. Therefore, our patient is retrospectively considered as having pressure ulcer complicated with critical colonization but not deep infection, as these criteria were not available when we treated this patient. For diagnosing critical colonization, the 10^5 bacterial growth guideline [1] is widely appreciated but the patient's severe mental condition prevented us from performing skin biopsy in our patient. In such instances the UPPER and LOWER criteria were useful to evaluate critical colonization. Because the result of swab cultures decreased from the quadrant III to the quadrant I culture using the cadexomer-iodine ointment in our case, this reduction of the bacterial burden due to critical colonization supposedly exerted preferential effect on the healing process.

CONFLICT OF INTEREST

The authors confirm that this article content has no conflict of interest.

ACKNOWLEDGEMENTS

Declared none.

REFERENCES

[1] Bowler PG. The 10^5 bacterial growth guideline: reassessing its clinical relevance in wound healing. Ostomy Wound Manage 2003; 49: 44-53.

[2] Smith DM. Pressure ulcers in the nursing home. Ann Intern Med 1995; 123: 433-42.

[3] Nicolle LE, Orr P, Duckworth H, *et al.* Prospective study of decubitus ulcers in two long term care facilities. Can J Infect Control 1994; 9: 35-8.

[4] Woo KY, Coutts PM, Sibbald RG. A randomized controlled trial to evaluate an antimicrobial dressing with silver alginate powder for the management of chronic wounds exhibiting signs of critical colonization. Adv Skin Wound Care 2012; 25: 503-8.

23

The Natural History of Food Sensitization in Children With Atopic Dermatitis and the Prognostic Role of Specific Serum IgE

Arianna Giannetti[1], Giampaolo Ricci[*,1], Arianna Dondi[1,2], Valentina Piccinno[1], Federica Bellini[1], Roberto Rondelli[1], Annalisa Patrizi[2] and Andrea Pession[1]

[1]*Pediatric Unit, Department of Gynecologic, Obstetric and Pediatric Sciences University of Bologna, Bologna, Italy*

[2]*Dermatology Unit, Department of Specialist, Diagnostic and Experimental Medicine, University of Bologna, Bologna, Italy*

Abstract: *Background*: The natural history and the prognostic factors for food tolerance in childhood atopic dermatitis (AD) are poorly understood.

Objective: We aimed at investigating the natural course of egg and milk allergy in children affected by AD and food allergy and identifying if the persistence of allergy is associated with high specific serum IgE (sIgE).

Methods: The retrospective study included 58 patients affected by AD, aged 9-16 months, with a first clinical examination between 1993 and 2002.

Results: Patients with AD and allergy to hen's egg (N=58) or cow's milk (N=44) were studied. In most patients milk and egg tolerance was reached before school age, but it was achieved later in children with severe AD and high egg sIgE.

Conclusions: The food tolerance is normally reached before school age and, at the time of diagnosis, levels of sIgE>5kU/L for hen's egg are risk factors for a later tolerance achievement.

Keywords: Atopic dermatitis, egg allergy, food allergy, milk allergy and specific serum IgE.

INTRODUCTION

Atopic dermatitis (AD) is a chronic inflammatory skin disease with specific immune and inflammatory mechanisms that affects between 15% to 30% of the pediatric population with an age dependency [1,2]. Food allergy is much more common in children with AD, with an association of 15-30% (even if some authors report it to be up to 80%) [3-6].

The main offending foods are cow's milk, hen's egg, peanuts and fish [7].

Sensitization to food occurs early, peaking at approximately 6 to 9 months of age [8] and generally does not increase later in childhood [9,10].

Three prospective studies showed that about two-thirds of children will outgrow their egg allergy by early school age [11-13]. However, a recent large, retrospective review by Savage *et al.* [14] of 881 egg-allergic individuals reported that a significant proportion of egg allergic patients was still allergic in their late childhood or adolescence.

The overall prognosis of cow's milk allergy is also good, with a total recovery of 56% at 1 year, 77% at 2 years, 87% at 3 years, 92% at 5 and 10 years and 97% at 15 years of age [15].

*Address correspondence to this author at the Pediatric Unit, Department of Gynecologic, Obstetric and Pediatric Sciences, University of Bologna, via Massarenti n° 11, 40138, Bologna, Italy;
E-mail: giampaolo.ricci@unibo.it

In a previous study which included children with a diagnosis of AD and first examined at an age of 9 to 16 months, our group showed that the presence of allergic sensitization at one year of age might predict the development of respiratory allergy [16].

The aim of the present study is to investigate the natural course of and acquisition of tolerance in hen's egg and cow's milk allergy in children with AD and to identify if allergy persistence is associated with high sIgE.

MATERIALS AND METHODS

Study Population and Inclusion Criteria

Patients included in this study represent a part of the cohort already analyzed in a previous retrospective study [16], in which children were enrolled according to the following criteria:

a. diagnosis of AD at an age of 9 to 16 months made at our Pediatric Allergology Outpatients Clinic, with a first clinical examination between 1993 and 2002;
b. availability of a detailed family and personal history;
c. performance of allergometric tests (skin prick tests (SPTs) and sIgE serum level for food and inhalant allergens);
d. telephone availability;
e. informed consent by the parents.

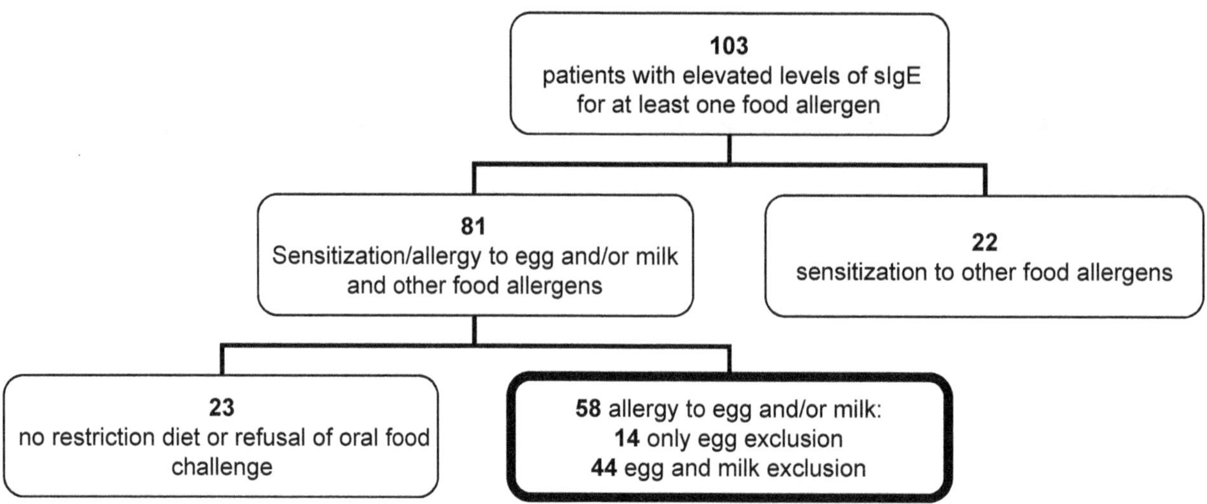

Fig. (1). Study population flow chart.

For the present analysis, we selected those patients with sIgE >0.35 kU/L for at least one food allergen at first observation (n=103), only 81 (78.6%) of whom with a sensitization and/or food allergy to cow's milk and hen's egg. Among them, 23 children were not on a restriction diet or refused to perform food challenge, whereas 58 were on hen's egg or cow's milk exclusion diet (Fig. **1**). Therefore, we performed our analysis on 58 children: 14 were allergic to hen's egg (with symptoms of urticaria in 11 patients and AD acute flares in 3) and on an egg-free diet; the others were allergic to milk and sensitized to egg, so that they followed a milk and egg restriction diet on the basis of milk-allergy symptoms, AD severity and elevated hen's egg sIgE. In the 44 children with cow's milk allergy the symptoms were: acute flares of AD (7 patients), urticaria (34 patients), respiratory (1 patient), gastrointestinal (2 patients) (Table **1**).

The patients were followed with periodic check-ups until AD was controlled and they had reached the tolerance for the food. Oral challenges were repeated every 6-9 months (mean: 8 months) for 24 months after a diagnostic challenge and on a yearly basis thereafter. Accidental ingestion of a considerable amount of the offending food without a clinical reaction was considered as a negative challenge: this happened in 5 children for cow's milk and in 6 children for hen's egg (Table **1**). If a reported accidental ingestion had produced clinical symptoms, the reported dose ingested was recorded. In this case, convincing symptoms were considered as positive oral food challenges and the scheduled follow-up was delayed of 6-12 months.

Milk/egg hypersensitivity was assumed to have resolved when a whole egg or an entire glass of milk (150 ml) could be eaten or drunk with no apparent symptoms.

Clinical Assessment

At the time of the first evaluation, the diagnosis of AD was made by the physicians on the basis of the criteria of Hanifin and Rajka [17] and the evaluation of the severity of AD was assessed by the SCORAD index [18]. SCORAD index < 25 shows a mild AD (8 patients, 14%), 25-50 a moderate form (39 patients, 67%), >50 a severe form (11 patients, 19%).

Allergometric Assessment

At the first evaluation (between 1993 and 2002) the determination of sIgE was performed by ImmunoCAP™ (Pharmacia, Sweden) in all patients for the following allergens: cow's milk, hen's egg, soybean, wheat, peanut, nut, codfish, apple. A patient was considered as sensitized to an allergen when having sIgE levels higher than 0.35 kU/L.

All the sera were tested for sIgE levels in the central laboratory of our hospital.

Statistical Methods

Standard statistical descriptions of parameters were used to characterize the data (mean, median and range).

The primary outcomes were tolerance onset to cow's milk and to hen's egg in children with AD and duration of intolerance to both food allergens.

Both outcomes were estimated using the method of Kaplan and Meier; comparison between probabilities in different patient groups was performed using the log-rank test [19].

Tolerance onset probabilities to cow's milk and to hen's egg were computed from the date of diagnosis to the date of tolerance onset to cow's milk and to hen's egg respectively, while duration of intolerance (or persistence of allergy) was calculated from the onset to the disappearing of the allergy or the last date of contact.

Results were expressed as probability (%). All P values are 2-sided and values less than 0.05 were considered as statistically significant.

The Statistical analysis was performed using the STATA package [20].

RESULTS

All the 58 patients (35 males, 23 females) were on an egg-free diet; 44 (76%) were also on a milk-free diet. The mean follow-up of these patients was 127.6 ± 24.7 months. The mean age of children at first observation was 11.2 months. At follow-up the mean age was 138.8 months.

Table 1. Characteristics of the Population

Patient Number	Food Allergy	Symtoms of Egg Allergy	Symtoms of Milk Allergy	sIgE Egg (kU/L)	sIgE Milk (kU/L)	OFC Egg	OFC Milk	OCF Egg Outcome	OCF Milk Outcome
1	Egg	U		100		Yes	Yes	T	T
2	Egg	U		64.1		Yes	Yes	T	T
3	Egg	U		44		Yes	Yes	T	T
4	Egg	U		25.4		Yes	Yes	T	T
5	Egg	U		30		Yes	Yes	T	T
6	Egg	U		26.8		Yes	Yes	T	T
7	Egg	U		21.8		Yes	Yes	T	T
8	Egg	U		39.3		Yes	Yes	T	T
9	Egg	U		21		Yes	Yes	T	T
10	Egg	U		15.9		Yes	Yes	T	T
11	Egg	U		19		Yes	Yes	T	T
12	Egg	ADaf		17		Yes	Yes	T	T
13	Egg	ADaf		15.1		Yes	Yes	T	T
14	Egg	ADaf		17.6		Yes	Yes	T	T
15	Egg+milk	N	U	15.3	23.6	A	Yes	T	T
16	Egg+milk	N	U	7.7	1	A	Yes	T	T
17	Egg+milk	N	U	6.6	7.3	A	Yes	T	T
18	Egg+milk	N	U	4.9	5.1	A	Yes	T	T
19	Egg+milk	N	U	3.7	5.7	A	Yes	T	T
20	Egg+milk	N	U	2.1	7.5	A	Yes	T	T
21	Egg+milk	N	U	13	4	Yes	A	T	T
22	Egg+milk	N	U	3.4	17.3	Yes	A	T	T
23	Egg+milk	N	U	1.9	2.7	Yes	A	T	T
24	Egg+milk	N	U	4.9	3	Yes	A	T	T
25	Egg+milk	N	U	10	2.2	Yes	A	T	T
26	Egg+milk	N	U	5.4	16	Yes	Yes	T	T
27	Egg+milk	N	U	1.7	2.7	Yes	Yes	T	T
28	Egg+milk	N	U	7.5	4.5	Yes	Yes	T	T
29	Egg+milk	N	U	5.5	3.6	Yes	Yes	T	T
30	Egg+milk	N	U	4.9	8	Yes	Yes	T	T
31	Egg+milk	N	U	3.5	5.1	Yes	Yes	T	T
32	Egg+milk	N	U	10	3.2	Yes	Yes	T	T
33	Egg+milk	N	U	7.7	44.8	Yes	Yes	T	T
34	Egg+milk	N	U	4.8	3.4	Yes	Yes	T	T
35	Egg+milk	N	U	2.4	7.1	Yes	Yes	T	T
36	Egg+milk	N	U	6.3	5.5	Yes	Yes	T	T
37	Egg+milk	N	U	2.2	2.1	Yes	Yes	T	T
38	Egg+milk	N	U	12	2	Yes	Yes	T	T
39	Egg+milk	N	U	4.1	44	Yes	Yes	T	T
40	Egg+milk	N	U	1.6	1.2	Yes	Yes	T	T
41	Egg+milk	N	U	2.8	0.9	Yes	Yes	T	T

(Table 1) contd.....

Patient Number	Food Allergy	Symtoms of Egg Allergy	Symtoms of Milk Allergy	sIgE Egg (kU/L)	sIgE Milk (kU/L)	OFC Egg	OFC Milk	OCF Egg Outcome	OCF Milk Outcome
42	Egg+milk	N	U	1.3	57.8	Yes	Yes	T	T
43	Egg+milk	N	U	11.6	9.8	Yes	Yes	T	T
44	Egg+milk	N	U	1.3	1.2	Yes	Yes	T	T
45	Egg+milk	N	U	1.1	10	Yes	Yes	T	T
46	Egg+milk	N	U	10.6	0.9	Yes	Yes	T	T
47	Egg+milk	N	U	0.6	12	Yes	Yes	T	NT
48	Egg+milk	N	U	12.3	1.6	Yes	Yes	NT	T
49	Egg+milk	N	R	13.7	88.3	Yes	Yes	NT	NT
50	Egg+milk	N	G	5.1	0.4	Yes	Yes	T	T
51	Egg+milk	N	G	1.3	0.5	Yes	Yes	T	T
52	Egg+milk	N	ADaf	0.6	0.7	Yes	Yes	T	T
53	Egg+milk	N	ADaf	0.4	1.5	Yes	Yes	T	T
54	Egg+milk	N	ADaf	0.5	0.4	Yes	Yes	T	T
55	Egg+milk	N	ADaf	0.5	0.4	Yes	Yes	T	T
56	Egg+milk	N	ADaf	0.4	0.4	Yes	Yes	T	T
57	Egg+milk	N	ADaf	0.5	1.5	Yes	Yes	T	T
58	Egg+milk	N	ADaf	0.5	0.5	Yes	Yes	T	T

OCF: Oral food challenge; A: accidental ingestion of the offending food; U: urticaria; R: respiratory, G: gastrointestinal; ADaf: AD acute flares; N: none; T: tolerance, NT: No Tolerance/

Out of all the patients, 56 children (97%) developed tolerance to egg at a mean age of 46 months (range 13-156) and 42 (96%) to milk at a mean age of 37 months (range 10-115) (Fig. **2A**, **B**).

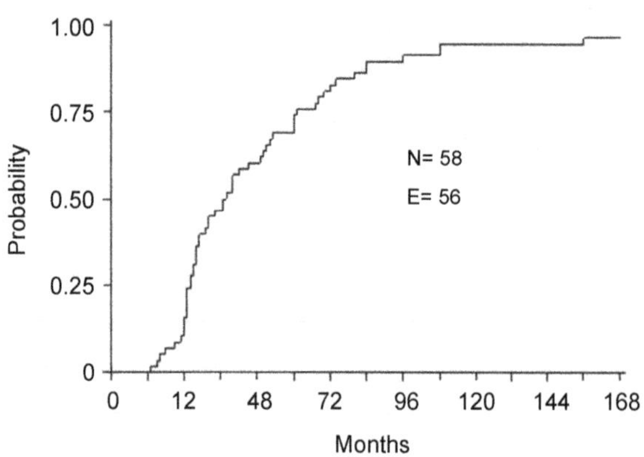

Fig. (2A). Tolerance onset to hen's egg in children with AD.

Furthermore, the patients with mild AD achieved the tolerance to milk and egg at a mean age respectively of 29 and 44 months, earlier than those with severe AD, who reached the tolerance respectively at a mean age of 53 and 57 months, although these differences were not statistically significant (Fig. **3A**, **B**).

Figs. (**4A**, **B**) show the Kaplan Meier curves for duration of the disease stratified according to the levels of sIgE.

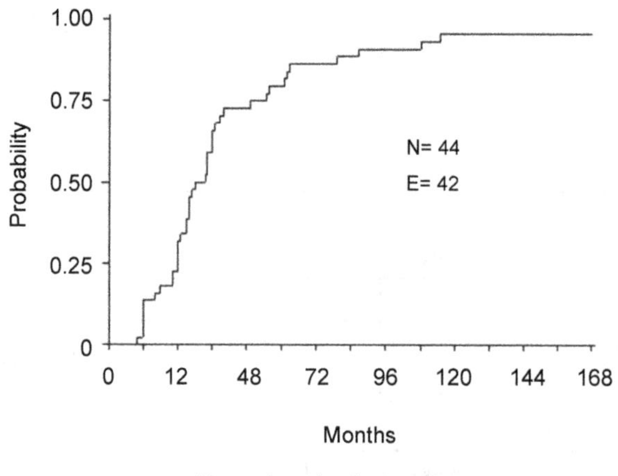

Fig. (2B). Tolerance onset to cow's milk in children with AD.

The patients were divided into two groups according to the median of sIgE (egg white: 5 kU/L, milk: 3 kU/L). Children with sIgE levels ≤5 kU/L for hen's egg white reached the tolerance significantly earlier than those with levels higher than 5 kU/L (*P=0.002*). Patients with cow's milk sIgE levels ≤3 kU/L apparently became tolerant earlier than those with sIgE >3 kU/L, but this difference was not statistically significant (Fig. **4A**, **B**).

DISCUSSION

The natural course of food allergy is different for each allergen. Allergies to peanuts, nuts, and seafood are more likely to persist, with a small fraction of patients developing tolerance, whereas allergies to milk, eggs, wheat, and soy generally resolve by childhood [21].

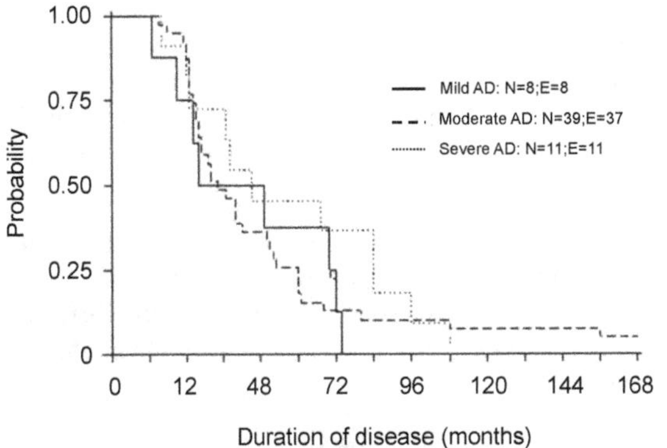

N= number of patients, E= events; Overall Log-rank p = 0.68

Fig. (3A). Curve for duration of hen's egg white intolerance stratified according to the severity of AD.

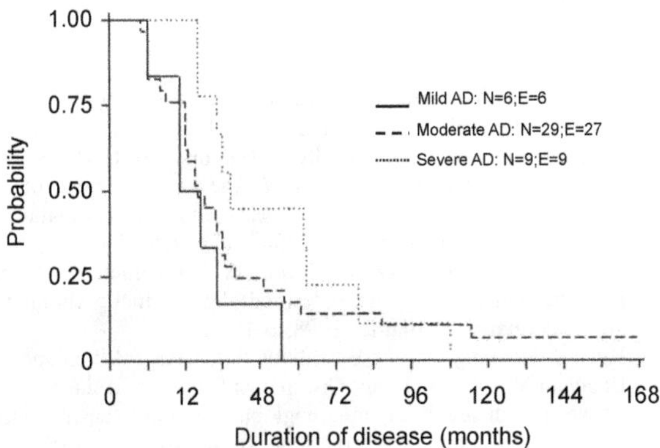

N= number of patients, E= events; Overall Log-rank p = 0.23

Fig. (3B). Curve for duration of cow's milk intolerance stratified according to the severity of AD.

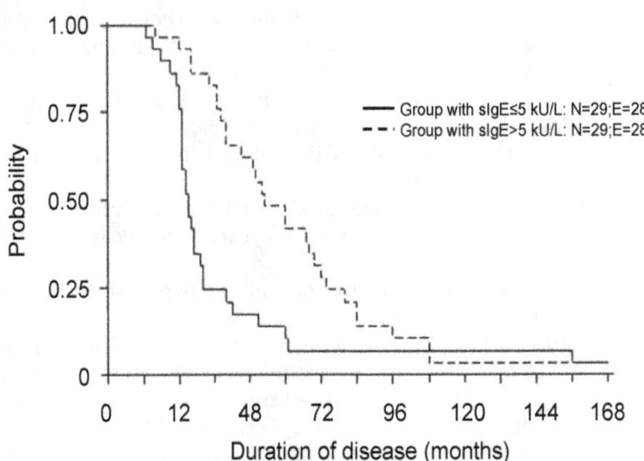

N= number of patients, E= events; Log-rank p = 0.0023

Fig. (4A). Curve for duration of the disease stratified according to the **hen's egg white** IgE levels. The patients were divided into two groups according to the median of sIgE (5 kU/L).

In the paper, we found that the tolerance for egg and milk was reached early: at 46 months to egg and at 37 months of age to milk (Fig. **2A**, **B**). Several studies report that most children with egg allergy outgrow their allergy by the early school-age years, whereas children affected by cow's milk allergy will probably tolerate the food by the age of 3[15, 10, 22-24].

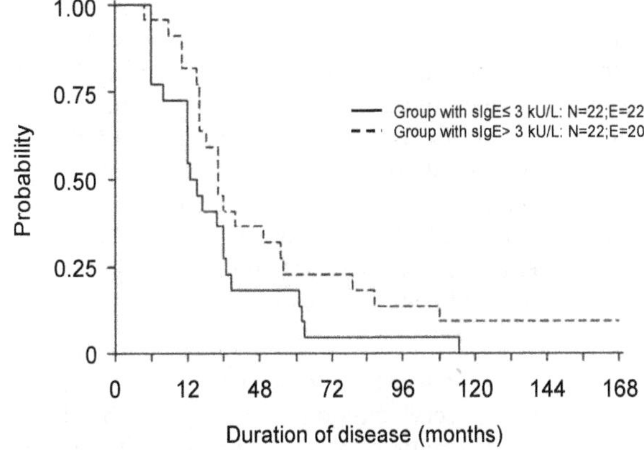

N= number of patients, E= events; Log-rank p = 0.095

Fig. (4B). Curve for duration of the disease stratified according to the **cow's milk** IgE levels. The patients were divided into two groups according to the median of sIgE (3kU/L).

Other studies report that between 31% and 51% of children allergic to egg usually overcome the problem [11,25-27]. According to Boyano-Martinez *et al.* [13], who studied 58 patients younger than 2 years of age with egg allergy, half of the children will tolerate the food at 35 months of follow-up and 66% after 5 years. In a prospective, birth cohort study on 1749 Danish children who were followed up to the age of 3, Høst and Halken [15] found that the prevalence of milk allergy was 2.2% and that, by the age of 3, most of the allergic children were able to tolerate milk.

However, other studies suggest a modification of the natural history of cow's milk and hen's egg allergy, with increasing persistence until a later age [14, 28]. In the large, retrospective review of 881 egg allergic individuals by Savage *et al.* [14], the rate of tolerance development, depending on the definition of egg allergy, was 36-66% by 10 years, 61-86% by 14 years and 80-95% by age 16 years. Skripak *et al.* [28] retrospectively analyzed 807 patients with IgE-mediated milk allergy and, despite the use of 3 sets of increasingly broad criteria to define tolerance, incidence rates of resolution at 4 years ranged from <1% to 26%, substantially lower than previously reported.

Unfortunately, it is difficult to compare results between studies because of different ages at study entry, different follow-up times and unlike populations; it is also possible that ethnic and genetic variations play a role in the development of oral tolerance. The main limitation of our study is that 44 patients were diagnosed with egg allergy on the basis of sIgE alone and did not have a history of reaction to food. This occurred because these children were being evaluated for AD before egg had been introduced into their diet, and then strict egg avoidance was instituted on the basis of a milk-free diet, the elevated sIgE and/or the severity of AD. An oral provocation test had not been proposed to the parents until the levels of sIgE were below the threshold of 7 kU/L, which predicts a high risk of reaction to food ingestion.

Although the natural history of egg and milk allergy has been thoroughly evaluated, previous results have been somewhat contradictory and an exact determination of when tolerance is acquired in each individual case is still not possible. Moreover, the prognostic factors for the development of tolerance in food allergy are poorly understood. Another aim of our study was to analyze the relationship between tolerance acquirement and the values of sIgE and AD severity as assessed at the time of the first examination. The predictive factors identified may help to define the prognosis of food allergy in each particular case and to answer parents' common questions about when their child will tolerate the ingestion of the offending food and when he or she will be able to reintroduce food in his or her diet.

Similarly to what has been reported by others [13, 29, 30], we found a very important role of high sIgE in predicting the persistence of allergy and, in particular, that patients with levels of sIgE for hen's egg white higher than 5 kU/L at diagnosis reach the tolerance later than those with lower levels (Fig. **4A**).

In a study which included children between 3 months and 14 years of age, 61% with AD and 90% with a family history of atopy [29], Sampson and Ho reported that in the presence of egg sIgE ≥7 kU/L, provocation testing would not be indicated, given the high probability that the test would prove positive. In the work by Boyano-Martínez *et al.* [13], the sIgE level is an important prognostic marker in children who only had cutaneous symptoms. Savage *et al.* [14], examining the relationship between the peak of egg sIgE level and the development of tolerance, have identified an egg sIgE level ≥50 kU/L as a marker of persistent egg allergy.

Montesinos *et al.* [30] performed a retrospective study of patients with egg allergy and found that the initial levels of sIgE for egg white were significantly lower in those patients who reached tolerance: sIgE levels of 1.52, 1.35 and 2.59 kU/L predicted clinical reactivity at the different follow-up timepoints analyzed (25-36, 37-48 and 49-60 months respectively).

Our study shows that high levels of sIgE for milk are not a risk factor for a later tolerance achievement.

However, in a recent study [31] on a population of 139 Portuguese children with milk allergy, higher sIgE levels to cow's milk (>17.5 kU/L) during the follow-up period were associated with a reduced likelihood of acquiring oral tolerance.

Also in the work of Vanto *et al.* [32] the milk sIgE levels >2 kU/L are useful prognostic indicators of the development of tolerance to milk in infants with milk allergy.

Levy *et al.* [33] compared patient with transient milk allergy with those with persistent milk allergy: no differences were found between the groups in mean age and symptoms and signs at the first allergic reaction and family history of atopy.

Food-sensitized children have been shown to have more severe and persistent AD [5,34,35]. The patients that develop AD before 3 months of age are at significantly greater risk of acquiring food allergies compared with those who develop AD after 12 months of age [5,36]. These data suggest that the presence of food sensitization and allergy earlier in life predicts a prognosis of severe AD, but conclusions about its role in the pathogenesis of AD cannot be drawn. In our study the patients with mild AD achieved the tolerance to milk and egg (with a mean respectively of 29 and 44 months) earlier than those with severe AD (with a mean respectively of 53 and 57 months) although not statistically significant (Fig. **3A, B**).

In conclusion, our study seems to highlight that, in the case of milk and egg allergy, food tolerance is normally reached before school age and that initial sIgE levels >5 kU/L for hen's egg white are risk factors for a later tolerance achievement.

CONFLICT OF INTEREST

The authors confirm that this article content has no conflict of interest.

ACKNOWLEDGEMENTS

Declared none.

REFERENCES

[1] Bieber T. Atopic dermatitis. N Engl J Med 2008; 358: 1483-94.

[2] Liu FT, Goodarzi H, Chen HY. IgE, Mast Cells, and Eosinophils in Atopic Dermatitis. Clin Rev Allergy Immunol 2011; 41: 298-310.

[3] Illi S, von Mutius E, Lau S, *et al.* The natural course of atopic dermatitis from birth to age 7 years and the association with asthma. J Allergy Clin Immunol 2004; 113: 925-31.

[4] Eigenmann PA, Sicherer SH, Borkowski TA, Cohen BA, Sampson HA. Prevalence of IgE-mediate food allergy among children with atopic dermatitis. Pediatrics 1998; 101: E8.

[5] Hill DJ, Hosking CS, De Benedictis FM, Oranje AP, Diepgen TL, Bauchau V; EPAAC Study Group. Confirmation of the association between high levels of immunoglobulin E food sensitization and eczema in infancy: An international study. Clin Exp Allergy 2008; 3: 161-8.

[6] Eller E, Kjaer HF, Host A, Andersen KE, Bindslev-Jensen C. Food allergy and food sensitization in early childhood: results from the DARC cohort. Allergy 2009; 64: 1023-9.

[7] Suh KY. Food allergy and atopic dermatitis: separating fact from fiction. Semin Cutan Med Surg 2010; 29: 72-8.

[8] Bath-Hextall F, Delamere FM, Williams HC. Dietary exclusion for improving established atopic eczema in adults and children: systematic review. Allergy 2009; 64: 258-64

[9] Brockow I, Zutavern A, Hoffman U, *et al.* Early allergic sensitizations and their relevance to atopic diseases in children aged 6 years: results of the GINI study. J Investig Allergol Clin Immunol 2009; 19: 180-7.

[10] Bock SA. Prospective appraisal of complaints of adverse reactions to foods in children during the first 3 years of life. Pediatrics 1987; 79: 683-8.

[11] Ford RP, Taylor B. Natural history of egg hypersensitivity. Arch Dis Child 1982; 57: 649-52.

[12] Dannaeus A, Inganäs M. A follow-up study of children with food allergy. Clinical course in relation to serum IgE- and IgG-antibody levels to milk, egg and fish. Clin Allergy 1981; 11: 533-9.

[13] Boyano-Martínez T, García-Ara C, Díaz-Pena JM, Martín-Esteban M. Prediction of tolerance on the basis of quantification of egg white-specific IgE antibodies in children with egg allergy. J Allergy Clin Immunol 2002; 110: 304-9.

[14] Savage JH, Matsui EC, Skripak JM, Wood RA. The natural history of egg allergy. J Allergy Clin Immunol 2007; 120: 1413-7.

[15] Høst A, Halken S, Jacobsen HP, Christensen AE, Herskind AM, Plesner K. Clinical course of cow's milk protein allergy/intolerance and atopic diseases in childhood. Pediatr Allergy Immunol 2002; 13 Suppl 15: 23-8.

[16] Ricci G, Patrizi A, Giannetti A, Dondi A, Bendandi B, Masi M. Does improvement management of atopic dermatitis influence the

appearance of respiratory allergic diseases? A follow-up study. Clin Mol Allergy 2010; 8: 8.

[17] Hanifin JM, Rajka G. Diagnostic features of atopic dermatitis. Acta Derm Venereol Suppl (Stockh) 1980; 92: 44-7.

[18] Consensus Report of the European Task Force on Atopic Dermatitis. Severiy scoring of atopic dermatitis: the SCORAD index. Dermatology 1993; 186: 23-31.

[19] Kaplan EL, Meier P. Nonparametral estimation from incomplete observations. J Am Stat Assoc 1958; 53: 457.

[20] StataCorp, STATA Statistical Software: Release 7.0. College Station, TX: Stata Corporation 2000.

[21] Lack G. Clinical practice. Food allergy. N Engl J Med 2008; 359: 1252-60.

[22] Saarinen KM, Juntunen-Backman K, Järvenpää AL, *et al.* Supplementary feeding in maternity hospitals and the risk of cow's milk allergy: A prospective study of 6209 infants. J Allergy Clin Immunol 1999; 104: 457-61.

[23] Schrander JJ, van den Bogart JP, Forget PP, Schrander-Stumpel CT, Kuijten RH, Kester AD. Cow's milk protein intolerance in infants under 1 year of age: a prospective epidemiological study. Eur J Pediatr 1993; 152: 640-4.

[24] Bishop JM, Hill DJ, Hosking CS. Natural history of cow milk allergy: clinical outcome. J Pediatr 1990; 116: 862-7.

[25] Sampson HA, Scanlon SM. Natural history of food hypersensitivity in children with atopic dermatitis. J Pediatr 1989; 115: 23-7.

[26] Bock SA. The natural history of food sensitivity. J Allergy Clin Immunol 1982; 69: 173-7.

[27] Boyano-Martínez MT, Martin Esteban M, Pascual C, Ojeda JA. Food allergy in children. II. Prognostic factors and long-term development. An Esp Pediatr 1987; 26: 241-5.

[28] Skripak JM, Matsui EC, Mudd K, Wood RA. The natural history of IgE-mediated cow's milk allergy. J Allergy Clin Immunol 2007; 120: 1172-7.

[29] Sampson HA, Ho DG. Relationship between food-specific IgE concentrations and the risk of positive food challenges in children and adolescents. J Allergy Clin Immunol 1997; 100: 444-51.

[30] Montesinos E, Martorell A, Félix R, Cerdá JC. Egg white specific IgE levels in serum as clinical reactivity predictors in the course of egg allergy follow-up. Pediatr Allergy Immunol 2010; 21: 634-9.

[31] Santos A, Dias A, Pinheiro JA. Predictive factors for the persistence of cow's milk allergy. Pediatr Allergy Immunol 2010; 21: 1127-34.

[32] Vanto T, Helppila S, Juntunen-Backman K, *et al.* Prediction of the development of tolerance to milk in children with cow's milk hypersensitivity. J Pediatr 2004; 144: 218-22.

[33] Levy Y, Segal N, Garty B, Danon YL. Lessons from the clinical course of IgE-mediated cow milk allergy in Israel. Pediatr Allergy Immunol 2007; 18: 589-93.

[34] Hill DJ, Hosking CS. Food allergy and atopic dermatitis in infancy: an epidemiologic study. Pediatr Allergy Immunol 2004; 15: 421-7.

[35] Tikkanen S, Kokkonen J, Juntti H, Niinimaki A. Status of children with cow's milk allergy in infancy by 10 years of age. Acta Paediatr 2000; 89: 1174-80.

[36] Lowe AJ, Abramson MJ, Hosking CS, *et al.* The temporal sequence of allergic sensitization and onset of infantile eczema. Clin Exp Allergy 2007; 37: 536-42.

Dermatologic Manifestations of the LEOPARD Syndrome

S. Cao and A.F. Nikkels*

Department of Dermatology, University Hospital of Liège, Sart Tilman, Liège, Belgium

Abstract: The LEOPARD syndrome is an exceptional autosomal dominant genetic disease with a missense mutation of the PTPN11 gene in more than 90% of the cases. The principal clinical manifestations include extensive lentiginosis, heart conduction abnormalities, hypertrophic obstructive cardiomyopathy, ocular hypertelorism, pulmonary stenosis, genital anomalies, mental retardation, growth retardation and deafness. A woman with a LEOPARD syndrome illustrates the progressive development of melanocytic nevi. In fact, the majority of lentigines are actually melanocytic nevi. Sequential digital dermoscopy evidences progressive growth of some melanocytic lesions. The ever-increasing number of melanocytic nevi in the LEOPARD syndrome is a risk factor for melanoma and full body photography and dermoscopy are recommended for follow-up.

Keywords: LEOPARD syndrome, melanocytic nevi, dysmorphism, lentiginosis, PTPN11.

INTRODUCTION

The LEOPARD syndrome is an exceptional dominant autosomal disease (**L**entiginosis, **E**CG conduction anomalies, **O**cular hypertelorism/hypertrophic **O**bstructive cardiomyopathy (HOCM), **P**ulmonary stenosis, **A**bnormalities of genitalia, growth **R**etardation and **D**eafness)[1]. The first case was described in 1936 but the LEOPARD term was first used in 1969 [2]. Up to date, about 300 cases have been reported [3]. Many synonyms exist: cardiomyopathic progressive lentiginosis, multiple lentigines syndrome, cardio-cutaneous syndrome or Moynahan syndrome [1]. The LEOPARD syndrome is currently also referred to as Noonan syndrome with multiple lentigines or NSML (OMIM 151100) [3]. A woman is presented to illustrate the highly polymorphous character of this genetic syndrome, insisting in particular on the progressive evolution of the dermatologic features and the importance of repetitive total body photography and dermoscopy in the dermatologic follow-up.

CASE REPORT

A 38-years-old woman patient presented at the dermatology ward for multiple pigmented lesions. Clinical examination showed multiple variable-sized lentigines and melanocytic nevi covering the entire body. The first lentigines appeared at the age of 6 on her face and the upper back (Figs. **1**, **2**). At puberty, the number and size of lesions increased and they became more pigmented (Figs. **1**, **2**). Previous total body photography and dermoscopy never identified any suspect pigmented lesion. Several "lentigines" were previously excised as they appeared atypical but histopathology always identified benign melanocytic nevi. The patient was born at term after a pregnancy without any significant complications. Her birth weight was 4.050 kg and the body length 54 cm. She did not present any neonatal problems. Nevertheless, she appeared hypotonic at birth. Rapidly, a bilateral strabismus with a congenital nystagmus was noticed. Her psychomotor development was relatively slow: walking and speech acquisition at 3 years and diurnal sphincter control at 2 years with persistent enuresis until 25 years. She has been epileptic with tonoclonic crises and absences since she was 11. Mild mental retardation was noted with an IQ at 74. She followed specialized education from 7 to 21 years. She is able to read, write and to perform simple calculations. Currently, she lives with her mother and spends the day in a specialized occupational center. Clinical examination revealed an increased interpupillary distance. Her length was 1m74 and her weight 53 kg. Further medical history revealed asthma, anorexia, a surgical intervention for strabismus, osteoporosis and a minor chronic peripheral polyneuropathy of the limbs in relation with an autoimmune hypothyroidism. The latter was revealed by a delayed puberty. No gynecologic problem has ever been detected. There was no previous family history of lentiginosis. Her present treatment includes carbamazepine (Tegretol°), montelukast (Singulair°), desloratadine (Aerius°), levothyroxine (Elthyrone°) and heptaminol. As she presented hypertelorism and delayed psychomotor development, a karyotype was requested in 1978 and did not detect any chromosomal abnormalities. In 1992, an autoimmune thyroiditis was evidenced with an exaggerated prolactin (PRL) reactivity to the TRH test, maybe related to her carbamazepine treatment. Later, a low ferritin level prompted oral iron supplementation. Because of persistent headaches and increased PRL level, a MRI of the sella turcica was performed in 2003 but did not reveal any abnormalities. The last cardiological exploration was performed in 2008. The ECG demonstrated a right-axis deviation and a left posterior fascicular block. Nevertheless, the whole examination was practically within the normal limits. In 2009, a hearing test didn't reveal any signs of deafness. Genetic analysis by molecular analysis did not identify any mutation in the PTPN11 and RAF1 genes.

*Address correspondence to this author at the Department of Dermatology, CHU - Sart Tilman, University of Liège, B-4000, Liège, Belgium;
E-mail: af.nikkels@chu.ulg.ac.be

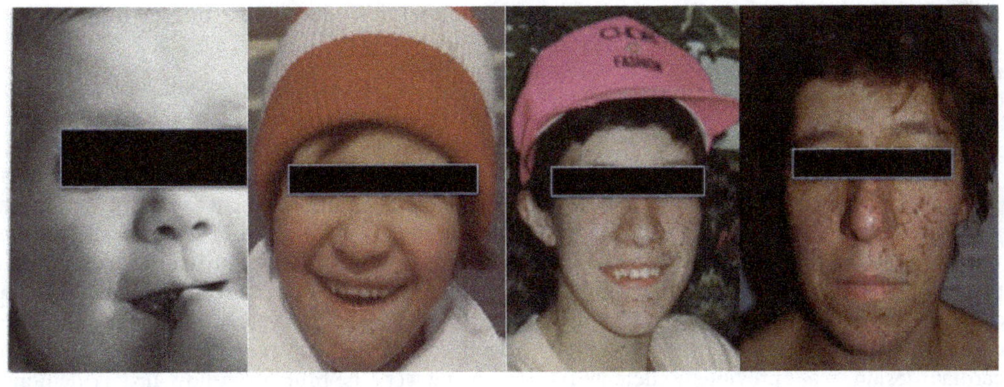

Fig. (1). Progressive appearance of the melanocytic lesions of the face.

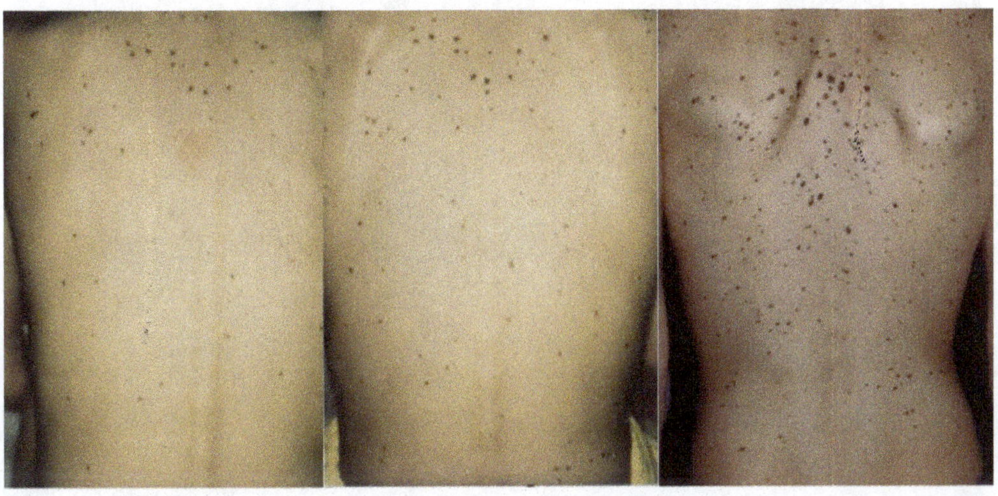

Fig. (2). Evolution of the melanocytic lesions of the back.

DISCUSSION

The LEOPARD syndrome is an exceptional disorder with an autosomal dominant transmission. The penetrance is very high and the expression highly variable. In about 90% of the cases, it is linked to a germline PTPN11 missense mutation with loss of function [1, 4]. The major clinical features are diffuse lentiginosis, ECG abnormalities, ocular hypertelorism, hypertrophic cardiomyopathy, pulmonary stenosis, genital anomalies, retardation of growth and deafness. Additional characteristics are a facial dysmorphism, skeletal abnormalities, neurological troubles, as observed in this case, hypotonia at birth, learning disabilities with mental retardation, oculomotor defects and EEG abnormalities [1, 5]. Rare cases of cancer, including melanoma, had been reported. Nevertheless, as total case number is so low, no particular cancer susceptibility is currently established [3].

The diagnosis of a LEOPARD syndrome requires diffuse lentiginosis and two other syndrome traits. If diffuse lentigines are absent, the presence of a first degree affected relative and three other distinct features are necessary. However the diagnosis is not always obvious, especially as some signs are lacking or only appear at an advanced age. Furthermore, it shares lots of characteristics with other genetic syndromes like the Noonan syndrome, also mediated by a PTPN11 mutation but of the gain function type [1]. Further differential diagnoses include type 1 neurofibromatosis, Costello syndrome, cardiofaciocutaneous syndrome, Peutz-Jeghers syndrome and Carney complex. All these syndromes, except the two latter, are in relation with a mutation in the RAS-MAPK signaling pathway that is involved in cellular proliferation, growth and differentiation [6,7]. In atypical cases of LEOPARD syndrome, a missense PTPN11 mutation confirms the diagnosis [4]. In case of negativity, a RAF1 mutation should be searched for that is present in 1/3 of the patients without a PTPN11 mutation [1]. In less than 5%, a BRAF mutation can be associated [8]. Molecular analysis provides additional interesting clinical information helping in the long-term management and follow-up of these patients. Indeed, the prevalence of cardiac conduction disorders, ventricular or left auricular hypertrophy and familial history of sudden death is significantly higher in PTPN11 mutation negative patients. On the other hand, among the PTPN11 mutations, those involving the exon 13 are associated with an increased risk of hypertrophic cardiomyopathy and severe cardiac complications whereas those involving exon 7 are more often linked to growth retardation and deafness compared to exon 12 mutations [1]. The presence of BRAF mutations are usually linked to moderate to severe cognitive impairment [9].

The mortality and morbidity predominantly depend on the extent of the cardiac abnormalities. A complete check-up, including rigorous clinical examination, growth parameters monitoring in children, hearing test (1/year until adulthood) and cardiological (1/year mainly when lentigines appear if none cardiac lesion was previously detected), neurological and urogenital evaluations, is highly recommended. In contrast, the management of other abnormalities does not differ from those in general population [1].

The multiple lentigines and melanocytic nevi require a regular follow-up because of their progressively increasing total number. A total UVA-UVB protection is advocated. Multiple melanocytic nevi are a significant risk factor for melanoma. As these patients steadily increase the number of lesion over lifetime, the potential risk for melanoma will theoretically increase. Until now, two cases of malignant melanoma have been reported in 300 reported cases [3,10,11]. Hence, a yearly total body photography [12], in addition to clinical examination and dermoscopic analysis can be very helpful for follow-up, as demonstrated in this patient. Dermoscopic follow-up with the Dermogenius°, a digitalized epiluminescence microscopy system clearly

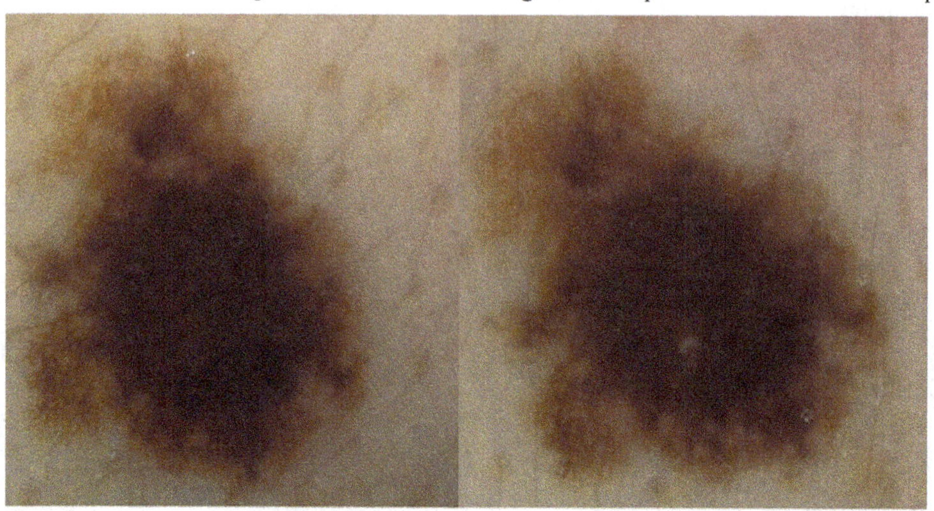

Pigmentary naevus 1. Increase in size over one year, note peripheral radial growth.

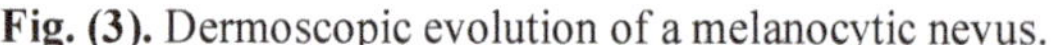

Fig. (3). Dermoscopic evolution of a melanocytic nevus.

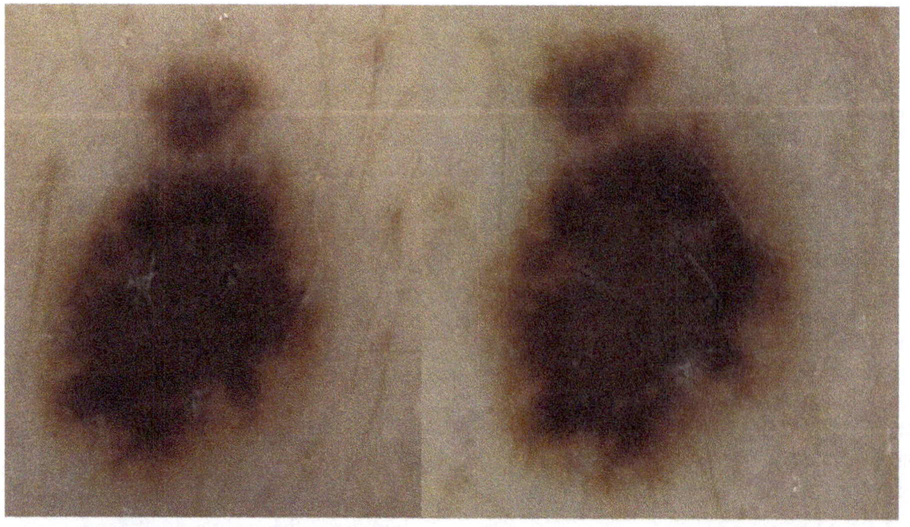

Pigmentary naevus 2. Increase in size over one year, note peripheral radial extension.

Fig. (4). Dermoscopic evolution of a melanocytic nevus.

reveals growth in size and increase of pigmentation in certain melanocytic nevi (Figs. **3**, **4**). For cosmetic reasons, some patients ask for treatment of the multiple lentigines. Many treatments are available including dermabrasion, electrodessication, cryotherapy, surgical excision, chemical peels, laser or intense pulsed light. One case was successfully treated by intense pulsed light [13].

CONCLUSION

LEOPARD syndrome is an exceptional autosomal dominant disorder with high penetrance and marked variable expression. It is frequently associated with a PTPN11 missense mutation. It is principally characterized by multiple lentigines and melanocytic nevi, cardiographic conduction defects, ocular hypertelorism, pulmonary stenosis, genital abnormalities, growth retardation and deafness. Repetitive total body photography combined with a thorough clinical and dermoscopic examination should help in the surveillance of the multiple lentigines and melanocytic nevi. The term NEOPARD (multiple nevi) is proposed as it suits more adequately the dermatologic alterations.

CONFLICT OF INTEREST

The authors confirm that this article content has no conflict of interest.

ACKNOWLEDGEMENTS

Declared none.

REFERENCES

[1] Sarkozy A, Digilio MC, Dallapiccola B. Leopard syndrome. Orphanet J Rare Dis 2008; 3: 13.

[2] Gorlin RJ, Anderson RC, Blaw M. Multiple lentigines syndrome. Am J Dis Child 1969; 117: 652-62.

[3] Kratz CP, Rapisuwon S, Reed H, Hasle H, Rosenberg PS. Cancer in Noonan, Costello, cardiofaciocutaneous and LEOPARD syndromes. Am J Med Genet C Semin Med Genet 2011; 157: 83-9.

[4] Kato H, Yoshida R, Tsukamoto K, *et al.* Familial cases of atypical clinical features genetically diagnosed as LEOPARD syndrome (multiple lentigines syndrome). Int J Dermatol 2010; 49: 1146-51.

[5] Coppin BD, Temple IK. Multiple lentigines syndrome (LEOPARD syndrome or progressive cardiomyopathic lentiginosis). J Med Genet 1997; 34: 582-6.

[6] Lodish MB, Stratakis CA. The differential diagnosis of familial lentiginosis syndromes. Fam Cancer 2011; 10: 481-90.

[7] Denayer E, Legius E. What's new in the neuro-cardio-facial-cutaneous syndromes? Eur J Pediatr 2007; 166:1091-8.

[8] Gelb BD, Tartaglia M. LEOPARD Syndrome. In: Pagon RA, Bird TD, Dolan CR, Stephens K, Adam MP, Eds. Seattle (WA): Gene Reviews 1993. Gene Rev 2007; 2010: 16.

[9] Koudova M, Seemanova E, Zenker M. Novel BRAF mutation in a patient with LEOPARD syndrome and normal intelligence. Eur J Med Genet 2009; 52: 337-40.

[10] Seishima M, Mizutani Y, Shibuya Y, Arakawa C, Yoshida R, Ogata T. Malignant melanoma in a woman with LEOPARD syndrome: identification of a germline PTPN11 mutation and a somatic BRAF mutation. Br J Dermatol 2007; 157:1297-9.

[11] Jurecka W, Gebhart W, Knobler R, Schmoliner R, Möslacher H. The leopard syndrome, a cardio-cutaneous syndrome. Wien Klin Wochenschr 1983; 95: 652-6.

[12] Salerni G, Carrera C, Lovatto L, Puig-Butille JA, Badenas C, Plana E, Puig S, Malvehy J. Benefits of total body photography and digital dermatoscopy ("two-step method of digital follow-up") in the early diagnosis of melanoma in patients at high risk for melanoma. J Am Acad Dermatol. 2012; 67: e17-27.

[13] Kontoes PP, Vlachos SP, Marayiannis KV. Intense pulsed light for the treatment of lentigines in LEOPARD syndrome. Br J Plast Surg 2003; 56: 607-10.

Chronic Idiopathic Penile Edema: Three Cases

L. Raty[1], V. Failla[1], R. Andrianne[2], M. Fillet[2], D. Waltregny[2] and A.F. Nikkels[*,1]

Departments of [1]Dermatology and [2]Urology, CHU du Sart Tilman, University of Liège, Belgium

Abstract: Chronic idiopathic penile edema (CIPE) is an exceptional entity with disabling persistent lymphedema of the penis, affecting accessorily the scrotum and the pubis. The onset presents with recurrent swelling of the external genitalia, regressing spontaneously. After 2-3 years the swelling becomes progressively persistent. Mictional and erectile dysfunctions are not uncommon. A thorough work-up including RX, ultrasound examination, CT scanning, MRI imaging, serology and extensive blood testing should be performed to exclude underlying causes, including neoplastic, infectious, vascular and inflammatory diseases. CIPE is associated with significant psychological and functional impact. Surgical correction is the sole therapeutic option. Three patients with CIPE and a review of the literature are presented in order to increase awareness of this rare condition.

Keywords: Lymphedema, male external genitalia.

INTRODUCTION

Lymphedema of the external male genitalia may be congenital or acquired [1]. Furthermore, acute episodes should be distinguished from chronic disease [2,3]. The onset may occur at any age. Acquired lymphedema may be due to fluid balance disorders, or vascular, neoplastic, infectious granulomatous and inflammatory diseases [4,5]. Only after a clueless extensive work-up, the longstanding acquired lymphedema is classified as chronic idiopathic penile edema (CIPE) [6,7]. CIPE is an exceptional entity with significant functional impotency and an important psychological impact. Three patients are presented as well as a comprehensive review of the literature.

CASE REPORTS

Case 1

A 59-year-old man without significant medical, urological or surgical history presented a sudden, non-painful, swelling of the external genitalia. There was no prior drug intake, nor traumatism. The patient did not complain of mictional or other functional disorders. There were no systemic signs. The swelling resolved spontaneously after 2 weeks. The second episode revealed an erythematous aspect of the skin and a pitting lymphatic infiltration (Fig. **1**). Palpation evidenced ill-defined subcutaneous, non-painful masses of the penis, extending towards the scrotum and the pubis. Two skin biopsies were performed under local anesthesia revealing a mixed type vasculitis and a spongiotic dermatitis. Rx work-up was not remarkable. Urologic examination showed no prostatism. The testes were normal and non-tender. Ultrasonography showed a marked echogenic thickening of the scrotal and penile subcutaneous tissue. A CT Scan did not reveal the presence of an inflammatory or neoplastic process, hence excluding a secondary lymphovascular swelling (Fig. **2**). No lymphadenopathy was palpated. MRI imaging also showed a thickening of the subcutaneous layer of the penis. Hepatic, renal, thyroid and pancreatic functions were normal. Sedimentation rate, CEA, IgG, IgA, IgM, C3, C4, rheumatoid factor, antinuclear antibodies, ANCA, PSA and beta HCG were in normal range. CIPE was retained as final diagnosis. Currently, the swelling is stable since 2 years. There are no mictional problems but the patient suffers from erectile dysfunction and is severely bothered by his condition. Despite, the patient refused surgical intervention.

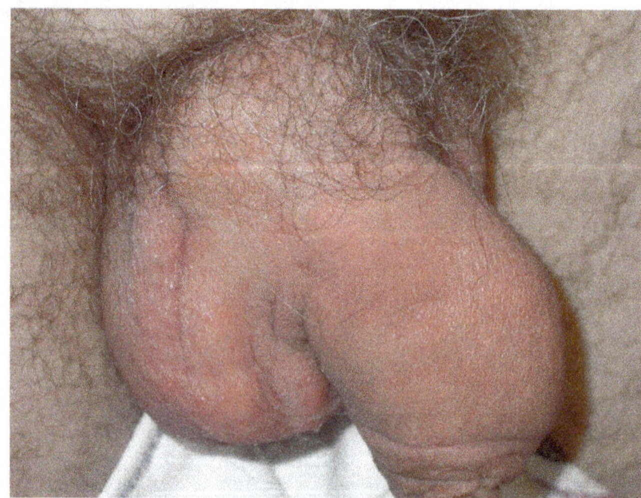

Fig. (1). Erythematous penile swelling.

Case 2

Since 3 years, a 49-year-old patient complained of recurrent episodes of painful diffuse swelling of the external genitalia. Progressively the swelling had become permanent, affecting the penis with an extension to the pubis and the

*Address correspondence to this author at the Department of Dermatology, University Hospital Center, University of Liège, B-4000 Liège, Belgium;

E-mail: af.nikkels@chu.ulg.ac.be

scrotum (Fig. **3**). No lymphadenopathy was observed. The skin was erythematous and itchy. There were no mictional problems. He presented erectile dysfunction with a significant impact on his quality of life. Urologic examination showed no prostatism. The testes were normal and non-tender. Furthermore, he presented a lupus-like syndrome with anti-cardiolipine antibodies and cutaneous IgG vasculitis. Previously, he had experienced 2 pulmonary embolisms and a deep venous thrombosis of the right leg. His medication consisted of salicylic acid 80 mg/day and chloroquine 200mg/day. The patient could not identify any triggering factor. Later, azathioprin 2x50mg/d and methylprednisolone 4 mg/d were required to treat the cutaneous vasculitis, as topical corticosteroids were non-effective. There was however no effect on the swelling. An extensive medical work-up, including CT scanner, MRI, ultrasonography and RX were unremarkable besides the subcutaneous swelling consistent with lymphedema. Extensive blood testing remained in the normal range. The CEA, CA 19.9 and CA 125 tumor markers were negative. As final conclusion, the diagnosis of CIPE was retained. Surgical correction was proposed but denied by the patient.

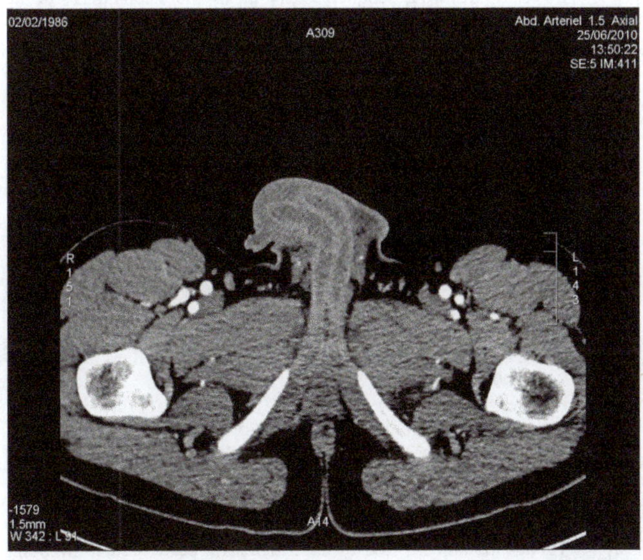

Fig. (2). CT scanning illustrating the penile lymphedematous swelling.

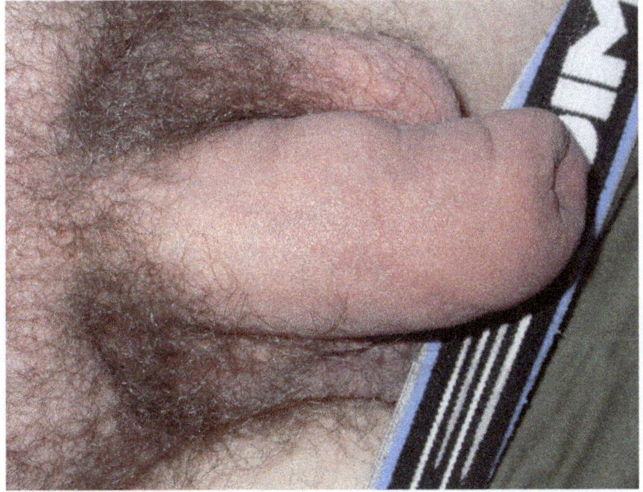

Fig. (3). Penile swelling.

Case 3

Since a year, a 54-year-old patient presented recurring, painless, swellings of the pubis, scrotum and penis, progressively becoming permanent (Fig. **4**). He presented mictional problems as well as erectile dysfunction. He also presented a deformation of the penile shaft. No adenopathy was present. The penile skin was itchy and erythematous. He had no remarkable medical or surgical history. The patient did not take any medication. An internal work-up including CT scanning and ultrasonography ruled out any obstruction. MRI revealed an irregular subcutaneous thickening of the pubis, scrotum and penis. The tumor markers PSA, CEA, CA 19.9 and CA 125 were in normal range. The B cell, CD4- and CD8-T lymphocytes, monocytes and myelocyte cell counts were unremarkable. Topical potent steroids reduced the erythematous aspect of the penis and partially improved the mictional problems, without however decreasing the swelling. CIPE was retained as working diagnosis.

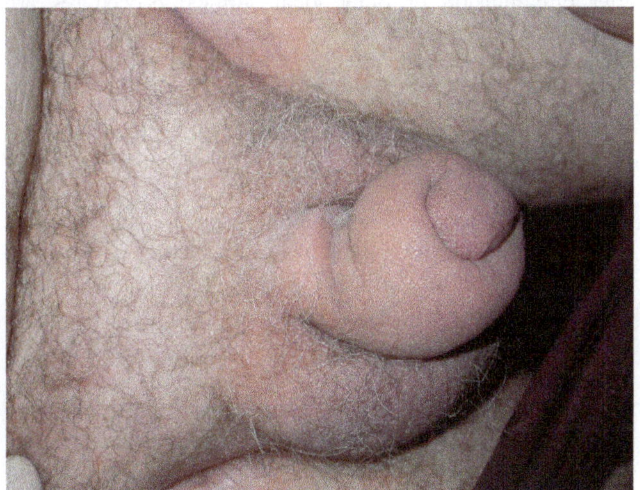

Fig. (4). Penile swelling with penile shaft deformation.

DISCUSSION

These cases illustrate typical examples of CIPE. CIPE is an exceptional disorder and epidemiological data are not available. CIPE affects preferentially the adult patient [8,9], but childhood cases have been reported [10].

The clinical course is stereotypic. The initial episodes are spontaneously resolving in 1-2 weeks. In children, the swelling usually disappears more rapidly. The swelling may be more or less diffuse and does not always recur at the same anatomical site. This initial phase can last for 1-4 years. Subsequently, there is a progressive organization of the lymphedema, similar to lymphedema of the lower extremities. At this stage, CIPE becomes extremely discomforting. All the three patients presented the particular disease progression. Clinical aspects vary from slightly indurate and moderate swelling to voluminous verrucous elephantiasis of the penis and scrotum [11]. Patients may suffer from recurrent pain, pruritus [12], chronic irritation, repeated infections, drainage, and sexual dysfunction, with limitation of local hygiene, ambulation and voiding in the standing position. CIPE represents an important functional, cosmetic, psychological and emotional problem [9], as illustrated by the presented cases.

Currently, CIPE is understood as a reduced lymphatic flow with subsequent enlargement of the penis, sometimes extending to the pubis and scrotum [8].

The diagnosis of CIPE can only be used after excluding all the potential causes of acquired chronic penile edema. In children, recurrent acquired swelling of the external genitals should exclude Crohn's disease [5]. In the adult patient, filariosis should be out ruled in endemic areas [8]. Prior surgery or radiotherapy-associated sequelae can also lead to lymphatic obstruction [13]. Congenital sequelae, neoplastic infiltration or inflammatory diseases should also be out ruled. Secondary peno-scrotal edema has also been described after amputation for septic diabetic foot [14]. Dengue hemorrhagic fever [15], acute necrotizing pancreatitis [16], hidradenitis suppurativa [13], foreign body injections or trauma with subsequent chronic infection [17] and continuous ambulatory peritoneal dialysis [18] are other rare causes. CIPE should also be distinguished from penile venereal edema [19]. Complications such as delayed healing after circumcision or other local surgical procedures are encountered. Long-term complications of CIPE include squamous cell carcinoma [9,20].

The diagnostic tools exploring acquired male genital swelling include color flow Doppler [10], lymphangiography [21], CT Scanner, or MRI. Histology is non-contributive as observed in patient 1 and 2. MRI is the preferential diagnostic method, accurately evidencing the subcutaneous lymphatic edema and ruling out other causes of eventual lymphatic obstruction [22].

No medical therapy exists for CIPE. Drainage has been proposed but is not feasible in real life. The sole definitive treatment is the surgical excision of the edematous and/or fibrotic tissues, together with reconstructive methods using local flaps and skin grafts [8,9,13,17,23,24]. Fasciocutaneous thigh flaps have been used for coverage of the scrotum, but these flaps can alter testicular thermoregulation, sometimes causing infertility. Full thickness skin grafts have also been used for coverage. The posterior based perineal flaps preserve perirectal lymphatics, a source of collateral lymphatic drainage. Another option is the modified Charles procedure, excising the involved skin followed by scrotoplasty and midline suture simulating the scrotal raphe. Afterwards, the penis is covered with a split-thickness skin graft with a zigzag suture on its ventral surface. This treatment option of CIPE is easily reproducible and allows better local hygiene, easier ambulation, voiding in the standing position, resuming sexual intercourse and better cosmetic results [25]. Other authors also related excellent cosmetic and functional results using this technique [22,24]. Wide excision of the involved area with subsequent coverage of exposed areas with split-thickness skin grafts in a single-stage procedure is another surgical technique. All the patients had excellent cosmetic results without recurrence of CIPE or compromise of sexual function postoperatively [23]. In short, once CIPE is a stable disease, surgical treatment is recommended and the functional and cosmetic results are excellent and patient rehabilitation is likely. It is however noteworthy that many patients refrain from surgical treatment, as in our cases.

In conclusion, CIPE is an exceptional and probably underrecognized entity, with disabling lymphedema affecting the penis, the scrotum and the pubis. The resolving episodes become progressively permanent. Mictional problems are rare but erectile dysfunction is usual. MRI is the preferential diagnostic method. Surgical correction is the only curative option.

REFERENCES

[1] Smeltzer DM, Stickler GB, Schirger A. Primary lymphedema in children and adolescents : a follow-up study and review. Pediatrics 1985; 76: 206-18.

[2] McDougal WS. Lymphedema of the external genitalia. J Urol 2003; 170: 711-6.

[3] van Langen AM, Gal S, Hulsmann AR, De Nef JJ. Acute idiopathic scrotal oedema: four cases and a short review. Eur J Pediatr 2001; 160: 455-6.

[4] Geyer H, Geyer A, Schubert J. Erysipelas and elephantiasis of the scrotum. Surgical and drug therapy. Urologe-Ausgabe A 1995; 34: 59-61.

[5] Murphy MJ, Kogan B, Carlson JA. Granulomatous lymphangitis of the scrotum and penis. Report of a case and review of the literature of genital swelling with sarcoidal granulomatous inflammation. J Cutan Pathol 2001; 28: 419-24.

[6] Thomas JA, Matanhelia SS, Rees RWM. Recurrent adult idiopathic penile oedema : a new clinical entity ? Hosp Update 1993; 667-8.

[7] Porter W, Dinneen M, Bunker C. Chronic penile lymphedema: a report of 6 cases. Arch Dermatol 2001; 137: 1108-10.

[8] Muehlberger T, Homann HH, Kuhnen C, Vogt PM, Steinau HU. Etiology, clinical aspects and therapy of penoscrotal lymphedema. Chirurg 2001; 72: 414-8.

[9] Halperin TJ, Slavin SA, Olumi AF, Borud LJ. Surgical management of scrotal lymphedema using local flaps. Ann Plast Surg 2007; 59: 67-72.

[10] Brandes SB, Chelsky MJ, Hanno PM. Adult acute idiopathic scrotal edema. Urology 1994; 44: 602-5.

[11] Luelmo J, Tolosa C, Prats J, Bella MR, Saez A, Pellicé C Jr. Tumorous lymphedema of the penis. Report of verrucous elephantiasis. A brief case. Preliminary note. Actas Urol Esp 1995; 19: 585-7.

[12] Tebbe-Gholami M, Roest W. A man with acute scrotal swelling. Ned Tijdschr Geneeskd 2010; 154: A16.

[13] García-Tutor E, Botellé del Hierro J, San Martín Maya A, *et al.* Surgical treatment of penile lymphedema associated with hidradenitis suppurativa. Acta Urol Esp 2005; 29: 519-22.

[14] Fahal AH, Suliman SH, Sharfi AR, el Mahadi EM. Acute idiopathic scrotal oedema in association with diabetic septic foot. Diabetes Res Clin Pract 1993; 21: 197-200.

[15] Chen TC, Lu PL, Chen YH, Tsai JJ, Chen TP. Dengue hemorrhagic fever complicated with acute idiopathic scrotal edema and polyneuropathy. Am J Trop Med Hyg 2008; 78: 8-10.

[16] Choong KK. Acute penoscrotal edema due to acute necrotizing pancreatitis. J Ultrasound Med 1996; 15: 247-8.

[17] Malloy TR, Wein AJ, Gross P. Scrotal and penile lymphedema: surgical considerations and management. J Urol 1983; 130: 263-5.

[18] Abraham G, Blake PG, Mathews RE, Bargman JM, Izatt S, Oreopoulos DG. Genital swelling as a surgical complication of continuous ambulatory peritoneal dialysis. Surg Gynecol Obstet 1990; 170: 306-8.

[19] Wright RA, Judson FN. Penile veneral edema. JAMA 1979; 241: 157-8.

[20] Hadway P, Lynch M, Corbishley CM, Mortimer PS, Watkin NA. Squamous cell carcinoma of the penis in a patient with chronic isolated penile lymphedema. Urol Int 2006; 76: 87-8.

[21] Samsoen M, Deschler JM, Servelle M, Raiga JC, Lelièvre G, Tardieu JC. Lymphoedema of penis and scrotum: two observations. Ann Dermatol Venereol 1981; 108: 541-6.

[22] Garaffa G, Christopher N, Ralph DJ. The management of genital lymphoedema. BJU Int 2008; 102: 480-4.

[23] Morey AF, Meng MV, McAninch JW. Skin graft reconstruction of chronic genital lymphedema. Urology 1997; 50: 423-6.

[24] Zacharakis E, Dudderidge T, Zacharakis E, Ioannidis E. Surgical repair of idiopathic scrotal elephantiasis. South Med J 2008; 101: 208-10.

[25] Modolin M, Mitre AI, da Silva JC, *et al.* Surgical treatment of lymphedema of the penis and scrotum. Clinics 2006; 61: 289-94.

In Vitro Efficacy of Four Insecticides Against Eggs of *Tunga penetrans* (Siphonaptera)

Tim Kiesewetter[1], Liana Ariza[2], Maria M. Martins[3], Jean E. Limongi[4,5], Juliana Junqueira da Silva[5], Júlio Mendes[4], Cláudia M. Lins Calheiros[6], Heiko Becher[7] and Jorg Heukelbach[*,2,8]

[1]*School of Medicine, University of Cologne, Cologne, Germany*

[2]*Department of Community Health, School of Medicine, Federal University of Ceará, Fortaleza, Brazil*

[3]*Faculty of Veterinary Medicine, Federal Universidade of Uberlândia, Uberlândia, Brazil*

[4]*Institute of Biomedical Sciences, Federal Universidade of Uberlândia, Uberlândia, Brazil*

[5]*Centre of Control of Zoonotic Diseases, Municipal Health Secretariat of Uberlândia, Minas Gerais, Brazil*

[6]*Institute of Biological Sciences and Health, Federal University of Alagoas, Maceió, Brazil*

[7]*Institute of Public Health, University of Heidelberg, Heidelberg, Germany*

[8]*Anton Breinl Centre for Public Health and Tropical Medicine, School of Public Health, Tropical Medicine and Rehabilitation Sciences, James Cook University, Townsville, Australia*

Abstract: Systematic assessments of control measures against the jigger flea *Tunga penetrans* are scarce, and there are no published data available on the efficacy of environmental insecticides against immature stages. We tested four environmental contact insecticides used by Brazilian authorities for disease control (deltamethrin, bifenthrin, dichlorvos and etofenprox) against *T. penetrans* eggs. Eggs were reared *in vitro.* Hatch rates were observed under standardized conditions and compared to a control group (40 eggs in each group). No larvae hatched after treatment with the organophosphate dichlorvos (100% efficacy). The efficacies of the other products tested varied between 17% and 57%. The data show that the organophosphate dichlorvos had a good *in vitro* efficacy. The use of dichlorvos can be directed to typical spots where early stages of *T. penetrans* are expected, considering its toxicity. Disease control should also consist of prevention measures concerning housing and environmental conditions, veterinary and human health measures.

Keywords: chigoe flea, efficacy, insecticides, prevention, *Tunga penetrans.*

INTRODUCTION

Infestation with the jigger flea *Tunga penetrans* (tungiasis) is a Neglected Tropical Disease causing substantial health burden in endemic areas [1]. Though affecting many people in resource-poor communities in sub-Saharan Africa, the Caribbean and Latin America, systematic evaluations of control measures against tungiasis are scarce [2-4].

Control of tungiasis is complex and would need an interdisciplinary approach [5]. The prevalence in humans in endemic regions can easily reach more than 50% and cause considerable morbidity [6-12]. Domestic animals such as pigs and dogs are the main animal reservoirs, and control measures thus would need to consider domestic animals [4, 5, 13]. In addition, immature stages are found in the environment where they may survive for a prolonged period [14]. For emergency control measures, eggs may be treated with environmental insecticides, but there are no efficacy data available on these insecticides against immature stages of *T. penetrans*. For example, in Rio Grande do Sul State in the extreme south of Brazil, the State Health Secretariat regularly sprays compounds of affected houses with alpha-cypermethrin without any evidence.

To provide evidence for control measures, we tested four insecticides used in disease control programs in Brazil against *T. penetrans* eggs. Eggs were reared *in vitro,* and hatch rates were observed under standardized conditions.

MATERIALS AND METHODS

The study was carried out in the city of Uberlândia (Minas Gerais State), situated in Brazil's savannah region. To obtain fertile *T. penetrans* eggs, laboratory-raised Wistar rats were exposed according to procedures described previously on compounds in the outskirts of Uberlândia where tungiasis occurs [15-17].

From September to October 2010, a total of 25 rats were exposed at 11 different locations. Two in two days, the infestation status and general status of animals were

*Address correspondence to this author at the Departamento de Saúde Comunitária, Faculdade de Medicina, Universidade Federal do Ceará, Rua Professor Costa Mendes 1608, 5. andar, Fortaleza CE, 60430-140, Brazil;

E-mail: heukelbach@web.de

assessed. The rats were transported after 5 to 7 days to the laboratory of the Federal University of Uberlândia for a thorough examination. The lesions were counted and classified according to the Fortaleza Classification [18]. Infested rats with the embedded fleas expelling eggs (stage 3 according to Fortaleza Classification; Fig. **1**) were held over black cardboard for 3 to 5 hours to facilitate detection and collection of deposited eggs. Eggs were examined for physical integrity, counted and transferred to Petri dishes.

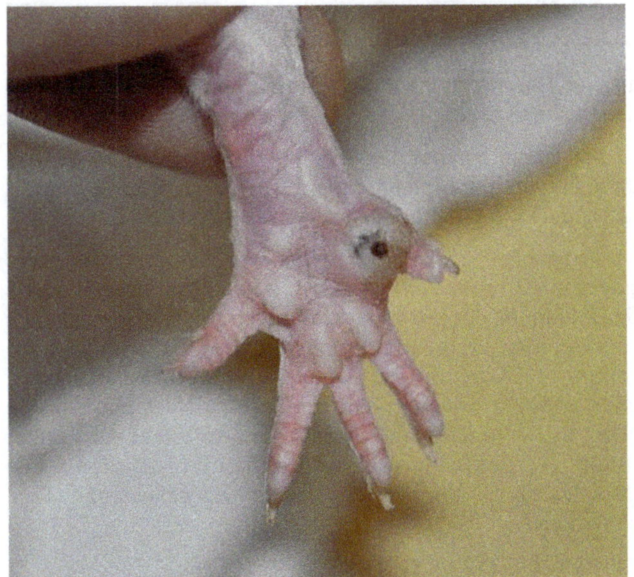

Fig. (1). Rat infested with *T. penetrans* (stage III according to Fortaleza Classification).

Environmental insecticides tested are given in Table **1**. All insecticides are registered by the Brazilian Ministry of Health for peridomestic and environmental spraying. The concentration was chosen as recommended in the product information for the control of small insects (Table **1**). These concentrations are also used by the centers for zoonosis control throughout Brazil. In each insecticide and control group, 40 eggs were tested. Batches of eggs were pooled and then randomized into one of the four treatment or control groups. 175 µl of the insecticide were applied from 5 cm distance using a standardized hand pump spray bottle. That equals an application of about 0.022 l/m^2. In the control group tap water was used.

The Petri dishes were placed in a polystyrene box and incubated at environmental temperature (24.7-27.8°C). To establish consistent humidity, damp cloth was placed inside the boxes. Relative humidity varied from 50.4% to 71%. After 3, 5 and 7 days the eggs were examined for hatching, and larvae counted. All procedures and examinations were conducted by a single observer to prevent inter-observer variation.

Data were entered using Excel spread sheets and checked for entry errors. Corrected hatch rates were calculated as: (crude hatch rate in test group) / (crude hatch rate in untreated control group). Efficacy of a product was defined as: (1 - corrected hatch rate). Negative values (hatch rate in intervention group higher than in control group) were considered as 0% efficacy. 95% confidence intervals for efficacy were calculated according to an asymptotic formula, as described by Rosenheim and Hoy [19]. Calculated values below 0% or above 100% in confidence intervals were set to 0% or 100%, respectively. Relative frequencies between groups were compared applying Fisher's exact test to evaluate statistical significance. Analysis was done using SAS (version 9.2, SAS Institute Inc., Cary, USA).

The study was approved by the Ethical Review Board for Animals (*Comissão de Ética na Utilização de Animais - CEUA*) of the Universidade Federal de Uberlândia, protocol no. CEUA/UFU 092/10.

RESULTS

The 25 rats were exposed to households expected to be infested with the jigger fleas twice or three times. In total, data of 67 exposures were collected. In eight cases (11.9%), tungiasis lesions were found. The number of lesions per rat ranged between 1 and 18 (mean: 8.5).

The numbers of hatched eggs and efficacies of the tested insecticides are shown in Table **2**. No larvae hatched after treatment with the organophosphate dichlorvos. The efficacies of the other products tested varied between 17% and 57%. Dichlorvos showed significantly higher efficacy than the other insecticides tested ($p<0.0001$). On day three, 21/29 (72%) larvae in the deltamethrin group showed spontaneous movement. No other larvae in the intervention groups showed vital signs. In the control group, all 35 hatched larvae were fully active.

DISCUSSION

This is the first systematic study on the efficacy of insecticides against immature stages of *T. penetrans.* The data show that at a concentration commonly used by Brazilian control programs, only the organophosphate dichlorvos had an acceptable ovicidal efficacy. As with the exception of deltamethrin, hatched larvae did not show vital signs for the other products, a residual larvicidal effect is possible.

The use of insecticides has been considered one of the means in an integrated approach to control tungiasis in affected regions [5]. In this context, environmental

Table 1. Details of Insecticides Tested Against Eggs of *Tunga penetrans*

Product	Producer	Active Ingredient	Tested Concentration
Deltametrina 25 ce	Fersol, Mairinque, SP, Brazil	25g/L Deltamethrin (type II Pyrethroid)	0.25g/L (5.5 mg/m^2)
Bifentol 200 sc	ChemoNE, Bezerros, PE, Brazil	200g/L Bifenthrin (type I Pyrethroid)	0.6g/L (13.2 mg/m^2)
DDVP 1000 ce	Fersol, Mairinque, SP, Brazil	825 g/L Dichlorvos	4.125g/L (90.75 mg/m^2)
Vectron 10 sc	Iharabras SA, Sorocaba, SP,Brazil	100 g/L Etofenprox	2 g/L (44 mg/m^2)

Table 2. Efficacy of Four Insectides Tested Against Eggs of *Tunga penetrans*

Insecticide	Number of Eggs	Number of Larvae (= Hatched Eggs)	Crude Hatch Rate	Corrected Hatch Rate	Efficacy (95% Confidence Interval)
Dichlorvos	40	0	0%	0%	100% (92.1-100)
Etofenprox	40	15	37.5%	42.9%	57.1% (29.3-75.1)
Bifenthrin	40	18	45.0%	51.4%	48.6% (30.0-67.2)
Deltametrin	40	29	72.5%	82.9%	17.1% 0-35.7
Control	40	35	87.5%	100%	0% (0-16.6)

insecticide spraying should be considered an emergency intervention and would need integration with other more sustainable measures. In fact, recent studies have shown that intermittent application of a plant-based repellent reduced morbidity significantly, but that transmission and subsequently morbidity increased rapidly after interruption of this intervention [20]. Control ideally should consist of individual therapeutic measures, and interventions concerning improved housing and environmental conditions, and veterinary measures to reduce animal reservoirs such as cats, dogs, pigs and rats [4, 21]. As off-host life stages of *T. penetrans* can be found indoors and/or outdoors (which may vary from setting to setting), the use of an efficacious insecticide such as dichlorvos may be performed in addition to these control measures, directed to typical areas where early stages are expected [14, 22, 23].

One matter of concern is the mammalian toxicity of dichlorvos, an organophosphate that is absorbed through skin, gastrointestinal tract and the respiratory system. The insecticide is highly volatile with a vapor pressure of 0.012 mmHg at 20°C [24], thus reasonable precautions have to be taken when used indoors. Organophosphates irreversibly inactivate the acetylcholine esterase. Overexposure may cause a variety of symptoms, according to the route of exposure. Whereas inhalation may cause ocular and respiratory symptoms, ingestion causes gastrointestinal discomfort. Dichlorvos may also lead to allergic contact dermatitis. In severe cases, paralysis of respiratory muscles can lead to death. Low-dose long-term effects are still discussed due to uncertainties in the study designs concerning dose and insecticide mixture [25].

Synthetic pyrethroids (deltamethrin, bifenthrin) are usually considered less toxic, but were less efficacious against eggs in our study. They block the voltage-dependent sodium channel resulting in a stable hyperexcitable state of tissues. Symptoms of acute pyrethroid intoxication include paraesthesia, nausea, headache, muscle fasciculation, dizziness, fatigue and convulsions. Only a few studies have been conducted concerning long-term toxicity of pyrethroids. The results support that there are limited effects in humans exposed to pyrethroids [26, 27].

Etofenprox is a non-ester synthetic pyrethroid with a similar mode of action. Yet its toxicity to humans and mammals is lower [28]. The main targets of acute intoxication are liver, kidney, thyroid and the hematopoietic system. The International Programme on Chemical Safety found no evidence for geno-toxicity [29]. The USEPA classified etofenprox as a possible human carcinogen. Mid- and long term data as to the chronic impact on humans still need to be evaluated.

As larvae hatched but did not show vital signs on day three in both, the Etofenprox and Bifenthrin group, a residual larvicidal effect of these compounds is possible.

In conclusion, we have shown that control of immature stages of *T. penetrans* with environmental insecticides is feasible in the context of an integrated control approach, at a concentration used currently by Brazilian authorities for the control of different insect species. Control measures against other endemic diseases using these insecticides may thus be integrated with tungiasis control in endemic settings. Further studies are needed to assess the efficacy of environmental insecticides of low toxicity under laboratory and field conditions.

CONFLICT OF INTEREST

The authors confirm that this article content has no conflict of interest.

ACKNOWLEDGEMENTS

We thank the Centro de Control de Zoonoses, Uberlândia and the Universidade Federal de Uberlândia, Uberlândia for support. The study was financed by a "Projeto Universal" grant from the *Conselho Nacional de Desenvolvimento Científico e Tecnológico* (CNPq). JH is research fellow from CNPq.

REFERENCES

[1] Heukelbach J, de Oliveira FA, Hesse G, Feldmeier H. Tungiasis: a neglected health problem of poor communities. Trop Med Int Health 2001; 6: 267-72.

[2] Buckendahl J, Heukelbach J, Ariza L, Kehr JD, Seidenschwang M, Feldmeier H. Control of Tungiasis through Intermittent Application of a Plant-Based Repellent: An Intervention Study in a Resource-Poor Community in Brazil. PLoS Negl Trop Dis 2010; 4: e879.

[3] Heukelbach J. Invited Review: Tungiasis. Rev Inst Med Trop Sao Paulo 2005; 47: 307-13.

[4] Pilger D, Schwalfenberg S, Heukelbach J, *et al.* Investigations on the biology, epidemiology, pathology, and control of *Tunga penetrans* in Brazil: VII. The importance of animal reservoirs for human infestation. Parasitol Res 2008; 102: 875-80.

[5] Heukelbach J, Mencke N, Feldmeier H. Editorial: Cutaneous larva migrans and tungiasis: the challenge to control zoonotic ectoparasitoses associated with poverty. Trop Med Int Health 2002; 7: 907-10.

[6] Collins G, Mcleod T, Konfor NI, Lamnyam C, Ngarka LE, Njamnshi NL. Tungiasis: A neglected health problem in rural Cameroon. Int J Collab Res Intern Med Public Health 2009, 1: 2-10.

[7] Ugbomoiko US, Ofoezie IE, Heukelbach J. Tungiasis: high prevalence, parasite load, and morbidity in a rural community in Lagos State, Nigeria. Int J Dermatol 2007; 46: 475-81.

[8] Joseph JK, Bazile J, Mutter J, *et al.* Tungiasis in rural Haiti: a community-based response. Trans R Soc Trop Med Hyg 2006; 100: 970-4.

[9] de Carvalho RW, de Almeida AB, Barbosa-Silva SC, Amorim M, Ribeiro PC, Serra-Freire NM. The patterns of tungiasis in Araruama township, state of Rio de Janeiro, Brazil. Mem Inst Oswaldo Cruz 2003; 98: 31-6.

[10] Muehlen M, Heukelbach J, Wilcke T, Winter B, Mehlhorn H, Feldmeier H. Investigations on the biology, epidemiology, pathology and control of *Tunga penetrans* in Brazil. II. Prevalence, parasite load and topographic distribution of lesions in the population of a traditional fishing village. Parasitol Res 2003; 90(6):449-55.

[11] Feldmeier H, Heukelbach J, Eisele M, Sousa AQ, Barbosa LM, Carvalho CB. Bacterial superinfection in human tungiasis. Trop Med Int Health 2002; 7: 559-64.

[12] Wilcke T, Heukelbach J, César Sabóia Moura R, Regina Sansigolo Kerr-Pontes L, Feldmeier H. High prevalence of tungiasis in a poor neighbourhood in Fortaleza, Northeast Brazil. Acta Trop 2002; 83: 255-8.

[13] Ugbomoiko US, Ariza L, Heukelbach J. Pigs are the most important animal reservoir for *Tunga penetrans* (jigger flea) in rural Nigeria. Trop Doct 2008; 38: 226-7.

[14] Linardi, PM, Calheiros CML, Campelo-Junior EB, Duarte EM, Heukelbach J, Feldmeier H. Occurrence of the off-host life stages of Tunga penetrans *(Siphonaptera)* in various environments in Brazil. Ann Trop Med Parasitol 2010; 104: 337-45.

[15] Calheiros, CML. Aspectos biológicos e ecológicos de *Tunga penetrans* (L.,1758) (Siphonaptera: Tungidae) em áreas endêmicas brasileiras. Ciencas: Instituto de Ciências Biológicas, Universidade Federal de Minas, Gerais 2007.

[16] Nagy N, Abari E, D'Haese J, *et al.* Investigations on the life cycle and morphology of *Tunga penetrans* in Brazil. Parasitol Res 2007; 101: 233-42.

[17] Witt LH, Linardi PM, Meckes O, *et al.* Blood-feeding of *Tunga penetrans* males. Med Vet Entomol 2004; 18: 439-41.

[18] Eisele M, Heukelbach J, Van Marck E, *et al.* Investigations on the biology, epidemiology, pathology and control of *Tunga penetrans* in Brazil: I. Natural history of tungiasis in man. Parasitol Res 2003; 90: 87-99.

[19] Rosenheim JA, Hoy MA. Confidence Intervals for the Abbott's Formula Correction of Bioassay Data for Control Response. J Econ Entomol 1989; 82: 331-5.

[20] Feldmeier HJ, Kehr D, Heukelbach J. A plant-based repellent protects against *Tunga penetrans* infestation and sand flea disease. Acta Trop 2006; 99: 126-36.

[21] Heukelbach J. Revision on tungiasis: treatment options and prevention. Expert Rev Anti Infect Ther 2006; 4: 151-7.

[22] Witt L, Heukelbach J, Schwalfenberg S, Ribeiro RA, Harms G, Feldmeier H. Infestation of Wistar rats with *Tunga penetrans* in different microenvironments. Am J Trop Med Hyg 2007; 76: 666-8.

[23] Ugbomoiko US, Ariza L, Ofoezie IE, Heukelbach J. Risk Factors for Tungiasis in Nigeria: Identification of Targets for Effective Intervention. PLoS Negl Trop Dis 2007; 1: e87.

[24] O'Neil MJ, Ed. The Merck Index: An Encyclopedia of Chemicals, Drugs, and Biologicals. Whitehouse Station, NJ: Merck & Co Inc. 2001; pp. 541-2.

[25] Costa LG. Current issues in organophosphate toxicology. Clin Chim Acta 2006; 366: 1-13.

[26] Bradberry SM, Cage SA, Proudfoot AT, Vale JA. Poisoning due to Pyrethroids Toxicol Rev 2005; 24: 93-106.

[27] Vijverberg HP, van den Bercken J. Neurotoxicological effects and the mode of action of pyrethroid insecticides. Crit Rev Toxicol 1990; 21: 105-26.

[28] United States Environmental Protection Agency. Etofenprox: Human Health Risk Assessment for Proposed Section 3 Uses on Rice and as ULV Mosquito Adulticide.. Washington D.C.: USEPA, USA 2008.

[29] International Programme on Chemical Safety. Etofenprox Pesticide residues in food: 1993 evaluations Part II Toxicology. Geneva, Switzerland: IPCS, World Health Organisation 1993.

Development of an Ultraviolet A1 Light Emitting Diode-based Device for Phototherapy

Shunko A. Inada[*,1,3], Satoshi Kamiyama[1], Isamu Akasaki[1], Kan Torii[3], Takuya Furuhashi[3], Hiroshi Amano[2] and Akimichi Morita[3]

[1]*Department of Materials Science and Engineering, Faculty of Science and Technology, Meijo University, 1-501 Shiogamaguchi Tempaku-ku, Nagoya 468-8502, Japan*

[2]*Graduate School of Engineering, Akasaki Research Center, Nagoya University, Furo-cho, Chikusa-ku, Nagoya 464-8603, Japan*

[3]*Department of Geriatric and Environmental Dermatology, Nagoya City University Graduate School of Medical Sciences, Nagoya 467-8601, Japan*

Abstract: We developed a novel phototherapy device based on an ultraviolet light emitting diode (UV LED) with a peak wavelength of 365 nm and the full width at half maximum of 10 nm. The equipment comprised a 16 x 16 (50 cm x 50 cm) UV LED matrix. The system was designed to irradiate only the diseased part of the skin. To evaluate the characteristics of this device, we compared consumed power, irradiation intensity, uniformity of the irradiation intensity, rise time and stability of the irradiation intensity, and *in vivo* irradiation of mice between a conventional UVA1 (340-400 nm) phototherapy device and the UV LED device. The UVA1 LED device exhibited more desirable characteristics than the UVA1 lamp device, i.e., fewer thermal effects on *in vitro* and *in vivo* systems. Furthermore, to evaluate the efficacy of both light sources, cultured T cells were irradiated and the induction of apoptosis was analyzed. Both light sources efficiently induced apoptosis.

Keywords: Apoptosis, phototherapy, ultraviolet light emitting diode (UV LED).

INTRODUCTION

Ultraviolet (UV) irradiation for phototherapy is commonly used to treat refractory skin disease. A fluorescent light bulb that emits a narrow-band wavelength between 311 and 313 nm (narrow-band UVB) is used to treat refractory skin diseases such as psoriasis vulgaris and vitiligo vulgaris [1, 2]. A wavelength range of 340-400 nm (UVA1) is used to treat atopic dermatitis and urticaria pigmentosa [3, 4]. The use of a fluorescent light bulb as the light source, however, has several disadvantages: (1) Phototherapy systems using a fluorescent light bulb require many square meters of floor space and consume approximately 3.5-5 KW of electricity; (2) The light source has a relatively short lifetime and contains toxic substances; (3) Irradiation of healthy tissue is difficult to avoid when using a large-area irradiation device, leading to unwanted exposure; (4) The heat radiating from the light source is uncomfortable for the patients; and (5) Medical workers are also exposed to UV irradiation while operating the system.

To address these problems, a device based on a newly-developed light emitting diode (LED) should be considered for UVA1 irradiation. The single-chip GaN-based UV LED is relatively small (350 μm x 350 μm) [5]. This UV LED can be operated with a dry battery and can be used to irradiate only the diseased skin. Moreover, the lifetime of the LED is three times longer than that of normal fluorescent light bulbs, and the LED contains no toxic substances [6]. In addition, the UV LED has a narrower spectrum range than the fluorescent light bulb. The development of a UV LED device based on a III-nitride semiconductor was reported [7-9]. The emission efficiency of the UV LED, however, is significantly decreased at emission wavelengths shorter than 360 nm [10]. Although a visible LED and laser diode have been used to treat acne and facial rejuvenation [11-13], to our knowledge there are no reports of UV LED-based phototherapy.

We previously compared the effects of UVA1 LED (wavelength 365 nm, full width at half maximum (FWHM) of 10 nm, output power 1400 W/cm^2; ANUJ5010, Panasonic Co., Ltd.) with conventional UVA1 fluorescent lamp (340-400 nm) phototherapy equipment (Partial Body UVA1 Irradiation Sellamed 2000 System; Sellas, Germany) [14]. Jurkat T cells, a leukemic T cell line, were used to evaluate the efficacy of phototherapy. Apoptosis and necrosis were induced in Jurkat T cells irradiated by the UVA1 LED and conventional UVA1 lamp devices. The two different light sources had similar biologic effects. Both UVA1 light sources induced similar levels of apoptosis and necrosis [14].

In the present study, we developed a phototherapy system using the UVA1 LED. The UVA1 LED phototherapy device comprised a 16 x 16 (50 cm x 50 cm) UV LED matrix. It can selectively irradiate the diseased skin without affecting

*Address correspondence to this author at the Department of Materials Science and Engineering, Faculty of Science and Technology, Meijo University, 1-501 Shiogamaguchi Tempaku-ku, Nagoya 468-8502, Japan;

E-mail: m0641503@ccalumni.meijo-u.ac.jp

neighboring healthy skin. The device takes a picture of the area of skin to be treated, and a computer program built into the device selects the areas to be irradiated.

We compared the consumed power, irradiation intensity, uniformity of the irradiation intensity, rise time and stability of the irradiation intensity, and temperature during *in vivo* exposure of irradiated mice between the UVA1 LED phototherapy device and conventional UVA1 lamp phototherapy device. We also compared the ability of the two devices to induce apoptosis.

MATERIALS AND METHODS

Development of the UV LED Phototherapy Device

We developed a phototherapy system containing UVA1 LEDs (wavelength 365 nm, FWHM 7 nm, output power 250 mW) obtained from Nichia Corporation (Fig. **1**). The device comprised a 16 x 16 (50 cm x 50 cm) UV LED matrix. The system takes a picture of the intended treatment area, and a computer program then selects the region to be irradiated. The energy efficiency of the UV LED is approximately 22%; therefore, an aluminum heat sink with cooling water was used to cool the system. To prevent accidents, the system was controlled by sensors that monitor electricity, water leakage, seismic intensity, and heat.

Evaluation of Irradiation Intensity

For all of the comparisons of the two devices, the number of LEDs used in the UV LED device was decreased to match the size of the UVA1 lamp (28 cm x 24 cm). To compare the irradiation intensity of the UV LED and UVA1 devices, the light source was fixed above the center of an irradiation detector (IL1700 Research Radiometer SED005, International Light Technologies, Peabody, MA). The height of the light source was varied from 1 cm to 50 cm and the mean irradiation intensity was measured at 5-cm intervals.

Evaluation Uniformity of the Irradiation Intensity

To compare the uniformity of irradiation intensity of the UVA1 LED phototherapy and UVA1 lamp phototherapy devices, the light source was fixed above the center of the irradiation detector and irradiation intensity was measured at 5-cm intervals across the diameter while the height of the light source was varied from 1 cm to 50 cm at 5-cm intervals.

To compare the uniformity of the irradiation intensity of the UV LED and UVA1 lamp devices at 10, 20, 30, 40, and 50 mW/cm^2, the light source was fixed above the center of the irradiation detector. Irradiation intensity was measured at 5-cm intervals across the diameter.

Evaluation of the Rise Time and Stability of the Irradiation Intensity

To compare the rise time of the irradiation intensity of the UV LED and UVA1 lamp devices, the light source was fixed above the center of the power meter (VEGA PD300-UV OPHIR, North Logan, UT). Rise time was measured until the irradiation intensity reached a steady state from the power input. The stability of the irradiation intensity was measured for 1 h.

Evaluation of Temperature Characteristics

To compare the temperature characteristics, mice (C57BL/6) were irradiated for 20 min at 3 irradiation intensities (10, 20, and 30 mW/cm^2, which corresponded to doses of 12, 24, and 36 J/cm^2, respectively), and the temperature of both the skin surface and body of the mice was measured every 2 min. The skin surface temperature was measured by thermography (CPA-0306 CHINO Co., Ltd., Tokyo, Japan) and the body temperature was measured using a thermoelectric couple (CT-470 Custom Laboratory Thermocouples, St. Francis, MN) placed in the rectum. The experiment was performed 3 times at each irradiation intensity.

Evaluation of Temperature Characteristics Using Selective Irradiation Function

To confirm the selective irradiation function of the UV LED device, mice with a body size of approximately 8 cm x 3 cm were irradiated at an intensity of 30 mW/cm^2 for 20 min. The experiment was discontinued if the state of the mice became unresponsive while being irradiated by the UVA1 lamp phototherapy device. The temperature of both the skin surface and body of the mice was measured every 2 min. To compare with the UVA1 lamp, the same experiment was performed using a board with an 8 cm x 3 cm hole placed between the light source and the mouse. The skin surface temperature and body temperature were measured as described above.

Evaluation of Temperature Characteristics Using Far-Infrared Resonance Filter

To determine if the increased temperature in the skin surface and body was due to the UV light or the far-infrared rays produced by the light source, the mice were irradiated using a far-infrared resonance filter (size: 5 cm x 5 cm, transparent wavelength: 250-2000 nm, HAF-50S-15H, SIGMA KOKI Co., Ltd., Tokyo, Japan). To compare the effect of the filter, a board with a 5 cm x 5 cm hole was placed between the light source and the mice. The mice were irradiated for 20 min at an intensity of 30 mW/cm^2 using the UVA1 LED phototherapy and UVA1 lamp phototherapy devices. The temperature of both the skin surface and body of the mice was measured every 2 min as described above.

Evaluation of Temperature Characteristics of Three Types Mediums

Three types of media: Dulbecco's Phosphate Buffered Saline (PBS), RPMI1640 (with phenol red), and RPMI1640 (without phenol red) (Sigma Aldrich Co., Ltd., St. Louis, MO) and dishes of three different diameters, 3.5 cm, 6 cm, and 10 cm, were used for temperature analysis. The temperature of the medium was measured every 2 min using a thermoelectric couple (CT-470 Custom). The number of the UVA1 LEDs was decreased to match the size of the UVA1 lamp. The amount of medium put into each dish was as follows: 3.5-cm dish = 2 mL, 6-cm dish = 5 mL, and 10-cm dish = 10 mL. The experiment was performed 3 times for each condition.

Evaluation of Cellular Apoptosis

To confirm the positive control of cellular apoptosis, Jurkat T cells were cultured with RPMI1640 (with phenol

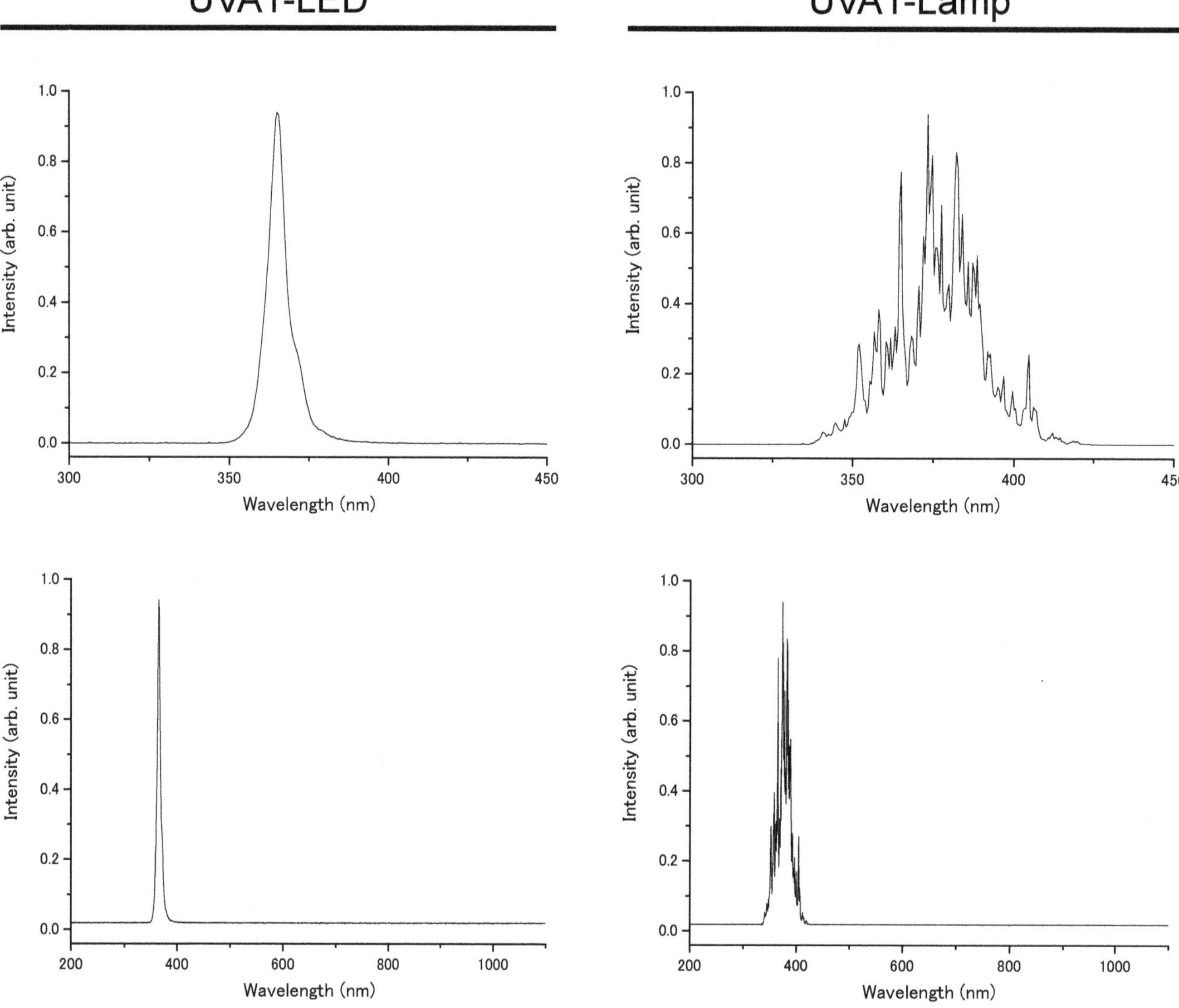

Fig. (1). UV LED and UVA1 lamp spectrums. The UV LED device has a peak wavelength of 365 nm and full width at half maximum (FWHM) of 7 nm. The UVA1 lamp has a peak wavelength of 373 nm and FWHM of 40 nm. The light source comprises UV, blue, and infrared filters. The top panels show only the UVA1 wavelength spectrum. The bottom panels show a larger spectrum (200 to 1000 nm).

red)/10% fetal bovine serum (Equitech Bio, Inc., Kerrville, TX)/50 mM HEPES buffer (Sigma-Aldrich)/5 mM sodium pyruvate (Sigma-Aldrich)/0.5 mM Minimal Essential Medium non-essential amino acids solution (GIBCO)/5x antibiotic-antimycotic (GIBCO) in 5% CO_2 at 37°C. Jurkat T cells were diluted to 0.5 x 10^6 cells/mL with PBS.

A broadband UVB (BB-UVB) light source (FL20S E-30/DMR, Toshiba Co., Ltd., Tokyo, Japan) was fixed at a height of 20 cm above the cultures and the irradiation intensity was 0.61 mW/cm^2. Twenty-four hours after either control, sham irradiation, or BB-UVB irradiation at doses of 20, 40, and 80 mJ/cm^2, the cells were collected to examine cellular apoptosis using a flow cytometer (BD FACS Canto II, Becton Dickinson Co., Ltd., Princeton, NJ). The cells were stained with propidium iodide and annexin V-fluorescein isothiocyanate (Medical & Biological Laboratories Co., Ltd., Nagoya, Japan).

Irradiation intensities of control, sham irradiation, and 10 J/cm^2, 20 J/cm^2, and 30 J/cm^2 UVA1 irradiation were applied to three dishes using the UVA1 phototherapy devices. The number of UVA1 LEDs was decreased to match the size of the UVA1 lamp. The UV LED was fixed at a height of 35 cm. The UVA1 lamp device was fixed at a height of 63 cm, and the irradiation intensity was 10 mW/cm^2.

Statistical Methods

We compared the UV LED and UVA1 devices using a two-tailed t-test. Results are expressed as the means ± SD. A P value of less than 0.05 was considered significant.

RESULTS

Evaluation of Consumed Power

The power consumed by the UVA1 LED phototherapy and UVA1 lamp phototherapy devices was measured using the same intensity and lamp size. The UVA1 LED consumed one-third the power of the UVA1 lamp (Fig. **2**).

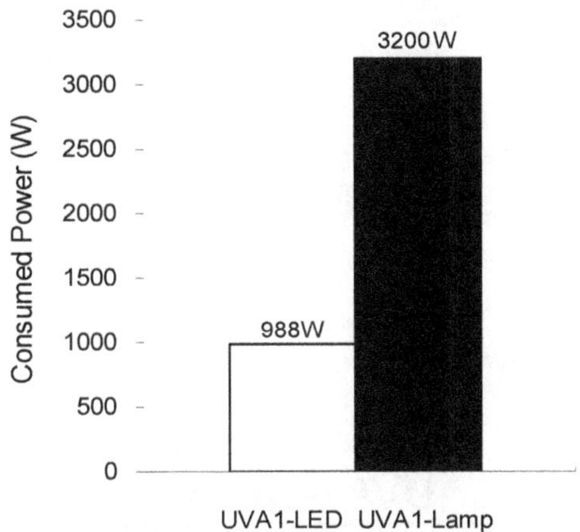

Fig. (2). Power consumption of the UV LED and UVA1 lamps was compared at the same intensity and dimension. The UV LED can irradiate at the same intensity and size using one-third the power required by the UVA1 lamp.

Evaluation of Irradiation Intensity

The irradiation intensity of both the UVA1 LED and UVA1 lamp devices was measured from a height ranging from 1 cm to 50 cm at 5-cm intervals. The UVA1 LED had lower intensity than the UVA1 lamp (Fig. **3a**). At a distance between 6 cm and 10 cm, the UVA1 LED produced uniform intensity.

Evaluation of Uniformity of Distance-Dependent Irradiation Intensity

Irradiation intensity was measured across the diameter at 5-cm intervals with the height of light source ranging from 1 cm to 50 cm at 5-cm intervals. The irradiation intensity of the UVA1 lamp decreased as the irradiation distance increased with a cosine function, and was uniform when the irradiation distance was smaller (Fig. **3b**). The UVA1 LED, however, produced uniform irradiation independent of the irradiation distance.

Evaluation of Irradiation Intensity Uniformity

The light sources were fixed above the center of the detector at distances that produced 10, 20, 30, 40, and 50 mW/cm^2 of irradiation. Irradiation intensity was measured across the diameter at 5-cm intervals. The intensity at 10 and 20 mW/cm^2 was uniform (Fig. **3c**). At 30, 40, and 50 mW/cm^2, however, the uniformity of the UVA1 lamp irradiation intensity decreased with a cosine function. In contrast, the UVA1 LED had a uniform intensity at each irradiation intensity.

Evaluation of the Rise Time and Stability of the Irradiation Intensity

Rise time was measured until the irradiation intensity reached a steady state. The intensity of the UVA1 lamp reached a steady state in approximately 1 min, and the intensity of the UVA1 LED reached a steady state within a few seconds (Fig. **4a**). The stability of irradiation intensity was measured for 1 h. While the UVA1 lamp irradiation intensity fluctuated over the course of 1 h of observation, that of the UVA1 LED was stable (Fig. **4b**).

Evaluation of Skin and Body Temperature

The temperature characteristics of mice were measured every 2 min for 20 min irradiation with the UVA1 LED and UVA1 lamp devices at intensities of 10, 20, and 30 mW/cm^2 (corresponding to irradiation intensities of 12, 24, and 36 J/cm^2) and compared. By the end of the observation period, body temperature was not significantly different between mice irradiated with the two devices (Fig. **5**). With increasing irradiation intensity, however, the skin surface temperature of mice irradiated with the UVA1 lamp increased 8°C to 10°C. In contrast, the skin surface temperature of mice irradiated with the UVA1 LED increased only 3°C to 4°C. In the experiment using an irradiation intensity of 30 mW/cm^2 with the UVA1 lamp, the state of the mouse became unresponsive after 18 min and the experiment was discontinued. At that time, the body temperature was 40.5°C, and the skin surface temperature was 60°C.

Evaluation of Temperature Characteristics Using the Selective Irradiation Function

To confirm the selective irradiation function of the UVA1 LED phototherapy device, mice were irradiated at 30 mW/cm^2 for 20 min, which was an intensity that could not be tested using the UVA1 lamp phototherapy device (see above). The temperature of both the skin surface and body as measured every 2 min. To compare with the UVA1 lamp, the same experiment was performed using a board with an 8 cm x 3 cm hole placed between the light source and the mouse. The body and skin surface temperatures of mice irradiated using the UVA1 LED barely changed (Fig. **6**). The body and skin surface temperatures of the mice irradiated with the UVA1 lamp, however, increased rapidly. Compared to the UVA1 LED, the UVA1 lamp increased the body temperature 5.1°C and the skin surface temperature 13.8°C. These results suggest that the UVA1 LED can treat affected skin more intensively without heating the skin than the conventional UVA1 lamp.

Evaluation of Temperature Characteristics Using a Far-Infrared Resonance Filter

The mice were irradiated with the UVA1 LED and UVA1 lamp devices using a far-infrared resonance filter and the temperature of both the skin surface and body of the mice was measured to determine if the increase in the skin surface and body temperature was due to UV or far-infrared irradiation. The far-infrared resonance filter did not affect the body or skin surface temperatures in mice irradiated with the UVA1 LED device (Fig. **7**). With the UVA1 lamp, however, the filter prevented an increase in the body (3.4°C without filter) and skin surface (13.7°C without filter) temperature. Thus, the increase in the body and skin surface temperature in mice irradiated with the UVA1 lamp was due to the emission of far-infrared rays.

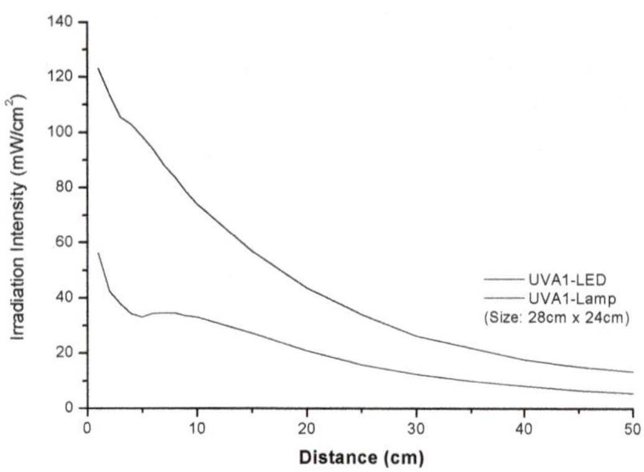

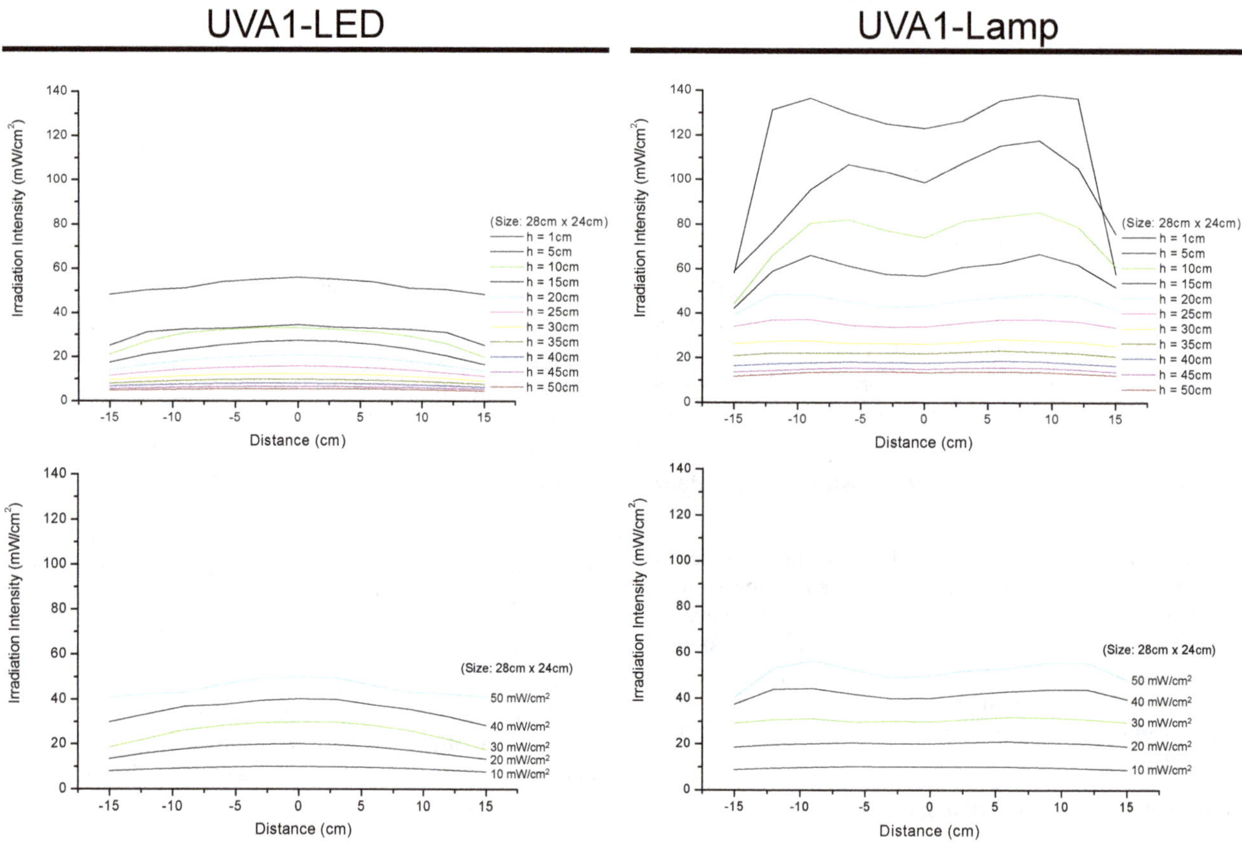

Fig. (3). The irradiation intensity and uniformity of irradiation intensity at 10, 20, 30, 40, and 50 mW/cm^2 of the UV LED and UVA1 lamp devices. (a) The UVA1 lamp had higher irradiation intensity than the UV LED device. From 6 cm to 10 cm, however, the UV LED device exhibited uniform intensity. (b) At short irradiation distances, the UVA1 lamp irradiation intensity tended to vary with a cosine function. UV LED produced uniform irradiation intensity independent of the irradiation distance. (c) The UVA1 lamp intensity at 10 and 20 mW/cm^2 was uniform, but the irradiation intensity at 30, 40, and 50 mW/cm^2 varied with a cosine function. The UV LED at each irradiation intensity was uniform.

Evaluation of Temperature Characteristics of Three Different-Sized Dishes

We analyzed the thermal effects of UV irradiation on culture plates with diameters of 3.5, 6, and 10 cm. The plates were irradiated at intensities of 10, 20, and 30 mW/cm^2 for 30 min with either the UVA1 LED or UVA1 lamp devices. The UVA1 lamp increased the temperature of the dishes, especially the 3.5-cm dish, more than the UVA1 LED device (Fig. **8**). The larger the dish, the smaller the thermal effects of the UVA1 devices.

Evaluation of Cellular Apoptosis

Jurkat T cells were irradiated with a BB-UVB light source as a positive control. After irradiation with BB-UVB (20, 40, or 80 mJ/cm^2), the Jurkat T cells underwent apoptosis (Fig. **9**). At a dose of 20 mJ/cm^2, the amount of apoptosis differed significantly between the 3.5 cm and 10

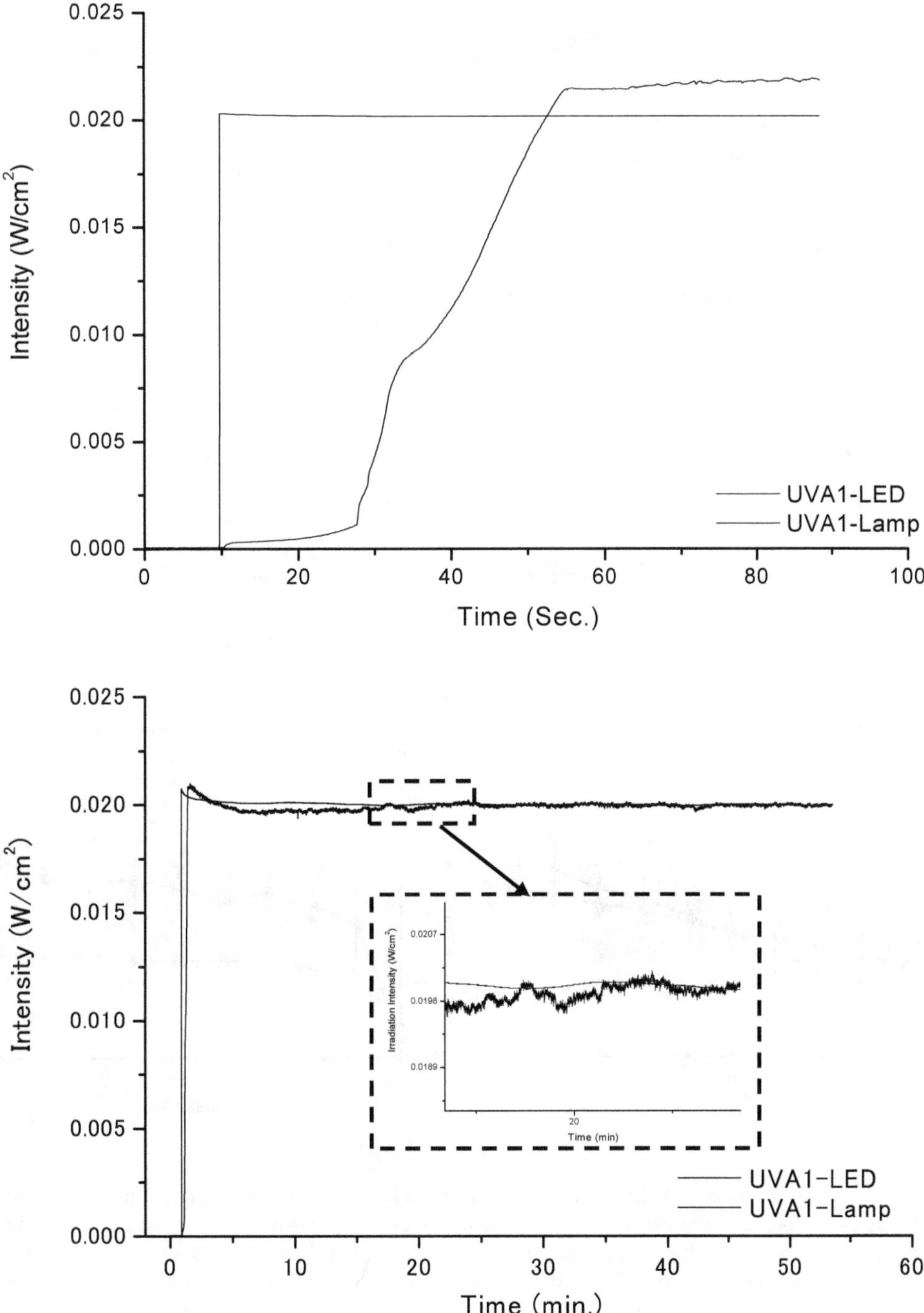

Fig. (4). Irradiation intensity rise time and stability produced by the UV LED and UVA1 lamp devices. (a) Irradiation intensity of UVA1 lamp reached a steady state in approximately 1 min. The irradiation intensity of the UV LED reached a steady state within a few seconds. (b) The UV LED produced more stable irradiation intensity than did the UVA1 lamp.

cm dishes (16% more apoptotic cells in the 3.5-cm dishes than in the 10-cm dishes). The percentage of apoptosis increased with an increase in irradiation, but the difference in apoptosis between 3.5 cm and 10 cm dishes was no longer significant.

To confirm that the UVA1 LED and UVA1 lamp devices induced apoptosis, control, sham irradiation, 10 J/cm^2, 20 J/cm^2, and 30 J/cm^2 UVA1 irradiation doses were applied to Jurkat T cells (Fig. **10**). As the irradiation dose increased, the percentage of apoptotic cells increased. In the 3.5-cm dishes, an irradiation dose of 30 J/cm^2 significantly increased the number of apoptotic cells. The UVA1 lamp significantly induced 3% more apoptotic cells than the UVA1 LED. In the 10-cm dishes, all three UVA1 doses (10, 20 and 30 J/cm^2) significantly induced apoptosis. The UVA1 lamp produced a higher percentage of apoptotic cells than the UVA1 LED device (10 J/cm^2,14.9%; 20 J/cm^2, 21.4%; and 30 J/cm^2, 3%). We initially assumed that, due to thermal effects, more apoptosis would be induced in the 3.5-cm dishes. Instead, the 10-cm dishes exhibited a higher percentage of apoptosis than the 3.5-cm dishes. Although the same concentration of cells was placed in each dish, the thickness of the cell layer

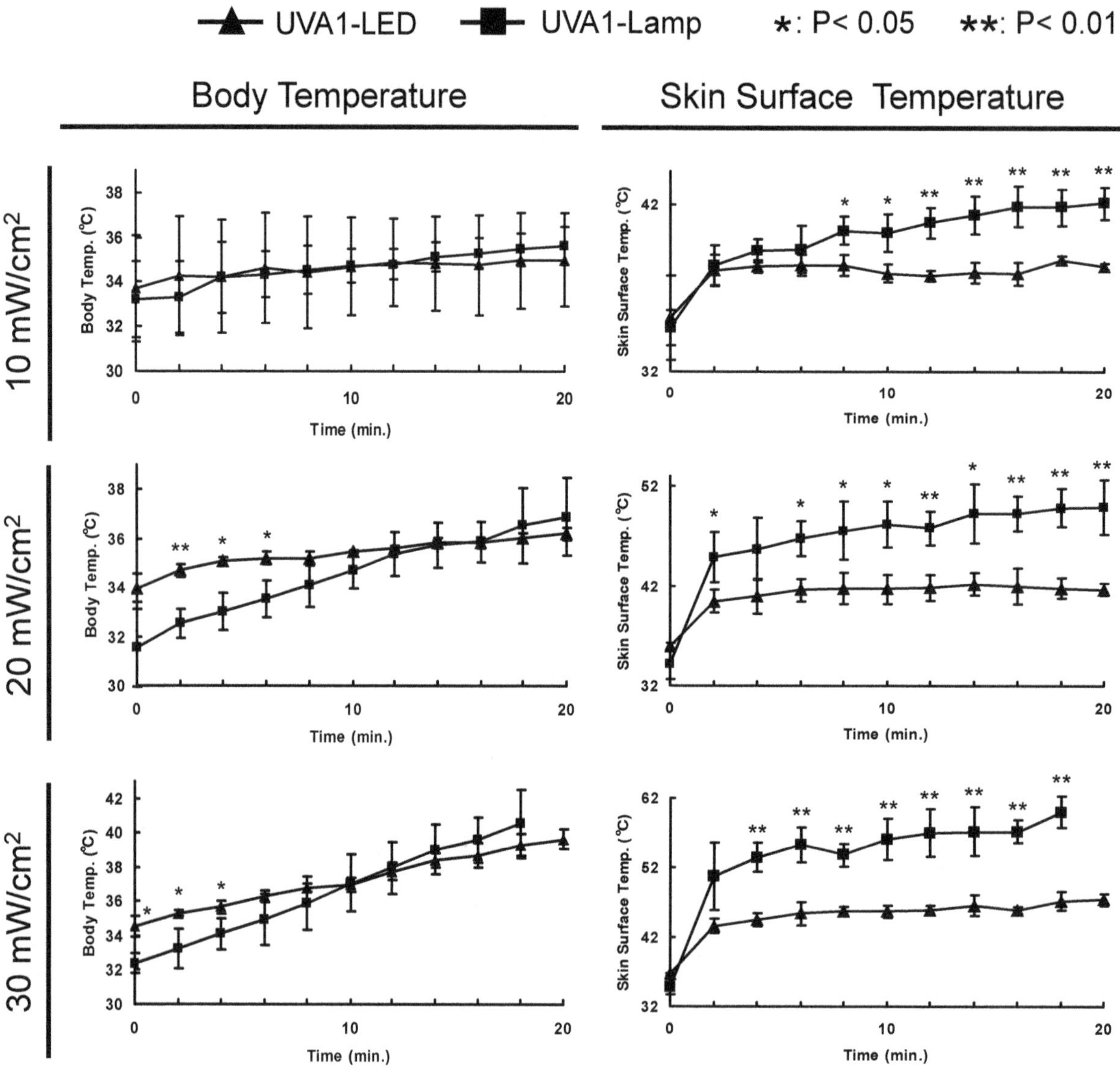

Fig. (5). The temperature characteristics of the UV LED and UVA1 lamp devices were measured using mice. The body and skin surface temperature of mice was measured for 20 min at irradiation intensities of 10, 20, and 30 mW/cm^2. At 8 min, the body temperature did not differ significantly between light sources. The skin surface temperature of mice irradiated with the UVA1 lamp increased 8°C to 10°C. The UV LED increased skin surface temperature 3°C to 4°C. At 30 mW/cm^{2}with the UVA1 lamp, the state became unresponsive at 18 min. At this time, the body temperature was 40.5°C, and the skin surface temperature reached 60°C. Results are expressed as means ± SD of three independent experiments.

differed. In the 3.5-cm dishes, the cell layer was 1-mm thick, and in the 10-cm dishes the cell layer was 0.2-mm thick. This difference in the surface area is thought to account for the differences in the effect of the UVA1 irradiation on the various plate sizes.

DISCUSSION

The longer wavelengths of UVA1 phototherapy (340-400 nm), which penetrate the dermal layers more deeply that shorter wavelength UVB radiation (290-320 nm), effectively treat atopic dermatitis by inducing apoptosis of skin-infiltrating T helper cells [15]. *In vitro*, the induction of T helper cell apoptosis is mediated through activation of the FAS/FAS-ligand system in irradiated cells as a consequence of singlet oxygen generation. The generation of singlet oxygen is considered to have a central role in inducing apoptosis and is an underlying mechanism of UVA1 phototherapy [16].

UVA1 was first used to treat patients with atopic dermatitis. The therapeutic efficacy of UVA1 therapy was evaluated in an open study in patients with acute severe exacerbations of atopic dermatitis. UVA1 is highly effective for rapidly inducing clinical improvement in patients exposed to 130 J/cm^2 UVA1 daily for 15 consecutive days

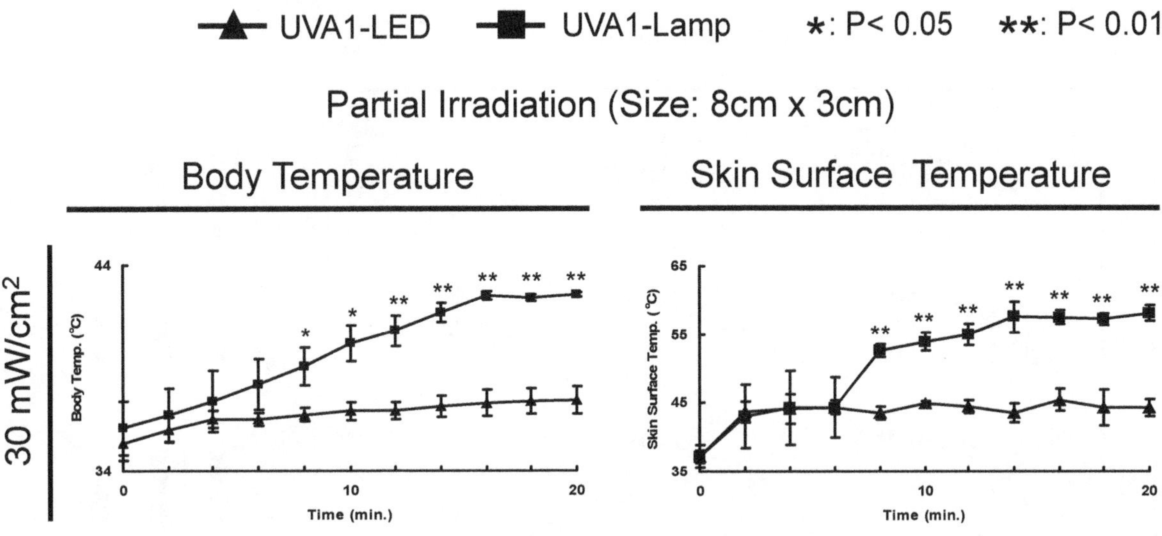

Fig. (6). The selective irradiation function was evaluated. Mice with a body size of approximately 8 cm x 3 cm were irradiated at an intensity of 30 mW/cm^2 for 20 min with the UV LED and UVA1 lamp devices. The temperature of both the skin surface and body was measured. The body and skin surface temperature of mice irradiated using UV LED increased very little. The body and skin surface temperatures of mice irradiated with theUVA1 lamp sharply increased. The UVA1 lamp increased the body temperature 5.1°C and the skin surface temperature 13.8°C more than the UV LED. Results are expressed as means ± SD of three independent experiments.

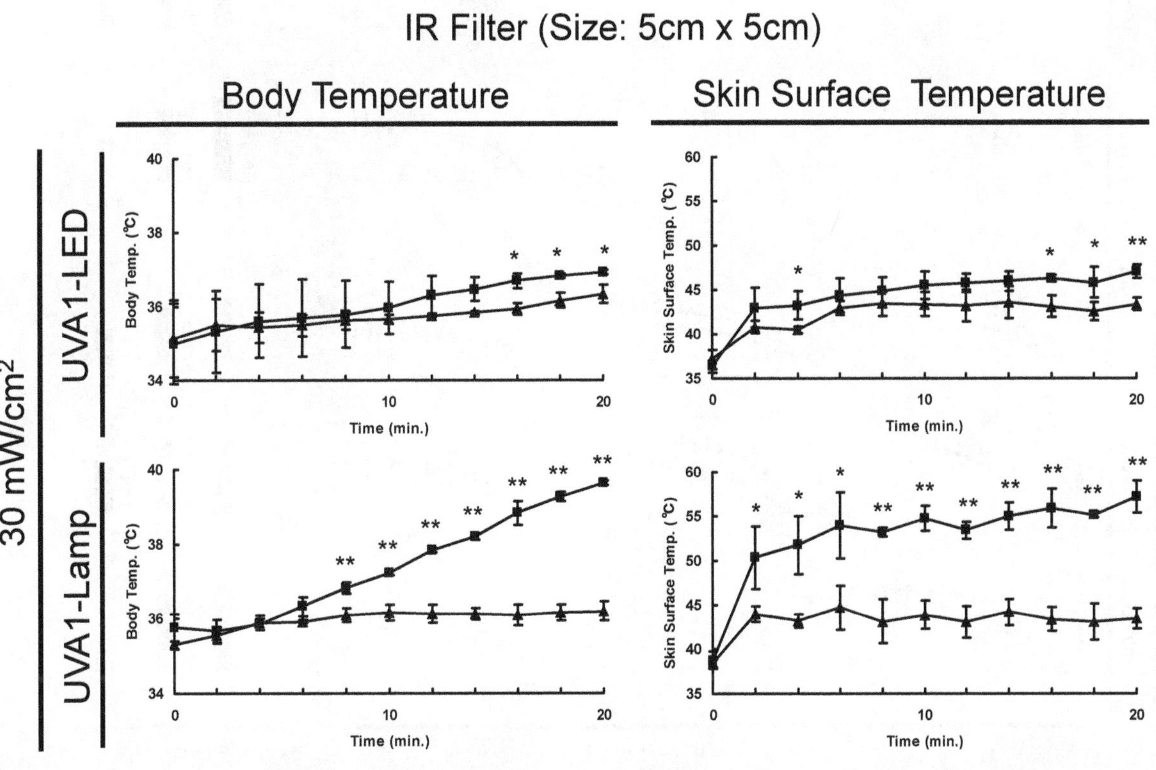

Fig. (7). Mice were irradiated using a far-infrared resonance filter (size: 5 cm x 5 cm, transparent wavelength: 250-2000 nm) for 20 min at an intensity of 30 mW/cm^2 using the UV-LED and UVA1 lamp devices. The temperature of both the skin surface and body was measured with and without the filter to show the effect of the filter on temperature. With the UV-LED device, the differences in the temperature of both the body and the skin surface did not differ significantly with or without the filter. With the UVA1-lamp, the body temperature increased 3.4°C more without filter than with the filter, and the skin surface temperature increased 13.7°C more without the filter than with the filter. Results are expressed as means ± SD of three independent experiments.

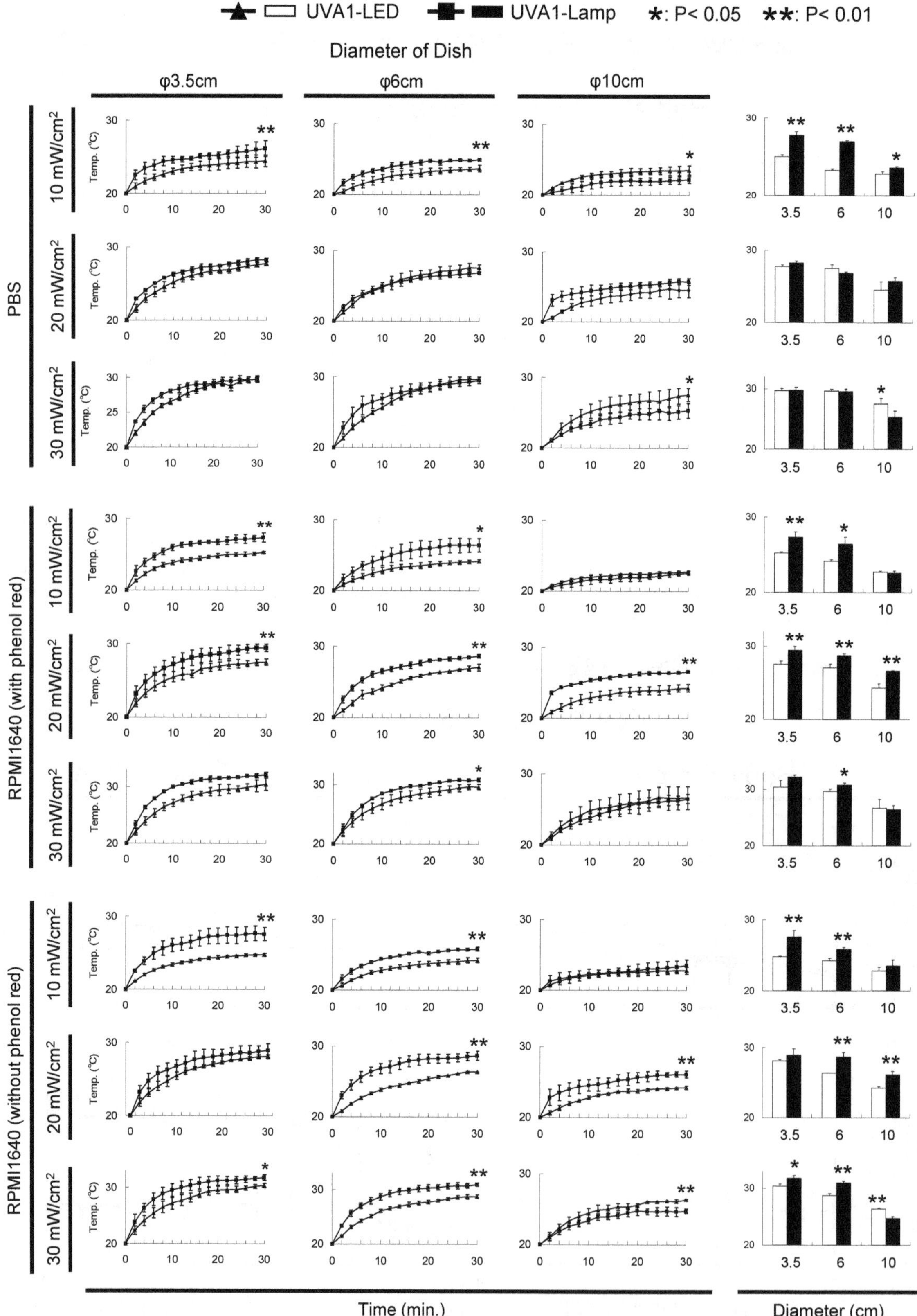

Fig. (8). Phosphate-buffered saline (PBS), RPMI1640 (with phenol red), and RPMI1640 (without phenol red), were placed in culture dishes of various diameters (3.5, 6, and 10 cm) and evaluated. The amount of medium placed into each dish was: 3.5 cm = 2 mL, 6 cm = 5 mL, and 10 cm = 10 mL. Each dish was irradiated with UVA1 (10, 20, and 30mW/cm^2) for 30 min using either the UV LED and UVA1 lamp device and the temperature of the medium was measured. The conditions used for measuring the irradiation intensity of UV light only were: 10mW/cm^2, 10mL PBS medium, and dish diameter of 10cm. The conditions used for measuring UV light intensity as well as heat were: 10mW/cm^2, 2mL PBS medium, and dish diameter of 3.5 cm. Results are expressed as means ± SD of three independent experiments.

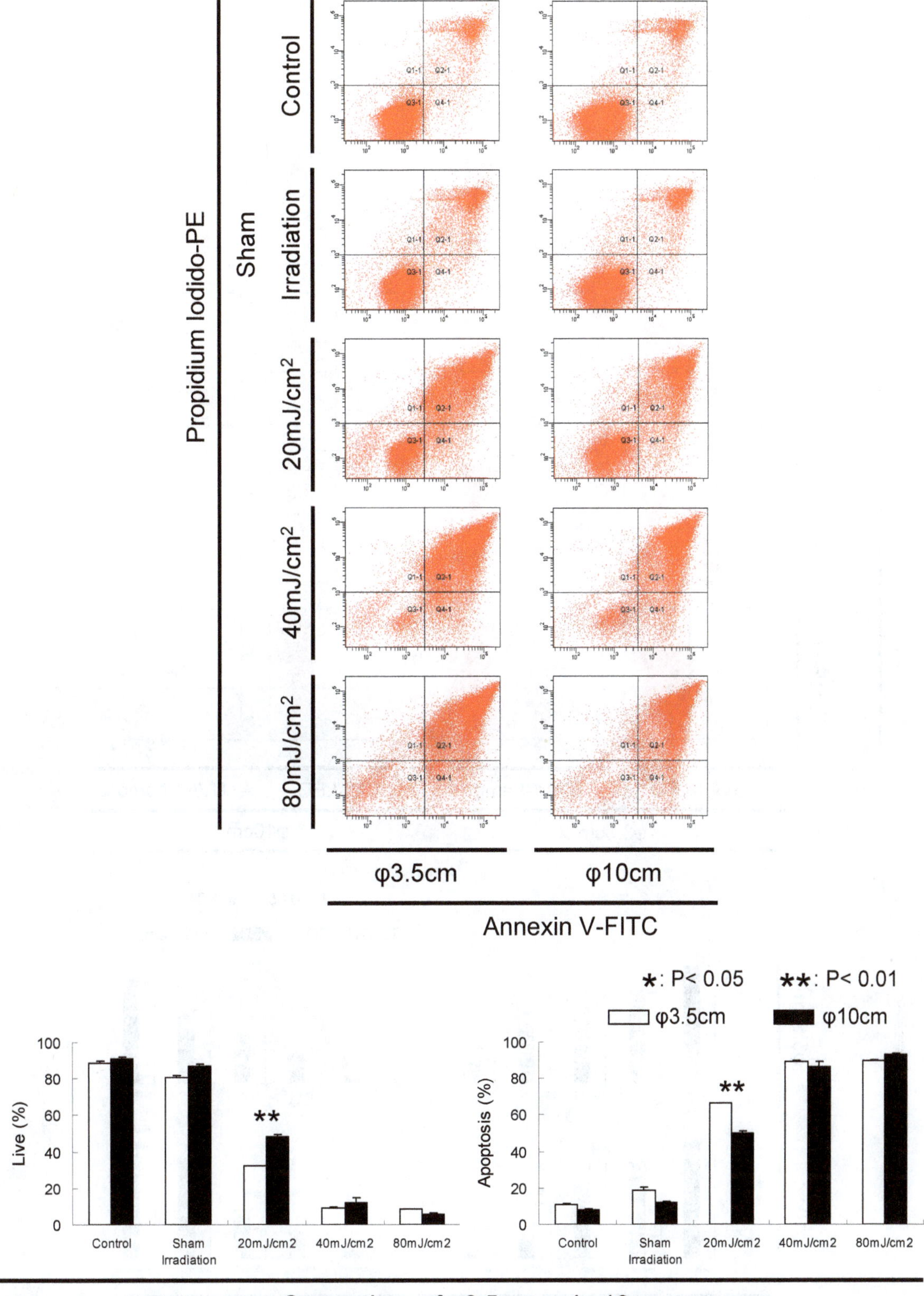

Fig. (9). Control, sham irradiation, 20 mJ/cm^2, 40 mJ/cm^2, and 80 mJ/cm^2 BB-UVB irradiation was applied to Jurkat T cells to induce cellular apoptosis. Jurkat T cells (0.5 x 10^6 cells/mL) were placed in either a 3.5-cm diameter dish (1 mL medium) or in a 10-cm dish (3 mL medium). At 20 mJ/cm^2 BB-UVB, the percentage of apoptotic cells differed significantly between the 3.5-cm and 10-cm dishes. The difference in percent apoptosis was no longer significant between the 3.5-cm and 10-cm dishes at BB-UVB doses of 40 mJ/cm^2 and 80 mJ/cm^2. The means ± SD (triplicate determinations) for one representative of three independent experiments is given.

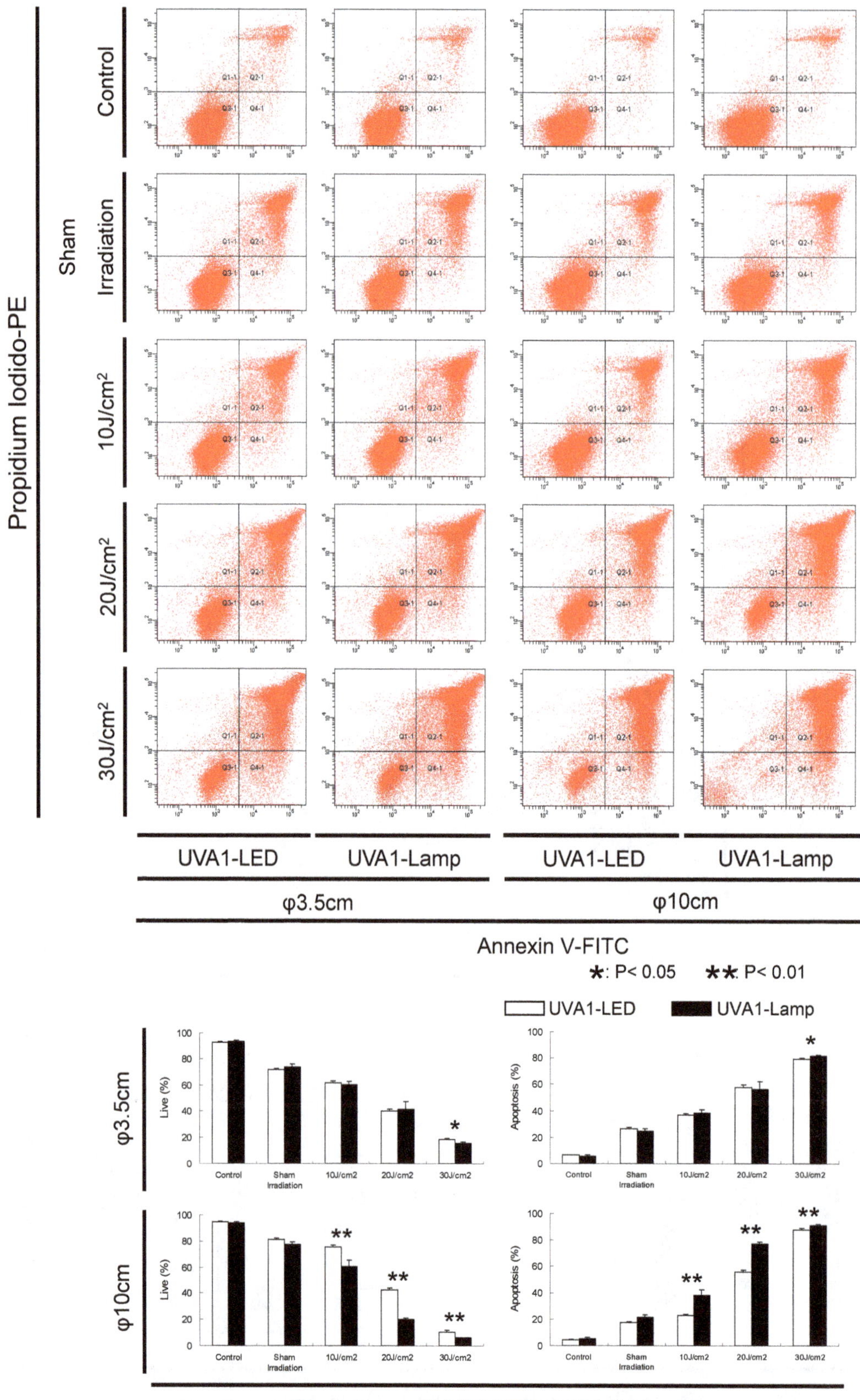

Fig. (10). Control, sham irradiation, 10 J/cm^2, 20 J/cm^2, or 30 J/cm^2 UVA1 irradiation was applied to Jurkat T cells using either the UV LED or UVA1 lamp devices to investigate cellular apoptosis. The Jurkat T cells (0.5 x 10^6 cells/mL) were placed in a 3.5-cm dish (1 mL) or in a 10-cm dish (3 mL). In the 3.5-cm dish, the irradiation dose of 30 J/cm^2 induced significantly more apoptosis, and the UVA1 lamp induced 3% more apoptosis than the UV-LED device. In the 10-cm dish, significantly more apoptosis was induced at doses of 10, 20, and 30 J/cm^2. At all three doses, the UVA1 lamp induced a higher percentage of apoptosis than did the UV LED. The means ± SD (triplicate determinations) for one representative of three independent experiments is given.

[17]. UVA1 is also an effective treatment for morphea (localized scleroderma), a disorder characterized by the overproduction of collagen by fibroblasts in affected tissues leading to thickening of the dermis. UVA1 irradiation disturbs cellular responsiveness to tissue growth factor-β1 through the induction of non-functional latent tissue growth factor-β and the downregulation of tissue growth factor-β receptors, which is a possible mechanism underlying the efficacy of UVA1 treatment [18]. Systemic sclerosis is also treated using UVA1 phototherapy. Direct irradiation of the skin with UV rays activates matrix metalloproteinase, reduces the types of cytokines involving T cells, and inhibits T cell activation [19]. UVA1 depletes skin-infiltrating T cells through the induction of T cell apoptosis and upregulation of matrix metalloproteinase-1 (collagenase-1) expression in dermal fibroblasts [19].

In the present study, we developed a phototherapy device that utilizes UV LEDs to treat refractory skin disease. The UV LED emits UV rays with a peak wavelength of 365 nm and FWHM of 7 nm. The equipment comprises a 16 x 16 UV LED matrix, which can irradiate the diseased part of the skin without affecting the neighboring healthy skin.

To evaluate the performance of the new device, we compared the consumed power, intensity and uniformity of the irradiation, and rise time and stability of the irradiation intensity with that of the conventional UVA1 lamp phototherapy device. In all comparisons, the UVA1 LED device exhibited more favorable characteristics than the UVA1 lamp device. Moreover, the temperature characteristics of both light sources were compared by measuring the body and skin surface temperatures of mice irradiated by the two devices. Although the body and skin surface temperature of mice irradiated with the UVA1 lamp increased sharply, the body and skin surface temperature of mice irradiated with UVA1 LED did not change remarkably. These findings indicate that the UVA1 LED device can be used to treat affected areas of the skin more intensively with less heat compared to the conventional UVA1 lamp.

To confirm that the UVA1 LED and UVA1 lamps could induce cellular apoptosis, Jurkat T cell cultures were irradiated with BB-UVB, sham irradiation, and 10 J/cm^2, 20 J/cm^2, and 30 J/cm^2 intensities. The experiment was performed in culture dishes with a diameter of 10 cm to evaluate the effect of UV light only on the cells, or a diameter of 3.5 cm to evaluate the effect of UV light and heat. The UVA1 lamp induced more cellular apoptosis than the UVA1 LED in each experiment. The UVA1 LED, however, effectively induced apoptosis in the cancer cells.

The findings of the present study demonstrated that the UVA1 LED phototherapy device possibly overcomes problems of conventional UVA1 lamp phototherapy devices. Based on these findings, a clinical study for the efficacy of UVA1 LED phototherapy device has been initiated.

ACKNOWLEDGMENTS

This work was financially supported by a Grant from the Ministry of Education, Culture, Sports, Science, and Technology, Japan. We would also like to thank Dr. Takashi Mukai (Nichia Chemistry Industry Co, Ltd) for providing the UV LED.

CONFLICT OF INTEREST

Declared none.

REFERENCES

[1] Krutmann J, Morita A. Therapeutic photomedicine phototherapy. In: Freedberg IM, Eisen AZ, Wolff K, Austen KF, Goldsmith LA, Katz SI, Eds. Fitzpatrick's dermatology in general medicine. New York: McGraw Hill 2007; pp. 2243-9.

[2] Scherschun L, Kim JJ, Lim HW. Narrow-band ultraviolet B is a useful and well-tolerated treatment for vitiligo. J Am Acad Dermatol 2001; 44: 999-1003.

[3] Krutmann J, Czech W, Diepgen T, Niedner R, Kapp A, Schopf E. High-dose UVA1 therapy in the treatment of patients with atopic dermatitis. J Am Acad Dermatol 1992; 26: 225-30.

[4] Stege H, Schopf E, Ruzicka T, Krutmann J. High-dose UVA1 for urticaria pigmentosa. Lancet 1996; 347: 64.

[5] Mukai T, Morita D, Nakamura S. High-power UV InGaN/AlGaN double-heterostructure LEDs. J Cryst Growth 1998; 189/190: 778-81.

[6] Morita D, Yamamoto M, Akaishi K, *et al.* Watt class high-output-power 365 nm ultraviolet light-emitting diode. Jpn J Appl Phys 2004; 43: 5945-50.

[7] Amano H, Sawaki N, Akasaki I, Toyoda Y. Metalorganic vapor phase epitaxial growth of a high quality GaN film using an AlN buffer layer. Appl Phys Lett 1986; 48: 353-6.

[8] Akasaki I, Amano H. Crystal growth and conductivity control of group III nitride semiconductors and their application to short wavelength light emitters. Jpn J Appl Phys 1997; 36: 5393-408.

[9] Iwaya M, Takanami S, Miyazaki A, *et al.* High-power UV-light-emitting diode on sapphire. Jpn J Appl Phys 2003; 42: 400-3.

[10] Mukai T, Nakamura S. Ultraviolet InGaN and GaN single-quantum-well-structure light-emitting diodes Grown on epitaxially laterally overgrown GaN substrates. Jpn J Appl Phys 1999; 38: 5735-9.

[11] Gold MH, Andriessen A, Biron J. Self-diagnosis of mild-to-moderate acne for self-treatment with blue light therapy. J Clin Aesthet Dermatol 2009; 2: 40-4.

[12] Jih MH, Kimyai-Asadi A. Laser treatment of acne vulgaris. Semin Plast Surg 2007; 21: 167-74.

[13] Bowler PJ. Impact on facial rejuvenation with dermatological preparations. Clin Interv Aging 2009; 4: 81-9.

[14] Inada AS, Amano H, Akasaki I, Kobayashi K, Morita A. Effect of UV irradiation on the apoptosis and necrosis of jurkat cell using UV LED. Proc SPIE 2009; 7231: 72310J1-6.

[15] Krutmann J, Morita A. Mechanisms of ultraviolet (UV) B and UVA phototherapy. J Invest Dermatol Symp Proc. 1999; 4: 70-2.

[16] Morita A, Werfel T, Stege H, *et al.* Evidence that singlet oxygen-induced human T helper cell apoptosis is the basic mechanism of ultraviolet-A radiation phototherapy. J Exp Med 1997; 186: 1763-8.

[17] Krutmann J, Czech W, Diepgen T, Niedner R, Kapp A, Schopf E. High-dose UVA1 therapy in the treatment of patients with atopic dermatitis. J Am Acad Dermatol 1992; 26: 225-30.

[18] Yin L, Morita A, Tsuji T. The crucial role of TGF-beta in the age-related alterations induced by ultraviolet A irradiation, J Invest Dermatol 2003; 120: 703-5.

[19] Yin L, Yamauchi R, Tsuji T, Krutmann J, Morita A. The expression of matrix metalloproteinase-1 mRNA induced by ultraviolet A1 (340-400 nm) is phototherapy relevant to the glutathione (GSH) content in skin fibroblasts of systemic sclerosis. J Dermatol 2003; 30: 173-80.

28

IL-4 and IL-12 Polymorphisms are Associated with Response to Suplatast Tosilate, a Th2 Cytokine Inhibitor, in Patients with Atopic Dermatitis

Hideki Nagase[1], Yoshinori Nakachi[1], Keiji Ishida[1], Mamoru Kiniwa[*,1], Satoshi Takeuchi[2], Ichiro Katayama[3], Yoshinari Matsumoto[4], Fukumi Furukawa[5], Shin Morizane[6], Sakae Kaneko[7], Yoshiki Tokura[8], Motoi Takenaka[9], Yutaka Hatano[10] and Yoshiki Miyachi[11]

[1]*Tokushima Research Center, Taiho Pharmaceutical Co., Ltd., Tokushima, Japan*

[2]*Department of Dermatology, Graduate School of Medical Sciences, Kyushu University, Fukuoka, Japan*

[3]*Department of Dermatology, Osaka University Graduate School of Medicine, Osaka, Japan*

[4]*Department of Dermatology, Aichi Medical University School of Medicine, Aichi, Japan*

[5]*Department of Dermatology, Wakayama Medical University, Wakayama, Japan*

[6]*Department of Dermatology, Okayama University Graduate School of Medicine, Dentistry and Pharmaceutical Sciences, Okayama, Japan*

[7]*Department of Dermatology, Shimane University Faculty of Medicine, Shimane, Japan*

[8]*Department of Dermatology, University of Occupational and Environmental Health, Kitakyushu, Japan (Present affiliation: Department of Dermatology, Hamamatsu University School of Medicine, Hamamatsu, Japan)*

[9]*Department of Dermatology and Allergology, Nagasaki University Hospital, Nagasaki, Japan*

[10]*Department of Dermatology, Faculty of Medicine, Oita University, Oita, Japan*

[11]*Department of Dermatology, Kyoto University Graduate School of Medicine, Kyoto, Japan*

Abstract: Th2-related immune and inflammatory responses have been implicated in the pathogenesis of atopic dermatitis (AD), but few clinical lines of evidence have been reported regarding how and whether Th2-related responses are associated with other risk factors in the treatment of AD patients. In this study, the associations between the polymorphisms of genes related to the pathophysiology of AD and the efficacy of suplatast tosilate, an oral immune-modulator known to downregulate Th2-related allergic responses, were analyzed in adult patients with chronic AD. Patients were recruited from our previous study, where suplatast tosilate was evaluated for its efficacy when used in combination with topical steroids. The genotypes of 35 single nucleotide polymorphisms (SNPs) of 27 genes related to AD pathogenesis were then determined in 17 responders and 18 non-responders, as defined by the improvement rate in their AD skin scores. While no significant difference in the patient background was observed between responders and non-responders, significant associations were noted between the response to treatment with suplatast tosilate and three SNPs of IL-4 (-590C/T: P=0.04, -33C/T: P=0.04) and IL-12B (1188A/C: P=0.03), but not for the other SNPs. Of note, ethnic differences in the genotype frequencies of IL-4 -590C/T and IL-12B 1188A/C SNPs were found. In conclusion, the present results raise the possibility that AD patients who tend to produce more IL-4 and IL-12 may be susceptible to suplatast tosilate treatment and that ethnic variations should be considered to further understand the role of Th2-related responses.

Keywords: Atopic dermatitis, single nucleotide polymorphism, IL-4, IL-12B, Th1, Th2, suplatast tosilate, ethnic difference.

INTRODUCTION

AD is one of the most common chronic inflammatory diseases of the skin. While its causes and mechanisms have not yet been fully elucidated, its pathogenesis has been characterized by altered skin barrier function and immune dysregulation. Recent genome-wide association studies or polymorphism analyses of candidate genes have further extended the view that patients with AD have genetically determined risk factors that affect the skin barrier and immune responses [1-6]. It should be noted, however, that few clinical lines of evidence have been reported regarding how these factors interact with each other and, more importantly, whether the down- or up-regulation of any gene or factor may affect the treatment of AD patients.

*Address correspondence to this author at the Tokushima Research Center, Taiho Pharmaceutical Co., Ltd., 224-2, Ebisuno Hiraishi, Kawauchi-cho, Tokushima, 771-0194, Japan;
E-mail: makiniwa@taiho.co.jp

In the present study, we focused on suplatast tosilate, which has been approved in Japan as an oral immune-modulator for AD, allergic rhinitis, and asthma [7-10]. This agent has been used as an adjunct to or in combination with topical anti-inflammatory and immunosuppressive agents and has been shown to reduce the requirements for these agents [11, 12]. Suplatast tosilate has been referred to as a Th2 cytokine inhibitor because 1) it was discovered based on its capacity to suppress murine IgE formation without affecting cellular immune responses [13], 2) it suppressed IL-4 and IL-5 production by Th2 cells [14], 3) it suppressed allergic inflammation *via* indirect actions on Th2 cells as well as direct actions on eosinophils [15-19], and 4) it affected certain biomarkers such as Th1/Th2 ratio during the treatment of allergic asthmatic patients [20]. Although its mechanism of action remains to be identified at a molecular level, it is reasonable to assume that its efficacy in allergic patients may be ascribed to the modulation of the Th2-related immune and inflammatory responses.

We previously performed a clinical study investigating the efficacy of suplatast tosilate in adult chronic AD patients who also received topical steroids but had responded poorly to adjunct therapy such as antihistamines [21, 22]. This study revealed that suplatast tosilate markedly improved the AD skin symptom scores in a certain group of patients, but not in all patients, enabling us to recruit suplatast tosilate responders and non-responders and to analyze the polymorphism of genes related to the pathophysiology of AD retrospectively. The results implicated the efficacy of suplatast tosilate in the modulation of both Th1 and Th2 responses in AD therapy and suggested ethnic variations in the pathogenesis of AD.

MATERIALS AND METHODS

Study Subjects

One hundred and sixty-three patients with atopic dermatitis whose conditions had been poorly controlled by other anti-allergic drugs at 11 hospitals between 2004 and 2006 were enrolled in our previous study [21, 22]. The Th2 cytokine inhibitor suplatast tosilate (300 mg/day) was administered to these patients. After 4 weeks or more of treatment, the skin symptom score was determined to evaluate the usefulness of suplatast tosilate. The effectiveness of suplatast tosilate was evaluated by comparing the improvement rate relative to the baseline skin symptom score [21, 22]. To classify the patients into a highly effective group and a poorly effective group, we divided all the cases into three groups based on the improvement rate of the skin symptom scores. The one-third of cases with the highest improvement rates were defined as "responders", and the one-third of cases with the lowest improvement rates were defined as "non-responders". As a result, 54 "responder" patients had an improvement rate of more than 58%, and 53 "non-responder" patients had an improvement rate of less than 25%. From these patients, a total of 35 patients (17 responders and 18 non-responders) provided informed consent to undergo SNP genotyping using DNA from a blood sample. The improvement rate for the 17 high-responders with an improvement rate of more than 58% for their skin symptom scores was 68.8 ± 12.2%. On the other hand, that of the 18 non-responders with an improvement rate of less than 25% was 1.4 ± 22.8%. This study was approved by the ethics committees of Kyoto University Graduate School of Medicine, Kyushu University, Osaka University Graduate School of Medicine, Aichi Medical University School of Medicine, Wakayama Medical University, Okayama University Graduate School of Medicine, Shimane University, University of Occupational and Environmental Health, Nagasaki University, Oita University and Taiho Pharmaceutical Co., Ltd.

SNP Genotyping Analysis

In each patient, 8.5 mL of blood was collected into a PAXgene Blood DNA tube (Qiagen Inc. CA, USA). DNA from the blood sample was purified using a PAXgene Blood DNA kit (Qiagen Inc.). The genotypes of 35 single nucleotide polymorphisms (SNPs) of 27 allergy-related genes were determined using a TaqMan real-time polymerase chain reaction (PCR) (TaqMan SNP Genotyping Assays; Life Technologies, CA, USA) or direct sequencing methods. The following 27 genes were investigated in this study: Th2 cytokines or cytokines promoting Th2 cells (IL-4, IL-5, IL-13, and TSLP), Th1 cytokine (IFN-γ), cytokines promoting Th1 cells (IL-12B and IL-18), proinflammatory cytokine (IL-17), chemokines (CCL5, CCL11, and CCL17), some of their receptors (IL-4R, IL-5R, IL-12R, IL-22R, IL-23R, and IFN-γR), other genes related to the symptoms of AD or atopic disease (IL-31R, Chymase, NGF, NGFR, FcεR1α, FcεR1β, HRH1, HRH4, and LTC4S), and filaggrin (FLG). Thirty-one of the 35 SNPs were genotyped using the Applied Biosystems 7900HT Real-Time PCR System. The assay IDs of the 31 SNPs are shown in Table **1**. The remaining four SNPs without a commercial TaqMan SNP genotyping assay were genotyped by direct sequencing at Takara Bio Inc. (Mie, Japan).

Statistical Analysis

The associations between the clinical parameters and the response to treatment with suplatast tosilate were evaluated using a likelihood ratio chi-square test for categorical data or the Student t-test for continuous data. The effect of suplatast tosilate on the clinical parameters was evaluated using a paired *t*-test. Hardy-Weinberg equilibrium of the genotyping results was evaluated using a Pearson's chi-square test. A likelihood ratio chi-square test was used to analyze the associations between the genotype of each SNP and the response to treatment with suplatast tosilate. All the analyses were performed using the statistical software JMP 7.0.1 and the SAS statistical package, version 9.1.3 (SAS Institute Inc., Cary, NC, USA). Differences were considered significant when $P<0.05$. Because this was the study with a small sample size, a correction for multiple comparisons was not made.

RESULTS

Patient Characteristics and Effect of Suplatast Tosilate on Th2-Related Parameters

No significant differences between the responders and the non-responders were observed with regard to sex, age, and the pre-treatment values for the skin symptom scores, IgE levels or eosinophil counts (Table **2**). Note that suplatast tosilate treatment did not affect the serum IgE level or the

Table 1. SNP list and Genotyping Methods

Gene Symbol	SNP name	rs ID	Methods	Assay ID
IL4	-590C/T	rs2243250	RT-PCR*	C__16176216_10
	-33C/T	rs2070874	RT-PCR	C__16176215_10
IL4R	Gln551Arg	rs1801275	RT-PCR	C___2351160_20
	Ile50Val	rs1805010	RT-PCR	C___2769554_10
IL5	-703C/T	rs2069812	RT-PCR	C__16274150_10
IL5RA	-80G/A	rs2290608	RT-PCR	C__15885096_10
IL12B	1188A/C	rs3212227	RT-PCR	C___2084293_10
IL12RB1	-2C/T	rs436857	RT-PCR	C____795468_1_
IL13	2044G/A	rs20541	RT-PCR	C___2259921_20
	-1112C/T	rs1800925	RT-PCR	C___8932056_10
IL17F	7488T/C	rs763780	RT-PCR	C___2234166_10
IL18	113T/G	rs360718	RT-PCR	C___2898461_10
IL22RA1	Arg518Gly	rs3795299	RT-PCR	C____440166_10
IL23R	Gln3His	rs1884444	RT-PCR	C__11728603_10
IL31RA	Ser497Asn	rs161704	RT-PCR	C___2839337_10
IFNG	874T/A	rs2430561	DS†	-
IFNGR2	Arg64Gln	rs9808753	RT-PCR	C___2443413_1_
CCL5	-28C/G	rs2280788	RT-PCR	C__15874396_20
	-403G/A	rs2107538	RT-PCR	C__15874407_10
CCL11	-384A/G	rs17809012	RT-PCR	C___2590323_10
CCL17	-431C/T	rs223828	RT-PCR	C___2392392_10
TSLP	-847C/T	rs3806933	RT-PCR	C___3166722_10
NGFB	Ala35Val	rs6330	RT-PCR	C___2525309_10
NGFR	Ser205Leu	rs2072446	RT-PCR	C__15870920_10
FCER1A	-66T/C	rs2251746	RT-PCR	C___1840470_20
MS4A2	-109C/T	rs1441586	RT-PCR	C___1842226_10
	Glu237Gly	rs569108	RT-PCR	C____900116_10
CMA1	-1897G/A	rs1800875	RT-PCR	C___2796262_10
HRH1	-17C/T	rs901865	RT-PCR	C__25471612_10
HRH4	Ala138Val	rs11665084	RT-PCR	C___3161321_20
LTC4S	-444A/C	rs730012	RT-PCR	C____644967_10
FLG	Tyr2194His	rs2184953	DS	-
	Tyr3105Asp	rs2065958	DS	-
	13347G/A	rs12730241	RT-PCR	C__31910001_10
	13586C/T	rs11204976	DS	-

*RT-PCR: reverse transcription polymerase chain reaction,
†DS: direct sequencing.

eosinophil count in either the responders or the non-responders (Table **3**).

Genotype and Allele Frequencies

The genotyping results and the allele frequencies of the 35 SNPs are shown in Table **4**. Among 34 SNPs (excluding the Filaggrin Tyr3105Asp SNP), the genotype frequencies were the values expected under Hardy-Weinberg equilibrium, and no significant difference was observed between the minor allele frequencies reported in this study and those shown in the SNPper (http://snpper.chip.org/bio/snpper-enter) or NCBI databases (http://www.ncbi.nlm.nih.gov/snp/) (data not shown), indicating that the genotyping

Table 2. Clinical Characteristics of the Patients

Parameters	Responders (n=17)	Non-Responders (n=18)	*P*-Value*
Sex Male/Female	11/6	10/8	0.58
Age (Range)	37.1±17.5 (18-79)	32.3±12.6 (13-62)	0.36
Skin symptom score (Pre) (Range)	8.6±2.8 (4-12)	10.4±4.0 (3-17)	0.12
IgE level (Pre) (IU/mL)	8645±8429	16356±21988	0.20
Eosinophil count (Pre) (cells/mm^3)	615±387	581±329	0.80
Eosinophil count (Pre) (%)	10.3±5.1	8.6±3.6	0.34

*The *P*-values for categorical data and for continuous data were obtained using the likelihood ratio chi-square test and Student t-test, respectively.

Table 3. Effect of Suplatast Tosilate on Skin Symptom Score, Serum IgE Level, and Eosinophil Count in Atopic Dermatitis Patients

Parameters		N	Pre-Treatment	Post-Treatment	*P*-Value*
Skin symptom score	Responders	17	8.6±2.8	2.8±1.5	<0.001
	Non-responders	18	10.4±4.0	10.2±4.2	0.61
IgE level (IU/mL)	Responders	16	8645±8429	7935±8605	0.29
	Non-responders	14	16356±21988	15047±19624	0.09
Eosinophil (cells/mm^3)	Responders	15	615±387	591±306	0.72
	Non-responders	14	581±329	722±527	0.28
Eosinophil (%)	Responders	15	10.3±5.1	9.1±5.4	0.18
	Non-responders	13	8.6±3.6	10.4±6.4	0.29

**P*-values were obtained using a paired *t*-test.

analysis was performed accurately. Regarding the genotyping results for the Filaggrin Tyr3105Asp SNP, the genotype frequency deviated from the values expected from Hardy-Weinberg equilibrium, and the minor allele frequency was significantly higher than that shown in the SNPper database (data not shown). This analysis may not have been performed accurately because the primer design region for the Filaggrin Tyr3105Asp SNP was highly homologous with other genes.

Associations between Genotype and Response to Treatment with Suplatast Tosilate

Significant associations between the response to treatment with suplatast tosilate and three SNPs of IL-4 (-590C/T: *P*=0.04, -33C/T: *P*=0.04) and IL-12B (1188A/C: *P*=0.03) were observed among the 35 SNPs genotyped in this study (Table **4**). The genotyping results of two SNPs (-590C/T and -33C/T) within the IL-4 promoter region were perfectly identical among the 35 patients in this study. Therefore, the IL-4 -590C/T SNP, as a representative of the two SNPs of IL-4 that showed a significant association with the response, was used in further analyses. For the IL-4 -590C/T SNP, patients with a C/C genotype had a significantly lower response rate to suplatast tosilate than those with a T/T or T/C genotype (0.0% *vs* 53.1%, *P*=0.04) (Table **5**). On the other hand, for the IL-12B 1188A/C SNP, patients with an A/A genotype had a significantly lower response rate to suplatast tosilate than those with a C/C or C/A genotype (12.5% *vs* 59.3%, *P*=0.02, odds ratio=10.2) (Table **5**). In a combination analysis of the two SNPs (IL-4 -590C/T and IL-12B 1188A/C), patients with either IL-4 -590C/T C/C or IL-12B 1188A/C A/A had a significantly lower response rate than those with other genotype combinations (10.0% *vs* 64.0%, *P*=0.002, odds ratio=16.0) (Table **5**).

Ethnic Differences in Genotype Frequency of IL-4 -590C/T and IL-12B 1188A/C SNPs

The genotype frequencies of IL-4 -590C/T T/T and IL-12B 1188A/C C/C, which were associated with a strong response to suplatast tosilate, were significantly higher among Asians than among Europeans based on the results of the HapMap project (Table **6**, http://www.ncbi.nlm.nih.gov/snp/).

Table 4. Genotype Frequency and Association Between Genotype and Response to Treatment with Suplatast Tosilate

SNP Name (SNP ID)	Genotype	Frequency (%) Total (n=35)		*P*-Value*	Frequency (%) Responders (n=17)		Non-Responders (n=18)		*P*-Value†
IL4 -590C/T	T/T	13	(37%)		9	(53%)	4	(22%)	
(rs2243250)	T/C	19	(54%)		8	(47%)	11	(61%)	
	C/C	3	(9%)	0.28	0	(0%)	3	(17%)	0.04
IL4 -33C/T	T/T	13	(37%)		9	(53%)	4	(22%)	
(rs2070874)	T/C	19	(54%)		8	(47%)	11	(61%)	
	C/C	3	(9%)	0.28	0	(0%)	3	(17%)	0.04
IL4R	A/A	30	(86%)		13	(76%)	17	(94%)	
Gln551Arg	A/G	5	(14%)		4	(24%)	1	(6%)	
(rs1801275)	G/G	0	(0%)	0.65	0	(0%)	0	(0%)	0.12
IL4R Ile50Val	G/G	16	(46%)		7	(41%)	9	(50%)	
(rs1805010)	G/A	16	(46%)		9	(53%)	7	(39%)	
	A/A	3	(9%)	0.72	1	(6%)	2	(11%)	0.67
IL5 -703C/T	T/T	13	(37%)		8	(47%)	5	(28%)	
(rs2069812)	T/C	15	(43%)		6	(35%)	9	(50%)	
	C/C	7	(20%)	0.49	3	(18%)	4	(22%)	0.49
IL5RA -80G/A	G/G	21	(60%)		12	(71%)	9	(50%)	
(rs2290608)	G/A	12	(34%)		5	(29%)	7	(39%)	
	A/A	2	(6%)	0.87	0	(0%)	2	(11%)	0.17
IL12B	C/C	8	(23%)		6	(35%)	2	(11%)	
1188A/C	C/A	19	(54%)		10	(59%)	9	(50%)	
(rs3212227)	A/A	8	(23%)	0.61	1	(6%)	7	(39%)	0.03
IL12RB1	C/C	24	(69%)		12	(71%)	12	(67%)	
-2C/T	C/T	11	(31%)		5	(29%)	6	(33%)	
(rs436857)	T/T	0	(0%)	0.27	0	(0%)	0	(0%)	0.80
IL13 2044G/A	G/G	15	(43%)		7	(41%)	8	(44%)	
(rs20541)	G/A	16	(46%)		7	(41%)	9	(50%)	
	A/A	4	(11%)	0.93	3	(18%)	1	(6%)	0.51
IL13 -1112C/T	C/C	20	(57%)		11	(65%)	9	(50%)	
(rs1800925)	C/T	13	(37%)		5	(29%)	8	(44%)	
	T/T	2	(6%)	0.95	1	(6%)	1	(6%)	0.65
IL17F	T/T	27	(77%)		13	(76%)	14	(78%)	
7488T/C	T/C	8	(23%)		4	(24%)	4	(22%)	
(rs763780)	C/C	0	(0%)	0.45	0	(0%)	0	(0%)	0.93
IL18 113T/G	T/T	26	(74%)		14	(82%)	12	(67%)	
(rs360718)	T/G	8	(23%)		3	(18%)	5	(28%)	
	G/G	1	(3%)	0.69	0	(0%)	1	(6%)	0.37
IL22RA1	G/G	19	(54%)		10	(59%)	9	(50%)	
Arg518Gly	G/C	16	(46%)		7	(41%)	9	(50%)	
(rs3795299)	C/C	0	(0%)	0.08	0	(0%)	0	(0%)	0.60

(Table 4) contd.....

SNP Name (SNP ID)	Genotype	Frequency (%) Total (n=35)		P-Value*	Frequency (%) Responders (n=17)		Non-Responders (n=18)		P-Value†
IL23R	T/T	11	(31%)		4	(24%)	7	(39%)	
Gln3His	T/G	20	(57%)		10	(59%)	10	(56%)	
(rs1884444)	G/G	4	(11%)	0.26	3	(18%)	1	(6%)	0.40
IL31RA	G/G	9	(26%)		6	(35%)	3	(17%)	
Ser497Asn	G/A	17	(49%)		6	(35%)	11	(61%)	
(rs161704)	A/A	9	(26%)	0.87	5	(29%)	4	(22%)	0.27
IFNG 874T/A	A/A	24	(69%)		12	(71%)	12	(67%)	
(rs2430561)	A/T	9	(26%)		5	(29%)	4	(22%)	
	T/T	2	(6%)	0.38	0	(0%)	2	(11%)	0.24
IFNGR2	A/A	10	(29%)		3	(18%)	7	(39%)	
Arg64Gln	A/G	18	(51%)		9	(53%)	9	(50%)	
(rs9808753)	G/G	7	(20%)	0.83	5	(29%)	2	(11%)	0.23
CCL5 -28C/G	C/C	26	(74%)		12	(71%)	14	(78%)	
(rs2280788)	C/G	8	(23%)		5	(29%)	3	(17%)	
	G/G	1	(3%)	0.69	0	(0%)	1	(6%)	0.37
CCL5 -403G/A	C/C	16	(46%)		9	(53%)	7	(39%)	
(rs2107538)	C/T	14	(40%)		7	(41%)	7	(39%)	
	T/T	5	(14%)	0.51	1	(6%)	4	(22%)	0.34
CCL11	A/A	17	(49%)		9	(53%)	8	(44%)	
-384A/G	A/G	15	(43%)		6	(35%)	9	(50%)	
(rs17809012)	G/G	3	(9%)	0.90	2	(12%)	1	(6%)	0.61
CCL17	C/C	11	(31%)		8	(47%)	3	(17%)	
-431C/T	C/T	14	(40%)		5	(29%)	9	(50%)	
(rs223828)	T/T	10	(29%)	0.24	4	(24%)	6	(33%)	0.14
TSLP -847C/T	C/C	20	(57%)		11	(65%)	9	(50%)	
(rs3806933)	C/T	11	(31%)		4	(24%)	7	(39%)	
	T/T	4	(11%)	0.22	2	(12%)	2	(11%)	0.61
NGFB	C/C	17	(49%)		7	(41%)	10	(56%)	
Ala35Val	C/T	15	(43%)		7	(41%)	8	(44%)	
(rs6330)	T/T	3	(9%)	0.90	3	(18%)	0	(0%)	0.09
NGFR	C/C	29	(83%)		16	(94%)	13	(72%)	
Ser205Leu	C/T	5	(14%)		1	(6%)	4	(22%)	
(rs2072446)	T/T	1	(3%)	0.22	0	(0%)	1	(6%)	0.17
FCER1A	T/T	30	(86%)		16	(94%)	14	(78%)	
-66T/C	T/C	5	(14%)		1	(6%)	4	(22%)	
(rs2251746)	C/C	0	(0%)	0.65	0	(0%)	0	(0%)	0.15
MS4A2	T/T	19	(54%)		11	(65%)	8	(44%)	
-109C/T	T/C	13	(37%)		5	(29%)	8	(44%)	
(rs1441586)	C/C	3	(9%)	0.72	1	(6%)	2	(11%)	0.48
MS4A2	T/T	25	(71%)		14	(82%)	11	(61%)	
Glu237Gly	T/C	10	(29%)		3	(18%)	7	(39%)	
(rs569108)	C/C	0	(0%)	0.32	0	(0%)	0	(0%)	0.16

(Table 4) contd.....

SNP Name (SNP ID)	Genotype	Frequency (%) Total (n=35)	P-Value*	Frequency (%) Responders (n=17)	Non-Responders (n=18)	P-Value†
CMA1	G/G	17 (49%)		7 (41%)	10 (56%)	
-1897G/A	G/A	16 (46%)		9 (53%)	7 (39%)	
(rs1800875)	A/A	2 (6%)	0.48	1 (6%)	1 (6%)	0.69
HRH1 -17C/T	G/G	31 (89%)		15 (88%)	16 (89%)	
(rs901865)	G/A	4 (11%)		2 (12%)	2 (11%)	
	A/A	0 (0%)	0.72	0 (0%)	0 (0%)	0.95
HRH4	C/C	31 (89%)		16 (94%)	15 (83%)	
Ala138Val	C/T	4 (11%)		1 (6%)	3 (17%)	
(rs11665084)	T/T	0 (0%)	0.72	0 (0%)	0 (0%)	0.31
LTC4S	A/A	21 (60%)		11 (65%)	10 (56%)	
-444A/C	A/C	13 (37%)		5 (29%)	8 (44%)	
(rs730012)	C/C	1 (3%)	0.54	1 (6%)	0 (0%)	0.35
FLG	C/C	9 (26%)		4 (24%)	5 (28%)	
Tyr2194His	C/T	21 (60%)		10 (59%)	11 (61%)	
(rs2184953)	T/T	5 (14%)	0.20	3 (18%)	2 (11%)	0.85
FLG	G/G	9 (26%)		4 (24%)	5 (28%)	
Tyr3105Asp	G/T	26 (74%)		13 (76%)	13 (72%)	
(rs2065958)	T/T	0 (0%)	<0.001	0 (0%)	0 (0%)	0.77
FLG	A/A	9 (26%)		4 (24%)	5 (28%)	
13347G/A	A/G	21 (60%)		10 (59%)	11 (61%)	
(rs12730241)	G/G	5 (14%)	0.20	3 (18%)	2 (11%)	0.85
FLG 13586C/T	A/A	9 (26%)		4 (24%)	5 (28%)	
(rs11204976)	A/G	21 (60%)		10 (59%)	11 (61%)	
	G/G	5 (14%)	0.20	3 (18%)	2 (11%)	0.85

*P-values were obtained using the Hardy Weinberg equilibrium (HWE) test.
†P-values were obtained using the likelihood ratio chi-square test.

Table 5. Association Between Genotype Combinations and Response to Treatment with Suplatast Tosilate

IL4 -590C/T		IL12B 1188A/C	Response Rate, %	P-Value*	Odds Ratio (95%CI)
T/T, T/C			53.1 (17/32)		-
C/C			0.0 (0/3)	0.04	
		C/C, C/A	59.3 (16/27)		10.2
		A/A	12.5 (1/8)	0.02	(1.1-94.8)
T/T, T/C	and	C/C, C/A	64.0 (16/25)		16.0
C/C	or	A/A	10.0 (1/10)	0.002	(1.7-147.5)

*P-values were obtained using the likelihood ratio chi-square test.

DISCUSSION

AD is increasingly recognized as a complex disease, since multifunctional cells and factors interact with each other in its pathogenesis. In the present study, based on the down-regulation of the Th2 inflammatory response by suplatast tosilate, we performed a pilot study to implicate Th2 suppression in the pathogenesis of AD by retrospectively analyzing the polymorphisms of genes reportedly associated with AD or atopic diseases. To this end, patients were recruited from our previous study, in which the efficacy of suplatast tosilate was investigated in adult AD patients whose conditions had been poorly controlled by treatment with topical steroids and adjunct anti-allergic agents, including antihistamines. We then examined the association of suplatast tosilate efficacy and 35

Table 6. Distribution of IL-4 -590C/T and IL-12B 1188A/C Genotypes Among Japanese and European Populations

SNP	Response to Suplatast Tosilate	Japanese		P-Value† (vs Present Study)	European	P-Value† (vs Present Study)
		Present Study (n=35)	HapMap project* (n=85,86)		HapMap Project* (n=113)	
IL-4 -590C/T						
T/T	high	13 (37%)	45 (53%)		2 (2%)	
T/C	medium	19 (54%)	33 (39%)		27 (24%)	
C/C	low	3 (9%)	7 (8%)	0.26	84 (74%)	<0.001
IL-12 1188A/C						
C/C	high	8 (23%)	28 (33%)		1 (1%)	
C/A	medium	19 (54%)	40 (47%)		41 (36%)	
A/A	low	8 (23%)	18 (21%)	0.56	71 (63%)	<0.001

*http://www.ncbi.nlm.nih.gov/snp/
†*P*-values were obtained using the likelihood ratio chi-square test.

SNPs of 27 allergy-related genes. Of note, no significant difference was seen in the minor allele frequencies of each SNP, with the exception of one SNP (Filaggrin Tyr3105Asp) with a low reliability, based on a comparison with an SNP control database for the Japanese population (SNPper or NCBI). These findings suggest that no genetic polymorphisms associated with susceptibility to AD were observed among the SNPs investigated in this study.

The results of the present SNP genotyping analysis clearly indicated that suplatast tosilate efficacy was associated with IL-4 and IL-12B polymorphisms, but not with any of the others, indicating that patients with a T/T or T/C genotype for the IL-4 -590C/T SNP as well as a C/C or C/A genotype for the IL-12B 1188A/C SNP responded to suplatast tosilate treatment at a significantly higher rate. Moreover, patients with both the IL-4 -590 T/T or T/C genotype and the IL-12B 1188 C/C or C/A genotype had a significantly higher response rate than those with other genotype combinations. Of note, SNPs in the regulatory sequences of genes are associated with the varying production of relevant cytokines. In fact, the promoter sequence of IL-4 -590T was reported to show a greater binding to nuclear transcription factors than that of -590C [23, 24]. Nakashima *et al.*, reported that PBMC with a -590T/T or -590T/C genotype produced higher levels of IL-4 than those with a -590C/C genotype [25]. In general, IL-4 is a major Th2 cytokine that plays an essential role in the class-switching of B cells to IgE-producing cells, Th2 cell differentiation, and the initial phase of tissue inflammation during the Th2-dominant phase of atopic diseases. Recently, IL-4 has been also reported to play an important role in regulating skin homeostasis and innate barrier function in AD lesions [26]. In fact, Burchard *et al.*, has reported that the sequence variant in the IL-4 promoter region is associated with the asthma FEV1 (Forced expiratory volume in one second) [27]. It is reasonable, therefore, to assume that patients with the IL-4 -590T allele tend to develop a Th2-dominated immune response, leading to the susceptibility of these patients to suplatast tosilate which down-regulates Th2-related responses including skin manifestations.

Suplatast tosilate has been reported to suppress IgE formation and eosinophil counts presumably through inhibition of Th2 cytokine in basic experiments and in several clinical studies in patients with atopic asthma [13-20]. However, no significant decreases in Th2-related parameters, such as the total IgE level and the eosinophil count, were observed after suplatast tosilate treatment even among the responders in this study. The reason for this contradiction is clearly unknown, but, as a possibility, a Th2-dependency may be decreased during the chronic phase of AD by the effect such as infections. In this sense, of great interest is the observation that patients with the IL-12B -1188 C/C genotype responded to suplatast tosilate treatment at a high rate. The IL-12B -1188 C allele was reported to result in IL-12B mRNA with a lower transcriptional activity and stability than that for the A allele [28]. Although IL-12 p40 encoded by IL-12B is a component of IL-12 (a p40 and p35 heterodimer) [29], the IL-12 p40 homodimer was reported to function as an antagonist of IL-12 action [30, 31]. In fact, PBMC with a -1188IL-12B C/C genotype having a high response rate to suplatast tosilate reportedly produced significantly higher levels of biologically active IL-12 upon stimulation with LPS or PPD than those of other genotypes with the A allele [32]. IL-12 is known to induce IFN-γ production [33], to suppress IgE synthesis [34], and to promote Th1 cell maturation [33]. The results, therefore, suggest that the efficacy of suplatast tosilate is associated with the Th1-immune response that also underlies the AD symptoms. This finding is partly in accordance with an observation by Matsui *et al.*, [35], who reported that PBMC from suplatast tosilate responders with childhood asthma produced higher amounts of IFN-γ than those of suplatast tosilate non-responders. The findings are also more directly in accordance with those by Murakami *et al.*, [36], who found that suplatast tosilate treatment significantly suppressed the elevated expression of IL-4, IL-5, and IFN-γ mRNA in caspase-1 transgenic mice that spontaneously developed AD-like dermatitis. They also observed that suplatast tosilate treatment significantly decreased the expression of IL-18, which induced Th1 responses in synergy with IL-12, possibly explaining the mechanism of suplatast tosilate efficacy for Th1-related responses.

The present results suggest that both Th2- and Th1-related responses may play more important roles in AD patients who responded to suplatast tosilate treatment than other factors, and ethnic differences may exist in the mechanism of chronic AD, since the allele frequencies of the IL-4 and IL-12B polymorphisms associated with the efficacy of suplatast tosilate differ significantly in the Japanese population compared with the European population. It should be noted, however, that these data were based on a retrospective analysis of a small sample size. Therefore, these results have to be confirmed in a large-scale prospective study. Moreover, further large-scale investigations taking ethnic differences into account are also needed to clarify the exact mechanism of chronic AD.

CONFLICT OF INTEREST

This study was funded by Taiho Pharmaceutical Co., Ltd (Tokyo, Japan). Hideki Nagase, Yoshinori Nakachi, Keiji Ishida and Mamoru Kiniwa are employees of Taiho Pharmaceutical Co., Ltd. The other authors declare that they have no other relevant conflicts of interest.

ACKNOWLEDGEMENTS

We thank Mrs. Saori Inoue and Mr. Yoshihiro Okayama (Taiho Pharmaceutical Co., Ltd., Tokushima, Japan) for technical and statistical assistance, respectively.

REFERENCES

[1] Cao Y, Liao M, Huang X, Mo Z, Gao F. Meta-analysis of genome-wide linkage studies of atopic dermatitis. Dermatitis 2009; 20: 193-9.

[2] Esparza-Gordillo J, Weidinger S, Folster-Holst R, *et al.* A common variant on chromosome 11q13 is associated with atopic dermatitis. Nat Genet 2009; 41: 596-601.

[3] Holloway JW, Yang IA, Holgate ST. Genetics of allergic disease. J Allergy Clin Immunol 2010; 125: S81-94.

[4] Kawasaki H, Kubo A, Sasaki T, Amagai M. Loss-of-function mutations within the filaggrin gene and atopic dermatitis. Curr Probl Dermatol 2011; 41: 35-46.

[5] Lesiak A, Kuna P, Zakrzewski M, *et al.* Combined occurrence of filaggrin mutations and IL-10 or IL-13 polymorphisms predisposes to atopic dermatitis. Exp Dermatol 2011; 20: 491-5.

[6] Sun LD, Xiao FL, Li Y, *et al.* Genome-wide association study identifies two new susceptibility loci for atopic dermatitis in the Chinese Han population. Nat Genet 2011; 43: 690-4.

[7] Katayama I, Kohno Y, Akiyama K, *et al.* Japanese guideline for atopic dermatitis. Allergol Int 2011; 60: 205-20.

[8] Nishimuta T, Kondo N, Hamasaki Y, Morikawa A, Nishima S. Japanese guideline for childhood asthma. Allergol Int 2011; 60: 147-69.

[9] Ohta K, Yamaguchi M, Akiyama K, *et al.* Japanese guideline for adult asthma. Allergol Int 2011; 60: 115-45.

[10] Okubo K, Kurono Y, Fujieda S, *et al.* Japanese guideline for allergic rhinitis. Allergol Int 2011; 60: 171-89.

[11] Miyachi Y, Katayama I, Furue M. Suplatast/tacrolimus combination therapy for refractory facial erythema in adult patients with atopic dermatitis: a meta-analysis study. Allergol Int 2007; 56: 269-75.

[12] Tamaoki J, Kondo M, Sakai N, *et al.* Effect of suplatast tosilate, a Th2 cytokine inhibitor, on steroid-dependent asthma: a double-blind randomised study. Tokyo Joshi-Idai Asthma Research Group. Lancet 2000; 356: 273-8.

[13] Koda A, Yanagihara Y, Matsuura N. IPD-1151T: a prototype drug for IgE antibody synthesis modulation. Agents Actions Suppl 1991; 34: 369-78.

[14] Yanagihara Y, Kiniwa M, Ikizawa K, Shida T, Matsuura N, Koda A. Suppression of IgE production by IPD-1151T (suplatast tosilate), a new dimethylsulfonium agent: (2). Regulation of human IgE response. Jpn J Pharmacol 1993; 61: 31-9.

[15] Sano Y, Miyamoto T, Makino S. Anti-inflammatory effect of suplatast tosilate on mild asthma. Chest 1997; 112: 862-3.

[16] Agrawal DK, Cheng G, Kim MJ, Kiniwa M. Interaction of suplatast tosilate (IPD) with chloride channels in human blood eosinophils: a potential mechanism underlying its anti-allergic and anti-asthmatic effects. Clin Exp Allergy 2008; 38: 305-12.

[17] Sano Y, Suzuki N, Yamada H, *et al.* Effects of suplatast tosilate on allergic eosinophilic airway inflammation in patients with mild asthma. J Allergy Clin Immunol 2003; 111: 958-66.

[18] Myou S, Fujimura M, Kurashima K, *et al.* Effects of suplatast tosilate, a new type of anti-allergic agent, on airway cough hypersensitivity induced by airway allergy in guinea-pigs. Clin Exp Allergy 2001; 31: 1939-44.

[19] Shiga M, Horiguchi T, Kondo R, *et al.* Long-term monotherapy with suplatast tosilate in patients with mild atopic asthma: a pilot comparison with low-dose inhaled fluticasone. Asian Pac J Allergy Immunol 2011; 29: 134-42.

[20] Yoshihara S, Ono M, Yamada Y, Fukuda H, Abe T, Arisaka O. Early intervention with suplatast tosilate for prophylaxis of pediatric atopic asthma: a pilot study. Pediatr Allergy Immunol 2009; 20: 486-92.

[21] Kitaba S, Inui S, Matsumoto Y, *et al.* Examination of an Inhibitory Effect on the Immunoglobulin E Production by Th2 Cytokine Inhibitor on Atopic Dermatitis. Hifu no kagaku 2007; 6 (Suppl 8): 8-14 (in Japanese, with English abstract).

[22] Matsumura Y, Matsumoto Y, Kitaba S, *et al.* Efficacy of Suplatast Tosilate for Treatment of Atopic Dermatitis Poorly Controlled by Other Anti-allergic Drugs. Hifu no kagaku 2007; 6 (Suppl 8): 1-7 (in Japanese, with English abstract).

[23] Rosenwasser LJ, Klemm DJ, Dresback JK, *et al.* Promoter polymorphisms in the chromosome 5 gene cluster in asthma and atopy. Clin Exp Allergy 1995; 25 (Suppl 2): 74-8; discussion 95-6.

[24] Song Z, Casolaro V, Chen R, Georas SN, Monos D, Ono SJ. Polymorphic nucleotides within the human IL-4 promoter that mediate overexpression of the gene. J Immunol 1996; 156: 424-9.

[25] Nakashima H, Miyake K, Inoue Y, *et al.* Association between IL-4 genotype and IL-4 production in the Japanese population. Genes Immun 2002; 3: 107-9.

[26] Sehra S, Yao Y, Howell MD, *et al.* IL-4 regulates skin homeostasis and the predisposition toward allergic skin inflammation. J Immunol 2010; 184: 3186-90.

[27] Burchard EG, Silverman EK, Rosenwasser LJ, *et al.* Association between a sequence variant in the IL-4 gene promoter and FEV(1) in asthma. Am J Respir Crit Care Med 1999; 160: 919-22.

[28] Hirota T, Suzuki Y, Hasegawa K, *et al.* Functional haplotypes of IL-12B are associated with childhood atopic asthma. J Allergy Clin Immunol 2005; 116: 789-95.

[29] Kobayashi M, Fitz L, Ryan M, *et al.* Identification and purification of natural killer cell stimulatory factor (NKSF), a cytokine with multiple biologic effects on human lymphocytes. J Exp Med 1989; 170: 827-45.

[30] Heinzel FP, Hujer AM, Ahmed FN, Rerko RM. *In vivo* production and function of IL-12 p40 homodimers. J Immunol 1997; 158: 4381-8.

[31] Ling P, Gately MK, Gubler U, *et al.* Human IL-12 p40 homodimer binds to the IL-12 receptor but does not mediate biologic activity. J Immunol 1995; 154: 116-27.

[32] Yilmaz V, Yentur SP, Saruhan-Direskeneli G. IL-12 and IL-10 polymorphisms and their effects on cytokine production. Cytokine 2005; 30: 188-94.

[33] Trinchieri G, Wysocka M, D'Andrea A, *et al.* Natural killer cell stimulatory factor (NKSF) or interleukin-12 is a key regulator of immune response and inflammation. Prog Growth Factor Res 1992; 4: 355-68.

[34] Kiniwa M, Gately M, Gubler U, Chizzonite R, Fargeas C, Delespesse G. Recombinant interleukin-12 suppresses the synthesis of immunoglobulin E by interleukin-4 stimulated human lymphocytes. J Clin Invest 1992; 90: 262-6.

[35] Matsui E, Shinoda S, Fukutomi O, Kaneko H, Fukao T, Kondo N. Relationship between the benefits of suplatast tosilate, a Th2 cytokine inhibitor, and gene polymorphisms in children with bronchial asthma. Exp Ther Med 2010; 1: 977-82.

[36] Murakami T, Yamanaka K, Tokime K, *et al.* Topical suplatast tosilate (IPD) ameliorates Th2 cytokine-mediated dermatitis in caspase-1 transgenic mice by downregulating interleukin-4 and interleukin-5. Br J Dermatol 2006; 155: 27-32.

Towards Developing Strategies to Reduce Health Care Costs in Dermatology

Mahsa Amir[1,§], Jeffrey H. Dunn[1,§], Melanie R. Bui[1], P. Alex McNally[4], Laura Huff[1], Sofia Mani[1], Ashley Hamstra[5], Jodi Duke[2] and Robert Dellavalle[*,1,3]

[1] *University of Colorado School of Medicine, Aurora, CO, USA*

[2] *University of Colorado Skaggs School of Pharmacy and Pharmaceutical Sciences, Aurora, CO, USA*

[3] *Dermatology Service, Department of Veterans Affairs Medical Center, Denver, CO, USA*

[4] *University of Colorado School of Medicine, Department of Surgery, CO, USA*

[5] *Loma Linda University Medical Center, Department of Dermatology, CA, USA*

Abstract: *Background*: The American Board of Internal Medicine has challenged medical specialties to develop "Top Five" lists in order to identify potential areas of wasted health care resources. The American Academy of Dermatology has not yet developed a "Top Five" list.

Objective: To provoke discussion on the need for more evidence, guidelines, and quality measures to reduce waste in Dermatology.

Methods: Dermatologists and medical professionals attending the 2010 Cochrane Skin Group Annual meeting were invited to complete a short-answer survey.

Results: The study had a response rate of 39% (n=24). Most responses fit under a common theme related to the lack of, and poor adherence to evidence-based guidelines including lack of randomized controlled trials for treatment of prevalent skin disease, use of expensive biologics, antibiotics or procedures when cheaper treatment alternatives exist, the use of screening or diagnostic procedures for diseases for which no effective treatment exists, inappropriate diagnostics (biopsies, allergy tests) or treatments (excision of benign lesions, inappropriate Mohs surgery) of skin diseases and lastly, inappropriate dermatology referrals from PCPs.

Limitations: The survey sample is small and limited to a small subset of medical professionals familiar with dermatology. While not definitive the survey results inspired this commentary and provided an initial basis for further discussion.

Conclusion: This commentary and survey are intended to encourage discussion regarding development of a "Top Five" list of ways to improve dermatology quality and efficiency.

Keywords: Quality, efficiency, evidence-based medicine, health care reform, ethics, economics.

INTRODUCTION

In 2011, The American Board of Internal Medicine and National Physicians Alliance challenged primary care physicians to develop lists of five activities to promote more effective use of health care resources [1, 2]. Published in the Archives of Internal Medicine [2], these evidence-based lists promote affordable, high-quality health care by improving treatment, reducing risk, and, when possible, reducing costs [2]. Howard Brody's 2010 editorial in the New England Journal of Medicine simultaneously challenged each medical specialty to develop top-5 lists of the most wasteful diagnostic tests and treatments as a starting point for demonstrating to the public that quality and efficiency can be synonymous in healthcare [3]. These ongoing efforts are manifested online by the Choosing Wisely website [1], which aims to foster discussion between patients and physicians about the utilization of healthcare resources that are scientifically based, free from harm, and necessary [1].

Table 1. Demographics of Survey Participants

Dermatologists	15
Researchers	2
Medical Students	2
Rheumatologist	1
Primary Care Physician	1
Epidemiologist	1
Managing editor	1
Medical Social Worker	1

*Address correspondence to this author at the Department of Veteran Affairs Medical Center, 1055 Clermont Street, Box 165, Denver, CO 80220, USA;

E-mail: robert.dellavalle@ucdenver.edu

§The first two authors listed contributed equally to this work.

Table 2. Survey Results and Corresponding Categories

Survey Result	Category
Absence of good RCTs in prevalent skin disorders	Better Evidence Based Practice and Adherence to Existing Guidelines (21)
Inappropriate drug selection	
Failing to use epinephrine in distal locations to help control bleeding, extra time to contain bleeding	
Twice daily as opposed to once daily topical corticosteroids	
Ineffective treatments	
Stopping anticoagulation prior to surgery -- stopping it increases risk of adverse reaction, consult with PCP to stop it is a waste of time	
Medications with minimal benefit compared with cheaper alternatives	
Short term and not long term studies in psoriasis	
Treatment of most Actinic Keratosis	
Biologic drugs for psoriasis when retinoids, MTX... have not been tried	
Shotgun approach to therapy based on single case reports of diseases that may have spontaneous remissions as part of their clinical course	
Screening or diagnostic procedures where no effective treatment exists	
Most acne treatments - they don't clear acne apart from isotretinoin	
Use of biologics in psoriasis before less expensive alternatives have failed	
Branded topical drugs equivalent to generics	
Branded doxycycline and minocycline drugs for acne	
Biological agents	
Prescribing medications for which there is no evidence	
Wart treatment	
Treatment of toenail fungus	
PDT for AKs	
Research compliance requirements	Systemic Healthcare Inefficiencies: Insurance, Medicare, Research, Malpractice (16)
Discrepancies between practice and science	
Administrative tasks for insurance reimbursement	
Complying with regulations for lab, nursing, clerks	
Effort wasted in obtaining prior authorizations for topical meds	
Staff time re Obtaining insurance approval for Procedures	
Staff time re Rx changes due to insurance non-coverage	
Time spent on prior authorization	
Staff time with paper records	
Regulations concerning the use of Accutane	
Malpractice rates without Tort Reform	
Paper record storage	
Expensive gene rearrangement tests and other tests to secure a diagnosis of CTCL	
Contracts	
Defensive medicine	
Billing insurance	

(Table 2 contd…..)

Excision benign lesions	Fraud, Waste and Abuse (14)
Treatment of multiple benign actinic keratoses and pretending that they are skin cancer	
Mohs for low-risk NMSCs	
Greed in private practice	
Professional fees for dermatologists	
Unnecessary biopsies	
Treatment of AKs or NMSCs in elderly patients with low life expectancies.	
Routine allergy tests for people with chronic urticaria	
Unnecessary investigations	
Total body skin exams in individuals at low risk for skin cancer	
Mohs for small tumors	
Topical barrier devices for atopic dermatitis	
Complex surgical repairs (when simple ones would suffice)	
Biopsy of benign lesions	
Antiwrinkle creams	Cosmetic Emphasis in Dermatology (14)
Cosmetic procedures	
Training dermatologists (at great cost to the health system) who will ultimately spend large portions of their professional efforts doing cosmetic procedures	
Micro-dermabrasions	
Bleaching therapy people from African descent	
Lasers	
Cosmetic surgery	
Cosmetic procedures with minimal benefit	
Treatment of wrinkles	
Treatment of signs of natural aging process	
Cosmetics	
Multiple body washes	
Cosmeceuticals	
Cosmeceuticals	
Delayed referral to dermatologist- inpatient	Improved Patient and Primary Care Provider Education Regarding Screening, Medication, Procedure Use (8)
Mohs surgery for chest and back skin cancer	
Non-attendance OPD/therapy visits	
Prioritizing pigmented lesions from the worried well with a low diagnostic yield	
Unused medications	
Yearly visits to dermatologists specifically for total body skin examinations by people with no excess risk factors	
Over utilization for specialty service that should be handled in primary care	
Delayed referral to dermatologist- outpatient	
Revamping of old products into different % age combinations for business purposes rather than concentrating on new therapeutics.	Pharmaceutical Industry (6)
Research in wrinkles	
Money from companies given to marketing and not clinical independent research	
Overpriced drugs including topicals	
Medical conventions with bad information	
Pharmaceutical company spending	

In response to these challenges, nine US medical groups have developed "Top Five" lists to improve healthcare by use of high quality, efficient, and evidence-based medicine [1-3].

The American Academy of Dermatology has not yet taken up these challenges. As a means of exploring the "Top Five" ways to save money in dermatology, medical professionals including dermatologists attending a 2010 international conference on Comparative Effectiveness Research in Dermatology at the University of Colorado School of Medicine were invited to complete an online survey prior to attendance (Table **1**). One survey question asked participants to list the top five wastes of money in the field of dermatology. Twenty-four of 61 attendees replied, yielding a response rate of 39%. Responses were analyzed by three independent authors and catalogued into core themes based upon response frequency (Table **2**).

Lack of, and poor adherence to evidence-based guidelines was the highest response category. Since many of the treatments in dermatology are topical, with local side effects, dermatologists frequently try treatments and combinations of treatments, reaching conclusions on the basis of personal experience or uncontrolled trials [4]. These uncontrolled trials often lead to errors and substantial bias, which is passed onto the patient in the form of inferior healthcare. Specific responses in this category included the lack of randomized controlled trials for treatment of prevalent skin disease, use of expensive biologics, antibiotics or procedures when cheaper treatment alternatives exist, the use of screening or diagnostic procedures for diseases for which no effective treatment exists, inappropriate diagnostics (biopsies, allergy tests), or treatment (excision of benign lesions, inappropriate Mohs surgery) of skin diseases. Another important response involved inappropriate dermatology referrals from PCPs, which could be improved by patient and primary care provider (PCP) education regarding screening and management of skin disease.

In conclusion, there is a broad spectrum of quality and cost-related inefficiencies in dermatology. While our survey is small and limited to a self-selected sample, the results are meant to initiate a discussion of those areas of waste in dermatology that could be reasonably condensed into a "Top 5" list congruent with those of other medical organizations [1, 3]. For example, the American Academy of Allergy, Asthma, and Immunology (AAAAI) has developed a one-page list of "Five Things Physicians and Patients Should Question", which specifically identifies unnecessary tests and treatments common to this specialty [5]. This list was created by an AAAAI taskforce that incorporated scientific evidence, membership feedback, and expert opinions into its recommendations [5].

There will no doubt be objections that more research is needed before a list such as this can be developed for the field of dermatology. As Brody notes in his editorial, however, "...no matter how desirable more research is, we know enough today to make at least a down payment on medicine's cost-cutting effort...we should at least begin where we can.... A Top Five list also has the advantage that if we restrict ourselves to the most egregious causes of waste, we can demonstrate to a skeptical public that we are genuinely protecting patients' interests and not simply "rationing" health care, regardless of the benefit, for cost-cutting purposes" [3]. There is an urgent but achievable need for comprehensive health care reform in the United States [6]. Once a Top Five list has been agreed upon, plans for educating dermatologists can be created and encouraged by organizations such as the American Academy of Dermatology. Dermatologists contribute to this effort by advocating for better treatment guidelines, educating patients and PCPs, and implementing high quality, cost-effective, evidence-based treatment into their clinical practice.

CONFLICTS OF INTEREST

The opinions expressed in this article represent the views of the authors and not of the United States government.

ACKNOWLEDGEMENTS

The authors would like to thank Maggie Cook-Shimanek, MD, Rosemary Highart, MD, Lauren MacLaughlin, Chad Vogeler, Brian Petersen, Daniel Sugai, Jill Feetham, and Laurel Geraghty for their valuable comments and insight in reviewing the manuscript.

FINANCIAL DISCLOSURE

This study was funded by a $20,000 NIAMS R13 conference grant (R13AR059425). The Veterans' Administration provided financial support for the study (Dr. Dellavalle). The sponsors had no role in the design or conduct of the study; in the collection, analysis, or interpretation of data; nor in the preparation, review, or approval of the manuscript.

REFERENCES

[1] American Board of Internal Medicine (ABIM). Choosing Wisely. Reference Available from: http: //choosingwisely.org/ [Accessed on: April 8, 2012].

[2] Smith SR, Aguilar I, Berger ZD, *et al.* The "Top 5" Lists in Primary Care: Meeting the Responsibility of Professionalism. Arch Intern Med 2011; 171(15): 1385-90.

[3] Brody H. Medicine's ethical responsibility for health care reform -- the Top Five list. N Engl J Med 2010; 362: 283-5.

[4] Bigby M. Evidence-based medicine in dermatology. Dermatol Clin 2000; 18(2): 261-76.

[5] American Academy of Allergy, Asthma, and Immunology. Five Things Physicians and Patients Should Question. Reference Available from: http: //choosingwisely.org/wp-content/uploads/2012/04/5things_12_factsheet_AAAAI.pdf [Accessed on: June 19, 2012].

[6] Berwick DM, Hackbarth AD. Eliminating waste in US health care. JAMA 2012; 307(14): 1513-6.

Herpes Simplex Virus Infections of the Nipple

Lara El Hayderi, Marie Caucanas and Arjen F. Nikkels*

Department of Dermatology, University Hospital of Liège, Liège, Belgium

Abstract: The usual sites of herpes simplex virus (HSV) type 1 and 2 infections are orolabial and anogenital, respectively. HSV infection of the nipple and periareolar area is exceptional but probably underrecognized. Typical features include severe pain and erosive or ulcerated erythematous confluent clusters of lesions of the nipple and periareolar area. It is usually unilateral and not recurring. HSV infection of the nipple is originating from autoinoculation, sexual transmission or breastfeeding. Diagnosis is often delayed. The Tzanck smear is the most rapid and adequate method of diagnosis. Immunohistochemistry enables viral identification. The treatment relies on topical disinfection and oral antiviral therapy, such as aciclovir, famciclovir or valaciclovir. Scarring is uncommon.

Keywords: Herpes simplex virus, nipple, areola, aciclovir.

INTRODUCTION

Herpes simplex virus (HSV) type-I and -II are responsible for orolabial and anogenital herpes, respectively. HSV-I or -II infections of the pubis, the bursa, the finger or the hair follicle are more seldom [1-5]. HSV infections of the nipple and/or areola are rather exceptional.

Three patients are presented with HSV infection of the nipple, as well as a literature review.

CASE REPORTS

1. A 20-year-old woman presented at the emergency ward for a painful ulcerated lesion of her left nipple. There was no particular medical or surgical history other than a mild atopic dermatitis. She did not take any drugs. The lesion, affecting the entire areola and nipple (Fig. **1**), was erythematous, ulcerated and extremely painful. She applied a zinc paste to alleviate the erosions. A left axillar lymphadenopathy was palpated. She presented no fever. A Tzanck smear was performed to exclude a viral infection. The immunohistochemical identification [6,7] was positive for HSV-1, whereas the HSV-2 and varicella zoster virus (VZV) stainings were negative. Serology showed a past HSV infection (IgG: +, IgM: -). The patient was not breastfeeding but had oral/hand-nipple contact with her partner who regularly experienced recurrent orolabial herpes (RHL). The patient and her partner did not suffer from genital herpes. Oral aciclovir (5 x 200 mg/d) was initiated for 7 days and about 10 days later, there was a complete resolution with no residual scarring. She never presented any recurrent herpetic lesion at this site until today.

Fig. (1). Erythematous and infiltrated HSV-1 infection of the nipple and areola.

2. A 38-year-old woman was admitted at the emergency ward for very painful, eroded and soothing lesions of her left nipple. She never presented similar lesions previously. She was otherwise healthy and did not take any medication. She was non-lactating. Her partner presented RHL and the lesions presented 2 days after oral contact with the nipple. The breast was not swollen or painful and there was a unilateral axillar lymphadenopathy. The patient and her partner were not afflicted by genital herpes. Immunohistochemistry applied to a Tzanck smear revealed a positive signal for HSV-2 antigens (Fig. **2**), but no signal for HSV-1 or VZV antigens. A treatment with oral aciclovir (200 mg, 5 x/d) was given for 10 days. A topical disinfection treatment was applied. After two weeks, no residual lesions were noted and the pain had disappeared completely.

*Address correspondence to this author at the Department of Dermatology, CHU of Sart Tilman, University of Liège, B-4000 Liège, Belgium;
E-mail: af.nikkels@chu.ulg.ac.be

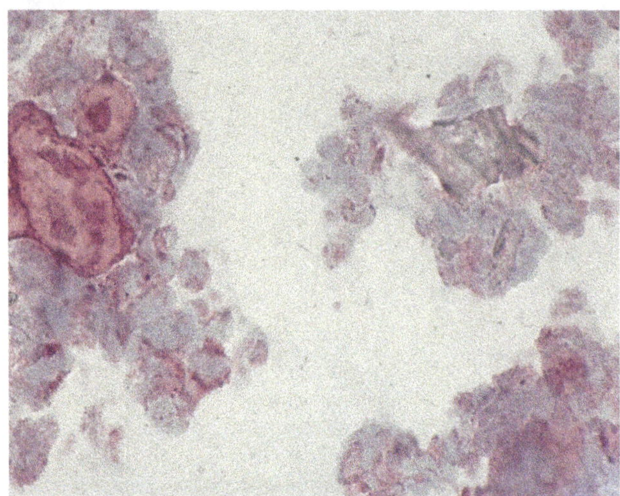

Fig. (2). HSV-2 positive immunostaining in multinucleated keratinocytes (Tzanck smear, Red signal, 100x).

3. A 48-year-old woman without any remarkable medical history presented a painful, soothing and eroded dermatosis on the right nipple and superior part of the areola. Bisoprolol was the only medication. This lesion appeared after a slightly traumatic oral/genital-nipple contact with her partner, who suffered from recurrent genital herpes. She presented a right axillar lymphadenopathy. The couple was known to be HSV-2 serodiscordant. A 2-mm punch biopsy was performed under local anesthesia and the histologic examination revealed the presence of intraepidermal blistering with eosinophilic, sometimes swollen keratinocytes. Some keratinocytes presented intranuclear inclusions. Immunohistochemical identification revealed the presence of HSV-2 antigens (Fig. **3**), but HSV-1 and VZV antigens were not detected. An initial treatment with topical antibiotics did not bring any relief. An oral treatment with aciclovir (2 x 500 mg/d, 7 days) was initiated. Complete healing without scarring occurred after 6 days. Since, she never experienced a recurrence of HSV-2 infection at this site.

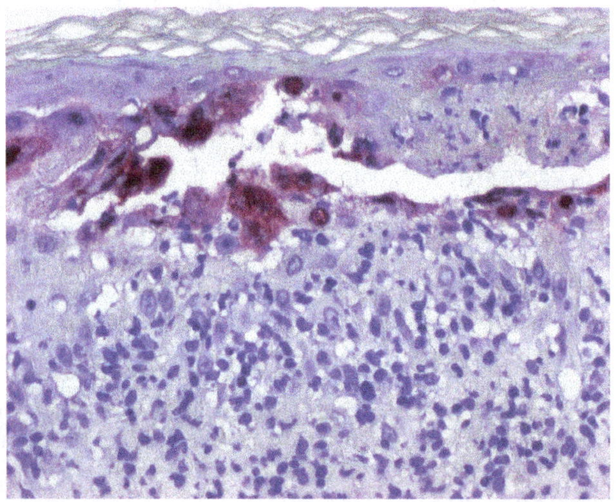

Fig. (3). HSV-1 positive immunostaining in epidermal keratinocytes (Skin biopsy, Red signal, 100x).

DISCUSSION

Incidence

HSV infection of the nipple and/or areola is very rare and has an estimated frequency of about 2% of all extragenital HSV lesions [8]. However, as the diagnosis is far from easy, it is probable that this entity is underdiagnosed. Up to date, only female patients have been reported in the literature [9-12]. All the patients were adults (19-48 years) and sexually active. All the publications reports single episodes and recurrent infections of the nipple were never mentioned.

Viral Type

The majority of infections are related to HSV-1 [11], whereas HSV-2 is more exceptional. However, viral identification is often not performed.

Clinical Manifestations

The dermatologic manifestations include small crops of blisters on an erythematous and slightly swollen base. Erosions, excoriations and ulcerations are often observed. Either the nipple is affected alone, but frequently the areola and periareolar area are also involved. Usually, these infections are unilateral [11,13], but bilateral infections have been reported [our case, 14-16]. Infections are usually restricted to the nipple and areola [8] although cutaneous dissemination may occur [10]. Some infections are accompanied by a locoregional lymphadenopathy [13] whereas others are not. The healing time is about 7 to 10 days and does not differ from other anatomical sites. No scarring has been reported after HSV infection of the nipple. A very characteristic feature is moderate to severe pain, probably related to the high degree of nerve supply of the nipple and the neurotropic character of the virus [17].

Risk Factors

No particular risk factors exist besides atopic dermatitis [12] and local trauma.

Complications

HSV mastitis is a rare but feared complication [11,13]. The breast is swollen and indurated with a local painful lymphadenopthy. Another complication is the risk of infecting a newborn during breastfeeding [18]. Disseminated neonatal herpes infection can originate from HSV infection of the nipple of the mother [19]. Hence, breastfeeding is absolutely contraindicated in case of breast lesions [20,21].

Transmission

HSV infection of the nipple can be the result of a reactivation of a previous local infection or *via* a new transmission.

At least three modes of transmission may explain HSV infection of the nipple. Transmission can occur from infant to mother, as demonstrated by the acquisition of nipple herpes, originating from a primary gingivostomatitis in a baby [14, 15, 22]. In the non-lactating woman, contamination may occur through oral sexual contact [10, 11, 16, 23], such as a partner with recurrent labial herpes. In this instance, HSV-1 is the usual culprit. The partner's hand to nipple contact is also possible [13]. Autoinoculation may also occur from a RHL or a recurrent genital HSV infection of the patient herself [4,13].

Reactivation has been suspected of an ancient local HSV infection of the nipple by a bite on the nipple by a new male partner without RHL whereas the former partner had RHL [11].

Diagnosis

The clinical diagnosis is very difficult as the disease is rare and is not part of the usual differential diagnoses.

The Tzanck test or cytodiagnosis, combined with immunohistochemistry (IHC), is the preferential method to identify HSV 1 or 2 in a very rapid, sensitive and specific way [6,9,13,24,25].

Sometimes a punch biopsy is performed, especially as mammary Paget's disease is suspected [10,13]. The cytology reveals a ground-glass appearance of the nuclei with multinucleated syncytial cells. Subsequenlty, either IHC [6] or in situ hybridization (ISH) [24] using DNA probes may be used to search for HSV antigens or DNA.

PCR is another highly sensitive and specific method to identify HSV in clinical specimens [10,11].

Mammography reveals dense fibroglandular tissue with increased density of the affected breast. Skin thickening may be present. Ultrasonography shows areas of diffuse skin thickening [13]. However, mammography and ultrasonography are not diagnostic in the case of herpes of the nipple.

Differential Diagnosis

Herpes zoster restricted to the nipple is a difficult clinical differential diagnosis, in particular as both entities are linked to pain [25]. However, extension beyond the nipple and a dermatomal distribution are favoring herpes zoster. Furthermore, bacterial infection, dermatomycosis, atopic dermatitis, Darier's disease, periareolar abscess [26] and allergic contact eczema have to be eliminated. Erosive adenomatosis and mammary Paget's disease have also to be ruled out, especially in the elderly patient.

Treatment

As these infections are uncommon, the treatment recommendations are expert based but not evidence based. Oral aciclovir was initiated at 200 mg 5 x/d, for 5 to 7 days in the majority of the patients [10,12,13]. All patients healed after 7 to 10 days and no residual scarring was ever mentioned in the literature. Newer thymidine kinase dependant antivirals such as famciclovir and valaciclovir may also be considered as treatment alternatives. Topical disinfection is recommended.

CONCLUSION

HSV infection of the nipple and the periareolar area are uncommon entities that may easily be misdiagnosed. Severe pain combined with an unilateral or bilateral acute erosive dermatosis should suggest the diagnosis. Sexual contact, autoinoculation and breastfeeding are recognized risk factors. Aciclovir, famciclovir and valaciclovir are the antiviral drugs of choice.

ACKNOWLEDGEMENT

Declared none.

CONFLICT OF INTEREST

The authors confirm that this article content has no conflict of interest.

REFERENCES

[1] Castronovo C, Lebas E, Nikkels-Tassoudji N, Nikkels AF. Viral infections of the pubis. Int J STD AIDS 2012; 23: 48-50.

[2] Nikkels AF, Pièrard GE. Treatment of mucocutaneous presentations of herpes simplex virus infections. Am J Clin Dermatol 2002; 3: 475-87.

[3] Nahmias AJ, Roizman B. Infection with herpes simplex viruses 1 and 2. N Engl J Med 1973; 2897: 19-25.

[4] Whitley RJ, Nahmias AJ, Visintine AM, Fleming CL, Alford CA. The natural history of herpes simplex virus infection of mother and newborn. Pediatrics 1980; 66: 489-94.

[5] Tyring SK, Carlton SS, Evans T. Herpes. Atypical clinical manifestations. Dermatol Clin 1998; 16: 783-8.

[6] Nikkels AF, Debrus S, Sadzot-Delvaux C, *et al.* Comparative immunohistochemical study of herpes simplex and varicella-zoster infections. Virchows Arch A Pathol Anat Histopathol 1993; 422: 121-6.

[7] Nikkels AF, Piérard GE. The Tzanck smear: heading the right way! J Am Acad Dermatol 2009; 61: 152-3.

[8] Corey L, Adams HG, Brown ZA, Holmes KK. Genital herpes simplex virus infections: clinical manifestations, course, and complications. Ann Intern Med 1983; 98: 958-72.

[9] Mardi K, Gupta N, Sharma S, Gupta S. Cytodiagnosis of herpes simplex mastitis: Report of a rare case. J Cytol 2009; 26: 149-50.

[10] Watanabe D, Kuhara T, Ishida N, Takeo T, Tamada Y, Matsumoto Y. Disseminated mucocutaneous herpes simplex virus infection in an immunocompetent woman. Int J STD AIDS 2010; 21: 213-4.

[11] Brown H, Kneafsey P, Kureishi A. Herpes simplex mastitis: case report and review of the literature. Can J Infect Dis 1996; 7: 209-12.

[12] Robinson GE, Underhill GS, Forster GE, Kennedy C, McLean K. Treatment with acyclovir of genital herpes simplex virus infection complicated by eczema herpeticum. Br J Vener Dis 1984; 60: 241-2.

[13] Soo MS, Ghate S. Herpes simplex virus mastitis: clinical and imaging findings. AJR Am J Roentgenol 2000; 174: 1087-8.

[14] Sealander JY, Kerr CP. Herpes simplex of the nipple: infant-to-mother transmission. Am Fam Physician 1989; 39: 111-3.

[15] Quinn PT, Lofberg JV. Maternal herpetic breast infection: another hazard of neonatal herpes simplex. Med J Aust 1978; 2: 411-2.

[16] Dekio S, Kawasaki Y, Jidoi J. Herpes simplex on nipples inoculated from herpetic gingivostomatitis of a baby. Clin Exp Dermatol 1986; 2: 664-6.

[17] Amir L. Test your knowledge. Nipple pain in breastfeeding. Aust Fam Physician 2004; 33: 44-5.

[18] Dunkle LM, Schmidt RR, O'Connor DM. Neonatal herpes simplex infection possibly acquired *via* maternal breast milk. Pediatrics 1979; 63: 250-1.

[19] Sullivan-Bolyai JZ, Fife KH, Jacobs RF, Miller Z, Corey L. Disseminated neonatal herpes simplex virus type 1 from a maternal breast lesion. Pediatrics 1983; 71: 455-7.

[20] Henrot A. Transmission materno-foetale et indirecte de l'infection HSV, traitement et prévention. Ann Dermatol Venereol 2002; 129: 533-49.

[21] Neifert MR. Returning to breast-feeding. Clin Obstet Gynecol 1980; 23: 1061-72.

[22] Gupta S, Malhotra AK, Dash SS. Child to mother transmission of herpes simplex virus-1 infection at an unusual site. J Eur Acad Dermatol Venereol 2008; 22: 878-9.

[23] Yoshida M. Herpetic pharyngitis with mammary and genital herpes due to sexual contact. Acta Derm Venereol 1999; 79: 250.

[24] Kobayashi TK, Okamoto H, Yakushiji M. Cytologic detection of herpes simplex virus DNA in nipple discharge by in situ hybridization: report of two cases. Diagn Cytopathol 1993; 9: 296-9.

[25] Watanabe D, Kuhara T, Ishida N, Takama H, Tamada Y, Matsumoto Y. Herpes zoster of the nipple: rapid DNA-based diagnosis by the loop-mediated isothermal amplification method. Int J STD AIDS 2010; 21: 66-7.

[26] Higgins SP, Stedman YF, Bundred NJ, Woolley PD, Chandiok P, Chandler P. Periareolar breast abscess due to Pseudomonas aeruginosa in an HIV antibody positive male. Genitourin Med 1994; 70: 147-8.

31

Serdev Suture for Buttock's Lift - Ambulatory Scarless Procedure

Nikolay P. Serdev[*,§]

Medical Centre "Aesthetic Surgery, Aesthetic Medicine", Sofia, Bulgaria

Abstract: *Background*: This article presents the author's technique and experience in the treatment of the flaccid "unhappy buttock" form with his surgical procedure of buttock lift by suture, without incision scars. The author first presented this new operation technique on a national level at the 2nd Annual Meeting of the National Bulgarian Society for Aesthetic Surgery and Aesthetic Medicine in Sofia on March 18, 1994 [1] and internationally at many scientific meetings over the world [2, 3, 4…]. The result is a visual change in the buttock position to a higher one, which elongates the lower limbs and changes the proportions between lower and upper half of the body.

Objective: The aim of this study is to describe a mini-invasive procedure of beautification of the buttock form without scars by creating a lifting effect on the buttock's subcutaneous tissue, using a suture that takes the inferiorly positioned deep fibrose tissue and fixes it upwards to the sacro-cutaneous fascia, discovered by the author. Aesthetic and technical considerations required properly sculpting the buttocks into a higher position, demonstrating nicely rounded form.

Methods: 1032 female patients, and 26 male patients aged 18-62 years, with ptosis and cellulite on the buttocks were treated since 1993 on an outpatient basis by the "Serdev suture technique without visible scars". Important instrumentarium is a long, curved, elastic needle and Polycon semi-elastic Bulgarian antimicrobial polycaproamide long term (in 2 years) absorbable surgical threads Polycon, produced in Bulgaria. This operation has been performed either alone or after ultrasonic assisted liposculpture (UAL) that reduces the amount of fat and heaviness.

Results: All patients reported a high degree of satisfaction. A stable improvement in the buttock position and form was observed for the period described. In the postoperative period the complication rate was minimal and resolved in the first 4-5 days post operative period. The skin puncture in the perianal zone makes antibiotic prophylaxis obligatory as well as a strict follow up for the first 7 days. Some pain in the sitting position was observed for at least 5 to 10 days, but all other social and professional duties and activities were possible.

Conclusions: This outpatient procedure is effective in the correction of buttock laxity and ptosis and creates a new form, universally accepted as "happy buttocks".

Keywords: Serdev Suture, Buttock's lift, Serdev needles, Semi-elastic Polycon thread.

INTRODUCTION

As more people seek body contour surgery, we should use our growing, developing knowledge and surgical experience to create new non-scaring surgical procedures for beautification, where formerly results of body contour surgery in areas like the buttocks have been less satisfying. A very small number of techniques are available for correction of the form and aesthetics of the buttocks, especially in cases of lax and ptotic buttocks. Non-scarring and sparing methods are preferred and requested by patients. So far, the minimally invasive technique most utilized for the fatty tissues has been liposuction exclusively. However the use of ultrasonic assisted liposculpture (U.A.L.) alone cannot lift or tighten up loose, lax and ptotic buttocks, and in our hands is combined with Serdev suture technique for buttock lift. In literature, liposuction is mostly followed by excision of tissue or other surgical methods. To improve the gluteal region in those patients whose problem is skin flabbiness rather than excessive fat, combinations of techniques are performed: liposuction, lipoinjections, implants for augmentation and lipectomy.

The aim of our paper is to present a new outpatient scarless buttock lift surgical procedure by closed approach suture that can meet patients requirements for beautification of buttocks form and position without scars, that has an uncomplicated, rapid post operative recovery period and is long lasting.

Special Threads and Needles

We present the Serdev[R] needles and the semi-elastic long-term absorbable Bulgarian threads that has made possible the introduction of a successful scarless, closed approach technique of Serdev Suture[R] buttock lift with almost no downtime.

Anatomy

The well accepted gluteal position is the position of the m. gluteus maximus. The musculo-sceletal framework is

*Address correspondence to this author at the Medical Center "Aesthetic Surgery and Aesthetic Medicine", 11, "20th April" St., 1606 Sofia, Bulgaria; E-mail: serdev@gmail.com

[§]President, The Bulgarian Society of Aesthetic Surgery and Aesthetic Medicine.

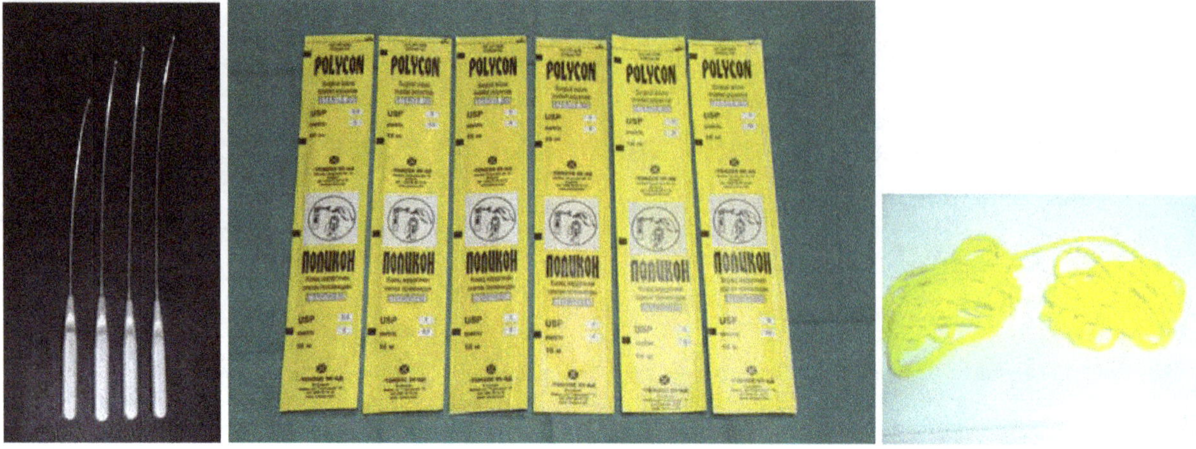

Fig. (1). Serdev[R] Needles and Bulgarian semi-elastic, anti-microbial, long term absorbable threads.

normally nicely formed. Unfortunately, female structure mostly includes an inferiorly positioned fatty tissue deposit, elongating ladies buttocks in lower aspect. These elongated hanging buttocks are visible from the frontal view as well that shortens the lengths of female lower limbs from the rear view. The hanging soft tissue is well known as "unhappy buttocks", different from the high gluteal position, called "happy buttocks".

The gluteal fatty tissue includes fibrotic fibres, fascial layers and trabecular system attaching the skin to the gluteus maximus fascia. The fascial tissue represents a flexible support for the soft framework of the human body. It forms a stable network for subdermal and deep fat layers, as well as cases for muscles, and sheaths for blood vessels and nerves. We use this stable fascial structure to fix higher the buttock soft tissue.

Serdev Fascia

Important anatomy landmark is the “Serdev fascia” or “sacro-cutaneous fascia” discovered by the author, fixing the skin to the lateral borders of the sacrum and the only safe fibrotic structure to hold the buttock’s heaviness in the new position. It is perpendicular to skin and sacrum and is located in the line between the Venera dimples at the sacroiliac joint and the upper point of the inter-gluteal fold at the sacrocococcygeal joint.

PATIENTS AND METHOD

The primary indication for buttock lift surgery by suture is the moderate to severe soft-tissue laxity in the lower trunk with minimal or mild residual fat deposits. If significant fat deposits are presented, we initially treat patients with UAL to reduce the volume and heaviness of the buttock fat tissue [2].

In selected cases, UAL was performed for body beautification and sculpturing, and to reduce the buttocks volume and heaviness.

The Serdev suture[R] was created for aesthetic purposes with the intention of creating a higher and more rounded attractive buttocks, at the same time creating a visible elongation of the legs and a change to the correlation of body to lower limbs length. True buttock sculpting demands a three-dimensional artistic understanding of the anatomic and surgical adipose layers of the central trunk, a stable immobile fixation to Serdev fascia and semi-elasticity of the suture to hold the mobile fibrotic buttocks tissue. This is essential in preventing complications from the buttock lifting such as trauma, inner tissue decubiti etc.

(A)

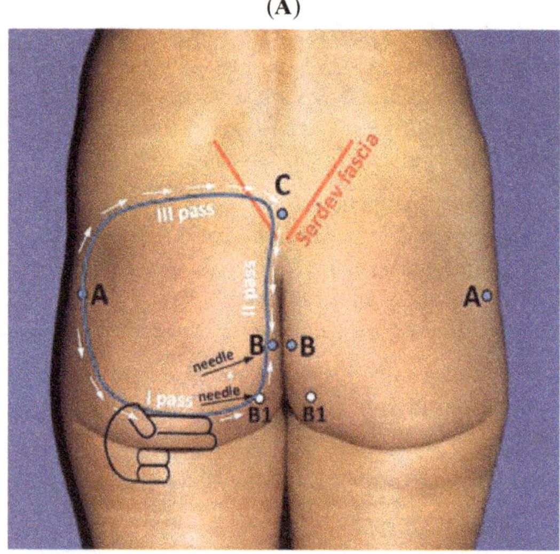

(B)

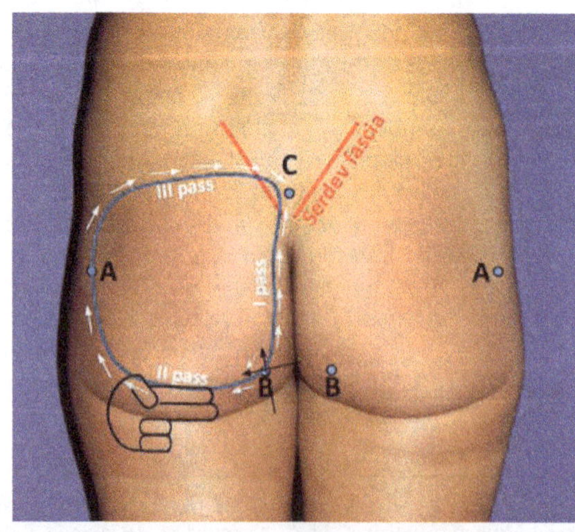

Fig. (2). A. Suture starting from lateral. **B.** Suture starting from medial. Arrows show needle direction. The Serdev sacro-cutaneous fascia perpendicular to sacrum and skin to hold the buttocks after the lift.

Our surgical technique contains a fixation of the complete supeficial fascial system of the buttock's soft tissue (2 fingers higher than the infra-gluteal fold – Fig. **2**) through a special long needle (Fig. **1**) and a suture technique including 3 steps: The first step for fixation of the subdermal fascial tissue could begin on the lateral aspect of the buttock – Point A (Fig. **3**) mostly using the same penetration point, like in liposuction, UAL or using an old one) and ends medial 2-3 cm higher and lateral from the anus at point B, while the second begins on the upper penetration point C and ends on the lower aspect of the inter-gluteal fold at B. The third fixation passes convex the upper part of gluteus maximus and ends at C, fulfilling the circular character of the suture. Elastic tightening of this suture assures a higher fixation of the gluteal fibrous layers of the lower part of the buttock to the Serdev sacro-cutaneous fascia. At the same time it corrects the trabecular system of the skin in a superficially convex "bucket". This superficial roundness is moved superiorly to its best position. The fixation of the suture to the stable inelastic Serdev fascia, maximally guaranties the longevity of the aesthetic effect. The elastic quality of the antimicrob polycaproamide Polycon that we use, reduces the possibility of decubiti of the fibrotic tissue and reduces complications.

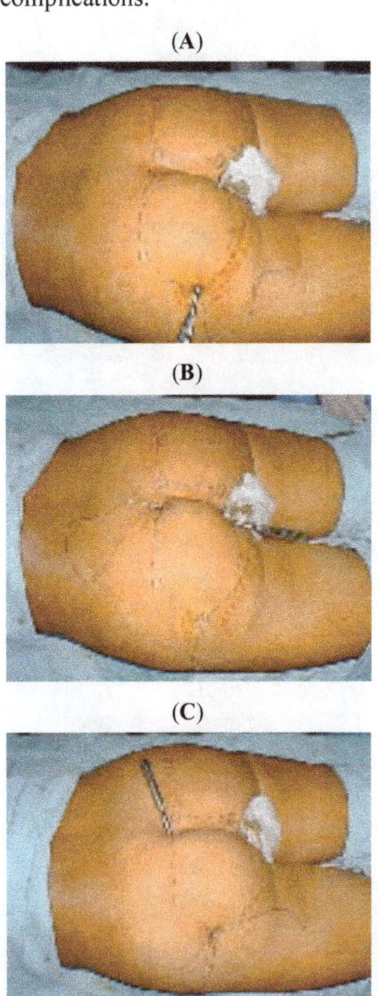

Fig. (3). **A**, **B**, **C**. Three steps minimum are necessary for a complete fixation of the buttock superficial fibrous system. It realizes a stable fixation of the lower buttock fibrotic soft tissue to the Serdev sacro-cutaneous fascia.

The 3 steps could be done in another order, starting from the medial lower aspect as shown on Fig. (**3**) without to exit at point B that is sometimes easier for beginners.

The buttock lift by suture requires 10 to 15 min of operating time per side, no blood transfusions, no stay at the clinic, no nursing care, and not more than a day or two off work.

More than thousand cases of laxity and ptosis in the gluteal area were operated during the years 1993-2012 to lift the buttocks for aesthetic reasons. This mini-invasive method, new in the beginning became fast a standard procedure internationally. It became very popular among patients and is accepted better than any excision surgery. Patients were informed about possible expected and unexpected risks of surgery and sign an informed consent. They were informed about the qualities of the Bulgarian semi-elastic antimicrobial thread, about the minimal trauma and the pain in sitting position in the first 3-6 days after the mini-invasive procedure, about the hygienic requirements and gradual exercise during the first month and a half after the procedure.

Positive fact is that the suture method for buttocks lift can be repeated and in 5 difficult cases of marked heaviness, and ptosis we have planed lifting in 2 steps. A second step could be planned at least after a year. In one patient we have done a second step after 19 months and a third step after another 18 months due to patients wish for beauty. We consider this case as an open door for suture lift repetition and possibility to maintain our patients in a good form with a short post operative downtime technique.

Our patients ranged in age from 18 to 62 years.

In the same session, patients who had moderate lower trunk and lower limb cellulite were treated with additional ultrasonic liposculpture of the lower body.

RESULTS

To judge a buttocks lift is difficult: UAL does not lift - it was used in our patients to reduce buttocks heaviness and to beautify the body shape around; A table is hard to be added because each patient's body changes much and differently during the years, some gain, other loose weight, body height reduces with time; both lower extremities and both gluteal folds are not equal; Sagging starts and is different in each patient and has no universal measure – but sagging after a suture lift starts from a higher (lifted) position; Gluteal fold is not exactly raised - the buttocks soft tissue is raised 2 fingers higher from the gluteal fold as drown in Fig. (**2**) to stretch and flatten a bit the fold; The suture material has a short elasticity to reduce trauma in fixation points, it is absorbable after final fibrosis1,5 – 2 years, because foreign bodies are unnecessary; The trauma of the blunt needle is minimal, the thread is antimicrobial, antibiotic for 7 days was administered; Follow up is strictly for the first 7 days post-op in the clinic, that reduces early post-op sequels; All these reduces risks; Effect is scarless and immediate and patients judge their satisfaction. Only complain was early post-op pain. We treat the early post-op possibilities for infection with daily showers, disinfection and change of bandages in the first seven days. Late post-op complains could appear as pain in a point after inadvisable exercising that appeared in 23 patients and was treated successfully in days with rest, repeated antibiotic for minimum 5 days and non-steroid anti-inflammatory suppositories.

The cosmetic results were evaluated with preoperative and postoperative photographs.

No patient was dissatisfied with the immediate and early result. Patients considered their results good, even in 21% excellent, during the first two years (Figs. **4-9**).

407 patients were followed for more than 15 years.

After 2 years, 74 patients report loosing the effect, the rest of the patients consider that the aging process of the buttocks is delayed in comparison to other body parts, form is still better than before, and even if normal ptosis is presented the postoperative ptosis is developing from a higher tissue level.

After 10 years, 174 patients still see preserving of some change in the buttocks form and projection, and better proportions in comparison with the pre-operative status.

On the 15th year, 138 patients still maintained their total body form and good shape and 76 of them were still satisfied with the buttock form, projection, and body proportions.

RISKS AND COMPLICATIONS

All surgical procedures are associated with risks. They may be divided into undesired sequelae, which are normal and expected, and complications, which are not normal or expected. The undesired sequelae of suction lipectomy are contour irregularities, hypaesthesia, oedema, ecchymosis, and pigmentary deposits. The potential complications are blood loss, haematoma, seroma, infection, greater saphenous vein thrombosis, fat emboli, and skin slough [3, 4]. In excision procedures additional complications are spreading scars as a result of tension, and occasional delayed healing of tense wounds. Excision buttock lifts has not gained widespread acceptance because of problems such as large trauma and blood loss, prolonged post op period, early inferior scar migration, and recurrence of ptosis. The most frequent complaint is unacceptable scarring and hypaesthesia [5, 6]. Lipoinjection complications are gluteal temporal hyperaemia and erythema, corresponding to fat necrosis [7-9].

Acceptance of bodily proportions in races different from those of Caucasians has to be foreseen. Furthermore, Afro-Americans and Japanese tend to hypertrophic scarring [10].

In our Patients we have not observed neurologic problems (ischiadic pain) because we do not touch the sacrococcygeal fascia, we use the Serdev fascia for suspension. Trauma is minimal and oedema is not visible for others. Ecchymosis are rarely presented.

We have had no thread expulsion. Sometimes we repeat the buttocks suture lift for beautification or in steps if too much heaviness and flabbiness are presented.

Infection: In our method we observed one case with a painful firmness around one of the entry points and another case with a local infection in one of the wounds. The cause for the first complication was the rigid nylon suture we have used in our first patient, causing a tissue decubitus in the point of tension on the soft tissue. After this complication

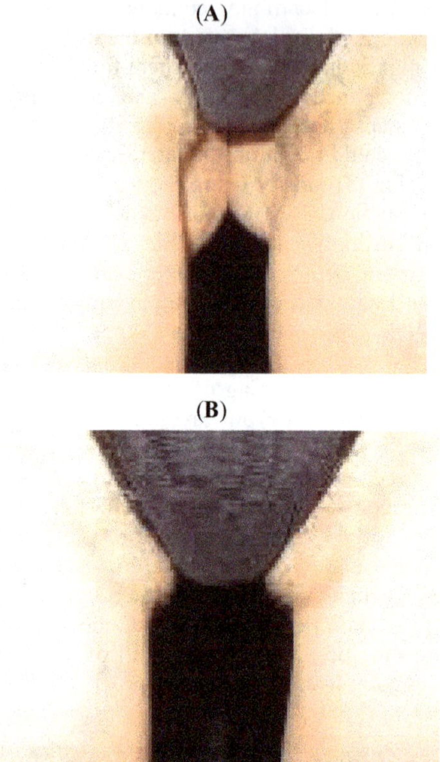

Fig. (4). **A**. Before. "Unhappy", sagging, loose buttock soft tissue, dropping between the thighs, often depresses ladies and they ask for buttock lift. **B**. After. "Happy" Buttocks after a suture lift. The idea to lift the hanging buttocks that optically elongates the legs is realized using the Serdev suture technique.

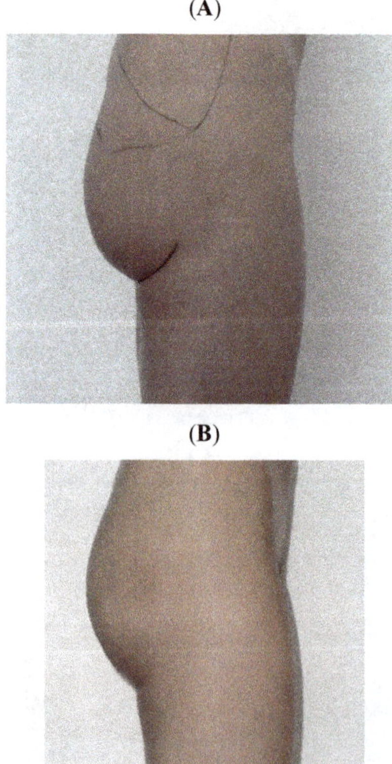

Fig. (5). Buttock lift in a young patient. **A**. Before, **B**. After. Young patients are mostly candidates for beautification and mini-invasive procedures.

occurred we changed the suture and now we use the Bulgarian antimicrobial one having a short elasticity. In the second case the Streptococcus local infection was easily treated.

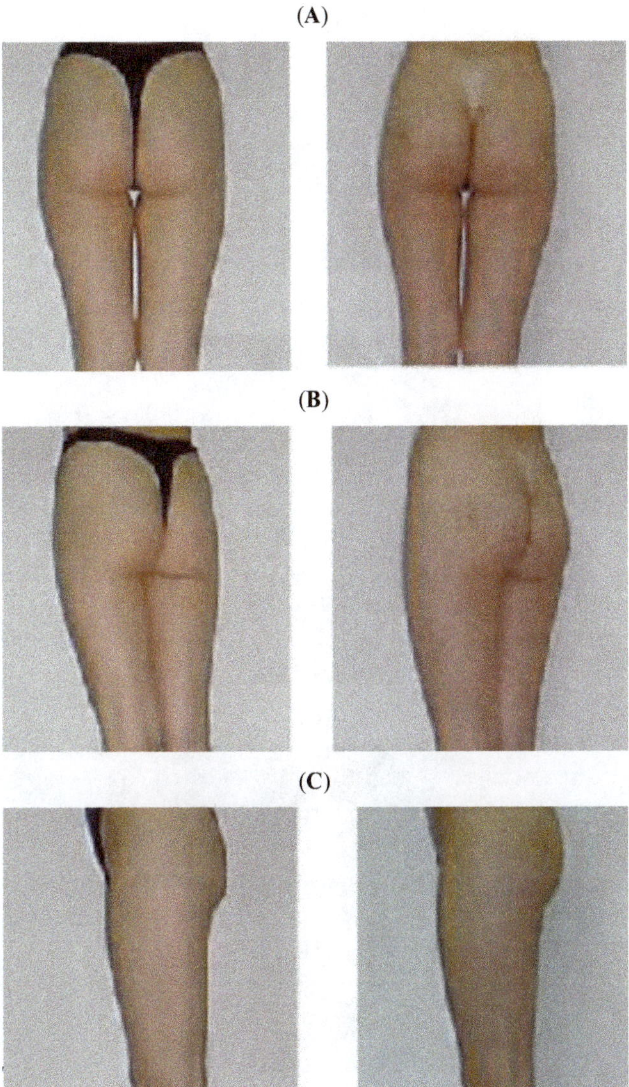

Fig. (6). Results after a buttock lift by suture only; **A**. Back view: before and after; **B**. Halfprofile: before and after; **C**. Profile view: before and after. Higher rounded buttock form is achieved. The only visible puncture scar of 1-2 mm could be visible in the lateral area of the buttock.

DISCUSSION

There is an increasing demand in modern society for surgical correction of the body contour. There are a limited number of operations specifically indicated for correction of non-aesthetic buttocks form, as a part of the totality of body appearance and proportion esthetics. The hips, thighs and the lower back frame the buttock contours. Buttock proportions are balanced by the anterior projection of the breasts. Ethnic differences in the shape and proportions of the buttocks create a variety of aesthetic variations in size and shape.

Flat and sagging buttocks without fat deposits are a common clinical condition, but there were no proven aesthetic and effective therapeutic options for buttocks lift and projection, previously to our technique.

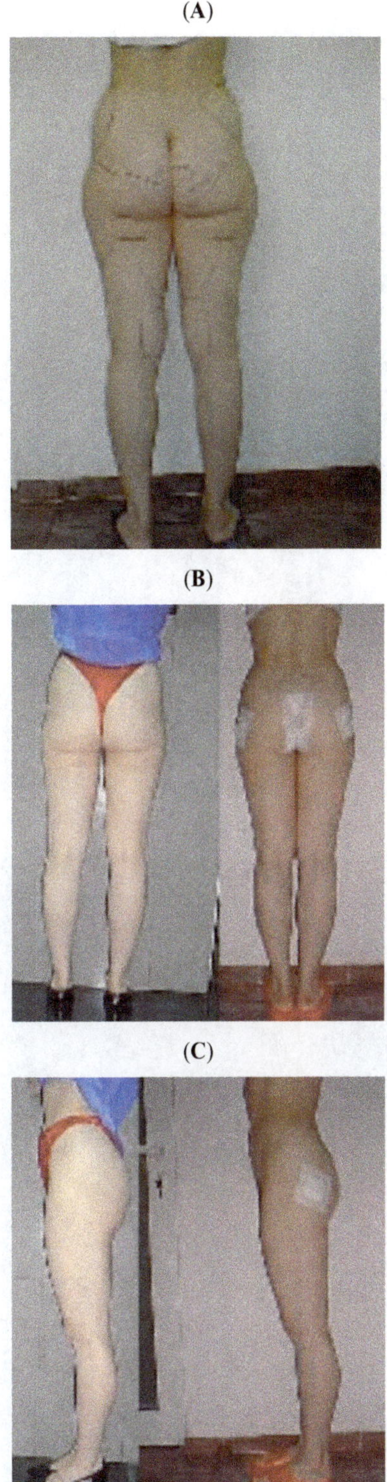

Fig. (7). A. The patient before total UAL of body and lower extremities. UAL was performed two months before the buttock lift by suture for total body and leg beautification as well as to reduce the heaviness of the hanging buttock soft tissue. Back view of the same patient before UAL of body and extremities; **B**. Buttock lift by suture: result on day one after surgery (back view): Buttocks are softly lifted, the subgluteal is raised and shortened; **C**. result on day first after surgery (profile view). "Happier" buttock form and elongation of the legs is visible. The closeness of the wounds to the anus area makes antibiotic prophylaxis and strict hygiene obligatory.

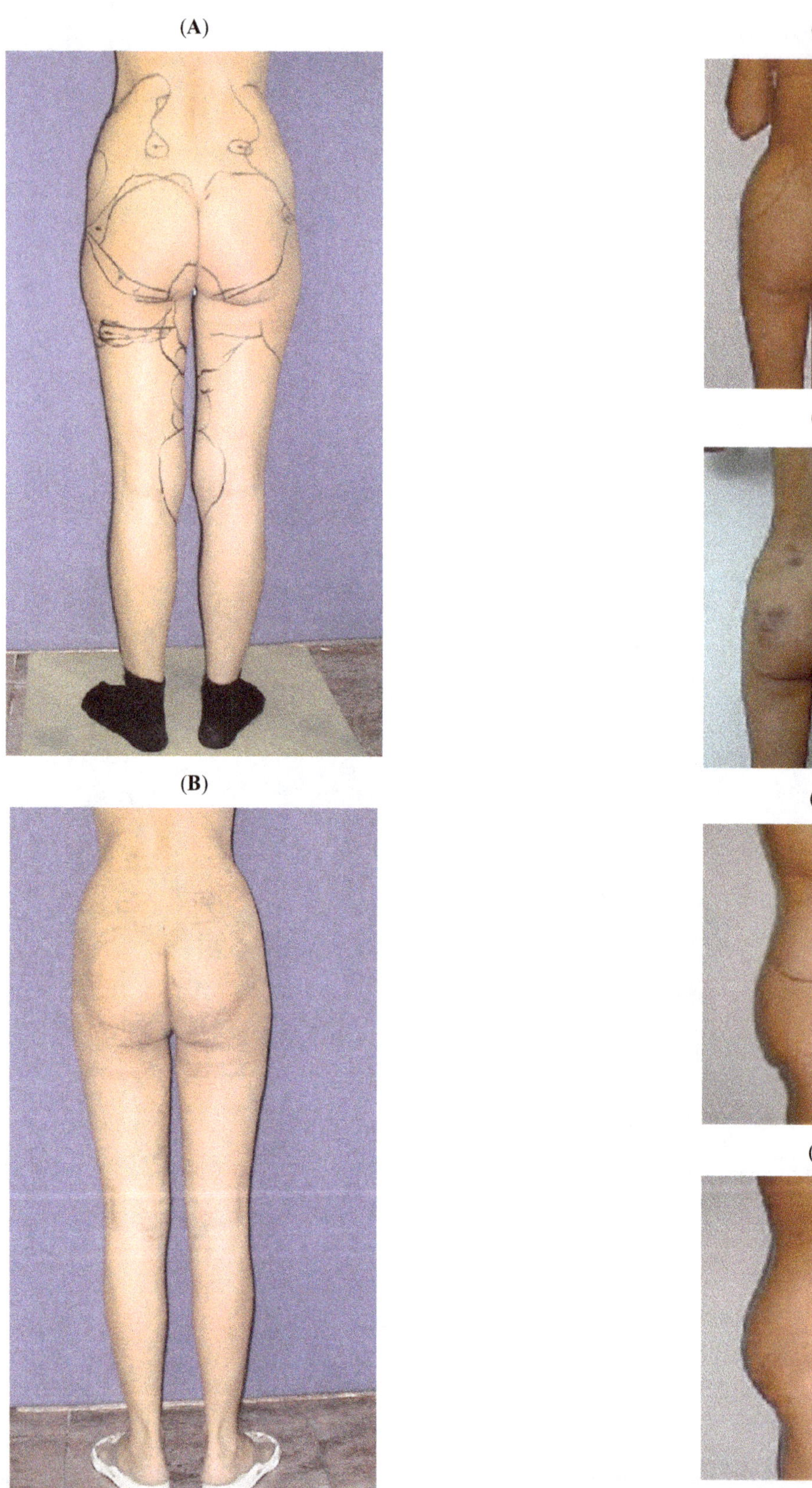

Fig. (8). **A**. Before, **B**. After a buttock lift combined with UAL lower limbs and trunk beautification. Result on day one. Drawings are still visible. Proportions are changed due to higher position of the buttocks. "Knee lifting" by UAL - creation of straight and elongated legs is one of the specialties of the author. Buttocks are lifted, infragluteal fold is lifted by 4-5 cm visibly elongating the lower limbs.

Fig. (9). **A**, **C**. A patient that was treated previously by excision lipoplasty of the inner, lateral thigh and buttocks (visible scars, irregularities and deformities). **B**, **D**. Result one day after buttock lift by suture and additional simultaneous UAL of flanks and abdomen. The buttocks are visibly lifted and a better-rounded form obtained. The use of UAL assured a body form beautification and at the same time a correction of irregularities and deformities.

Subcision is a surgical technique that is used in treating advanced degree cellulite [11]. To treat excesses of fat and skin tissue in that area, liposuction [12-14] and/or dermolipectomy [15, 16] are mostly used. Liposuction is performed through small skin incisions, which results in minimal scar formation and is associated with minimal complication rates. The indication for liposuction is restricted to the conditions in which the overlying skin is capable of retracting and adapting itself to the new contour. Otherwise, if excess skin is the cause of the deformity, a dermolipectomy is mostly performed. In these cases, the incisions have to be chosen in a way that the resulting scar may be hidden as well as possible.

Liposuction of the buttock area is less mentioned in the literature and for some authors it is a forbidden zone [17]. Two additional approaches in suction lipectomy of the buttock region are described: liposuction of the "banana" and liposuction of the "sensuous triangle" [13]. The banana is the highest part of the posterior thigh just below the buttock crease. It appears only in certain individuals and appears as a bulge. Controlled scar retraction of the thin cutaneous adipose flap allows for good results even in flaccid and aged skin due to some authors [14, 18]. A common complication of liposuction of this area is ptosis of the buttock crease The sensuous triangle is at the junction of the lateral buttock, lateral thigh, and posterior thigh. The use of ultrasound to improve the liposuction possibilities in body contouring [19, 20].

To improve buttock roundness and projection, fat transplantation and different implants, including mammary ones, were introduced [3,21,22]. An augmentation to sagging or hypertrophic buttocks similar to that of the breasts can be done [23].

Free fat graft has been used with success in cosmetic surgery to avoid the most common complications of doing a buttock augmentation with silicone prostheses and to find a better surgical procedure that is simpler, complementary with liposuction, and better able to deal with subtle body irregularities. In trying to achieve symmetry and better contour of the back torso and middle third of the body, the combination of liposuction and lipoinjection is rapidly becoming the procedure of choice for most of authors. Fat grafting is done in multiple tunnels in a deep plane [24], results are considered uniformly satisfactory. Liposuction is done with a tumescent technique in the lumbosacral, trochanteric, and subgluteal region to improve gluteal shape using additional lipofilling. Contour defects treated with autologus intramuscular fat graft injections need overcorrection by approximately 50 percent more volume. It is not an easy goal because of the high reabsortion of fatty tissue [25]. Delicate tissue handling and small total amount of fat transplanted by careful distribution in the recipient tissues are probably the factors responsible for longer lasting improvement in these patients [26]. Complications are minimal with enhanced satisfaction of both patients and surgeons.

In obese patients the functional benefits of a combination excision-suction lipectomy outweigh the disadvantages of the scarring [27]. If there is considerable excess of skin and tissue, excision procedures are performed to remove excess tissue by surgical resection *via* appropriately large incisions. Resulting scars from excision surgery are always visible (Fig. **9C**, **D**). Lipectomy with suction of the lower extremities has been of greater interest in recent years. Due to some authors the number of patients seeking dermolipectomy of the trunk and thighs is increasing. The so-called "lower body lift" combines the transverse flank/thigh/buttock lift and the fascial anchoring medial thigh lift in one operation [29]. Secondary high-buttock corrections pose difficult problems because of the poor vascularization of certain areas, the limited mobilization of the soft tissue, and the tendency toward poor scar formation. These factors limit the surgical techniques available. The tendency for the deformity to recur may necessitate several corrective procedures [4]. The deep planed torso-abdominoplasty is beneficial for treating gestation sequelae of the torso-abdominal wall, ptosis of the abdomen, vertical and horizontal enlargements of the musculoaponeurotic system, lipodystrophy, stretch marks, rhytidosis of the inguinal region, and ptosis of the external quadrant of the gluteus and the external trochanter area in one surgical procedure [30]. It creates pexy of the external quadrant of the gluteus region. Muscle strength is the limiting factor in repetitive squat lifting. Fatigue may be one of the determinants for changes in kinematics and choice of technique in lifting tasks. Lower body lift with superficial fascial system suspension is introduced to treat laxity of the entire lower trunk and thigh regions in one stage in selected patients This procedure needs 3 weeks off work and is expected to result in a tightening of the flank, buttocks, and total thighs. Minor complications are significantly higher than with the component procedures alone and occur in nearly 50 percent of patients [29]. Another surgical procedure, a circumferential torso excision was designed and utilized for minimal number of patients. This technique dramatically reduces the lateral flank and posterior tissue rolls to improve the operative results. Contour improvement of the buttocks and lateral thighs is produced as well [31]. A buried dermal-fat flap technique is particularly applicable to patients with asymmetry of the buttocks and thighs as well as those with ptosis of the buttocks. An advantage is that it creates a new gluteal fold at a predetermined higher level [16]. Belt lipectomy includes the traditional abdominoplasty or panniculectomy with excision extended laterally around the entire trunk. This technique yields a lateral thigh and buttock lift, and when combined with liposuction is used to improve contour of the thighs [32].

Correction of sequelae of primary hip-buttock-thigh plasty has become a common challenge in aesthetic plastic surgery. Due to some authors, suggested techniques for dealing with this problem include denuding the skin at the depressed area, pulling flaps upward and outward, using dermal buried flaps, and utilizing liposuction. Liposuction can be used successfully in combination with classic hip-buttock-thigh plasty to enhance the aesthetic result as well as to facilitate the surgical technique [28].

Excision body lifts are surgical procedures that are infrequently performed because the length of operating time increases the risk to the patient as well as the likelihood of surgeon fatigue. The other drawback of body lifts is the long incision line. However, these incisions are well accepted if they are well placed and if the results of body change are significant. Meticulous haemostasis, limited undermining, and the closure of dead space are factors that produce a more reliable procedure, both in terms of postoperative problems and the final results [33]. The transgluteal approach could be responsible, according to some authors for bad clinical results, due to injury of the nervus gluteus superius. Many anatomical variations are found concerning the point of the nerve's division into 2 branches, nearer or farther from the foramen ischiadicum [34].

CONCLUSION

Redundant tissue in sagging buttocks can be corrected by excision lifts. However, these are seldom used procedures because of postoperative problems such as unaccepted inferiorly displaced and wide scars, and early recurrence of ptosis, large trauma and blood loss, prolonged post op period.

In order to limit these complications in flat and sagging buttocks without remarkable fat deposits, we developed a surgical technique using a circumferential suture of the buttock's soft tissue. The fascial suspension gives strong vertical support with minimal tension on the skin, and reduces the complications traditionally associated with such procedures. The results of our operations are aesthetically compatible with and even much better than non-scarring techniques such as UAL and liposuction solely in young patient having strong and elastic skin and tissue, described in our presentations as well [19, 35]. Liposuction alone can not lift. The author's operation offers fewer complications than any other described.

In patients, whose problem was excessive fat in conjunction with skin flabbiness, UAL of the buttocks and surrounding tissues for beautification body contouring, combined with the buttock lift suture method, completed the main goals of the procedure.

Buttocks lift is an efficient and safe procedure to correct or enhance buttock contour. It has virtually eliminated blood transfusions and the major complications of dermolipectomies and liposuction under general anaesthesia.

The author's surgical procedure using a suture is simple, atraumatic and low in cost, with minimal morbidity and very good results. It is important to note that a good result does not depend on great surgery but rather on more simple, acceptable procedures for patients, resulting in harmonious structuring and positioning of the form, lifting of the lower portion of the buttocks, augmentation in the upper gluteus and better projection.

Complications are very few, and patient satisfaction is high.

CONFLICT OF INTEREST

The author confirms that this article content has no conflicts of interest.

ACKNOWLEDGEMENT

Declared none.

REFFERENCES

[1] Serdev NP. Suture suspensions for lifting or volume augmentation in face and body. 2nd Annual Meeting of the National Bulgarian Society for Aesthetic Surgery and Aesthetic Medicine; 1994 March 18th, Sofia, 1994; pp. 11-8.

[2] Serdev NP. Year 1994, Suture suspension for lifting or volume augmentation in face and body (English version). Int J Cosmet Surg 2001; 1(1): 2561-8.

[3] Cardenas-Camarena L, Lacouture AM, Tobar-Losada A. Combined gluteoplasty: liposuction and lipoinjection. Plast Reconstr Surg 1999; 104 (5): 1524-31.

[4] Regnault P, Daniel R. Secondary thigh-buttock deformities after classical techniques. Prevention and treatment. Clin Plast Surg 1984; 11(3): 505-16.

[5] Karnes J, Salisbury M, Schaeferle M, Beckham P, Ersek RA. Hip lift. Aesthetic Plast Surg 2002; 26(2): 126-9.

[6] Hagen K, Sorhagen O, Harms-Ringdahl K., Influence of weight and frequency on thigh and lower-trunk motion during repetitive lifting employing stoop and squat techniques. Clin Biomech (Bristol, Avon) 1995; 10(3): 122-7.

[7] Niechajev I, Sevcuk O. Long-term results of fat transplantation: clinical and histologic studies. Plast Reconstr Surg 1994; 94(3): 496-506.

[8] Guerrerosantos J. Autologous fat grafting for body contouring. Clin Plast Surg 1996; 23(4): 619-31.

[9] Peren PA, Gomez JB, Guerrerosantos J, Salazar CA. Gluteus augmentation with fat grafting. Aesthetic Plast Surg 2000; 24(6): 412-7.

[10] Ichida M, Kamiishi H, Shioya N. Aesthetic surgery of the trunk and extremities in the Japanese. Ann Plast Surg 1980 Jul; 5(1): 31-9.

[11] Hexsel DM, Mazzuco R., Subcision: a treatment for cellulite. Int J Dermatol 2000; 39(7): 539-44.

[12] Gargan TJ, Courtiss EH. The risks of suction lipectomy. Their prevention and treatment. Clin Plast Surg 1984; 11(3): 457-63.

[13] Schlesinger SL. Two arcane areas in liposuction: the banana and the sensuous triangle. Aesthetic Plast Surg 1991; 15(2): 175-80.

[14] Gasparotti M. Superficial liposuction: a new application of the technique for aged and flaccid skin. Aesthetic Plast Surg 1992; 16(2): 141-53.

[15] Pitanguy I. Surgical reduction of the abdomen, thigh, and buttocks. Surg Clin North Am 1971; 51(2): 479-89.

[16] Delerm A, Cirotteau Y. Cruro-femoro-gluteal or circumgluteal plasty. Ann Chir Plast 1973; 18(1): 31-6.

[17] Shaer WD. Gluteal and thigh reduction: reclassification, critical review, and improved technique for primary correction. Aesthetic Plast Surg 1984; 8(3): 165-72.

[18] Gasperoni C, Salgarello M. MALL liposuction: the natural evolution of subdermal superficial liposuction. Aesthetic Plast Surg 1994; 18(3): 253-7.

[19] Serdev NP. Buttock lift. Two own methods. 3rd International Congress of the South-American Academy of Cosmetic Surgery, Buenos Aires, Argentina, 2001; pp. 37-8.

[20] Serdev NP. Buttocks lift by ultrasonic assisted liposuction - My technique. Int J Aesthet Cosmet Beauty Surg 1991; 1(3): 130-54.

[21] Chajchir A. Fat injection: long-term follow-Up. Aesthetic Plast Surg 1996; 20(4): 291-6.

[22] Lack EB. Contouring the female buttocks. Liposculpting the buttocks. Dermatol Clin 1999; 17(4): 815-22.

[23] Lewis JR Jr. Body contouring. South Med J 1980; 73(8): 1006-11.

[24] Pereira LH, Radwanski HN. Fat grafting of the buttocks and lower limbs. Aesthetic Plast Surg 1996; 20(5): 409-16.

[25] Hanke CW, Bullock S, Bernstein G., Current status of tumescent liposuction in the United States. National survey results. Dermatol Surg 1996; 22(7): 595-8.

[26] de Pedroza LV. Fat transplantation to the buttocks and legs for aesthetic enhancement or correction of deformities: long-term results of large volumes of fat transplant. Dermatol Surg 2000; 26(12): 1145-9.

[27] Teimourian B, Adham MN. Anterior periosteal dermal suspension with suction curettage for lateral thigh lipectomy. Aesthetic Plast Surg 1982; 6(4): 207-9.

[28] (a) Guerrerosantos J. Secondary hip-buttock-thigh plasty. Clin Plast Surg 1984; 11(3): 491-503. (b) Lewis JR Jr. Body contouring. South Med J 1980; 73(8): 1006-11.

[29] Lockwood T. Lower body lift with superficial fascial system suspension. Plast Reconstr Surg 1993; 92(6): 1112-22.

[30] Gonzalez M, Guerrerosantos J. Deep planed torso-abdominoplasty combined with buttocks pexy. Aesthetic Plast Surg 1997; 21(4): 245-53.

[31] Carwell GR, Horton CE Sr. Circumferential torsoplasty. Ann Plast Surg 1997; 38(3): 213-6.

[32] Heddens CJ. Belt lipectomy: procedure and outcomes. Plast Surg Nurs 2001; 21(4): 185-9, 199.

[33] Pascal JF, Le Louarn C. Remodeling bodylift with high lateral tension. Aesthetic Plast Surg 2002; 26(3): 223-30.

[34] Lavigne P, Loriot de Rouvray TH. The superior gluteal nerve. Anatomical study of its extrapelvic portion and surgical resolution by trans-gluteal approach Rev Chir Orthop Reparatrice Appar Mot 1994; 80(3): 188-95.

[35] Lawrence N, Coleman WP 3rd. The biologic basis of ultrasonic liposuction. Dermatol Surg 1997; 23(12): 1197-200.

Quality and Efficacy of *Tribulus terrestris* as an Ingredient for Dermatological Formulations

Gian-Pietro Di Sansebastiano[*,1], Maria De Benedictis[1,#], Davide Carati[2], Dario Lofrumento[1], Miriana Durante[3], Anna Montefusco[1], Vincenzo Zuccarello[1], Giuseppe Dalessandro[1] and Gabriella Piro[1]

[1]*University of Salento, DiSTeBA, Campus Ecotekne, 73100 Lecce (LE), Italy*

[2]*EKUBERG Pharma s.r.l, Via Pozzelle n.36 73025 Martano (LE), Italy*

[3]*CNR, Istituto di Scienze delle Produzioni Alimentari (ISPA), Campus Ecotekne, 73100 Lecce (LE), Italy*

Abstract: *Tribulus terrestris* L. (Zygophyllaceae) is an annual plant commonly known as Puncture vine. It is dramatically gaining interest as a rich source of saponins. *T. terrestris* is a promising ingredient for many industries and recent patents on dermatological applications support the use of this plant for cosmetics and hygiene. Nonetheless problems arise in the selection of the material to be used. The extracts of different origins may differ substantially. Natural speciation processes normally influence 'variations' in wild-crafted medicinal plants. The genus *Tribulus* is emblematic. Taxonomic status of *T. terrestris* is complicated by the wide geographical distribution leading to high levels of genetic polymorphism. Being aware of such variability we selected 3 commercial *Tribulus* extracts and compared their biological effect on *Candida albicans* with the effect produced by an extract from local plants (South of Apulia, Italy). One of the commercial extracts with the best anti-*candida* performance was used to substitute triclosan in a detergent formulation and it proved to improve the product performance in the control of potentially pathogenic skin flora such as *C. albicans*.

Keywords: Anti-Candida effect, *Candida albicans*, intimate hygiene, skin flora, *Tribulus terrestris*.

INTRODUCTION

Tribulus terrestris L. (Zygophyllaceae) is an annual plant commonly known as Puncture vine [1, 2]. For centuries it has been used in the traditional medicines of China, India and several other regions. In the mid-1990s, the use of this plant became known in North America and Western Europe after Eastern European Olympic athletes said that taking *Tribulus* helped them in their performance [3].

It is gaining global interest as proven by the logarithmic growth in number of scientific publications observed from the 90s (5 publications per year) to the recent years (50 publications and over 400 citations in 2011; "Web of Science" Citation Report using Topic="*Tribulus terrestris*").

Extracts from the full plants or fruits are now used for a large number of applications ranging from skin care to human hormones regulation [4-6], as anti-bacterial [7], anti-inflammation [8], anti-virus and immuno-stimulant too. Biological activity (biocide and antioxidant) is clear in several studies but clinical, histological [9, 10] and cellular studies [11] are rare.

The reason for such a lack of information is probably due to the composition of the "extract". It is a "phytocomplex" rich in different compounds [12, 13], none of which can be found entirely responsible for the biological effect investigated.

The known active compounds in *Tribulus* are called steroidal saponins, primarily present in the leaf and fruit. The Bulgarian "Tribestan", from SOPHARMA, was the first standardized preparation [1] that has been initially described in Bulgarian patent applications [14, 15] and German articles [16]. More products were developed lately as preparations or food supplements. For examples we can list LIBILOV from USA, TRIBOSTIM TM and TRIBOVIT TM from Bulgaria, TRIBULUS-ZMB from Italy. All of them target impotence and libido disorders, in men and women. The product UNEX is proposed as diuretic [17].

Recent investigations focusing on the Bulgarian commercial products have indicated protodioscin and prototribestin as main components in the Bulgarian plant extracts [1], but the presence of many other components may be determined [18]. The extracts are rich of cinammic acid amides, lignanamides (tribulusamides A and B), alkaloids, flavonoids like rutin, quercetin and kaempferol, as well as steroidal saponins in many different forms: prototribestin, dioscin, protodioscin [19, 20] furostanol [21], spirostanol, sitosterol glucoside [22], terrestrosins A-E, desgalactotigonin, gitonin, tigogenin, gitogenin, beta-Sitosterol, spirosta-3,5-diene, stigmasterol, hecogenin, neohecogenin, ruscogenin [5, 23, 24] tribulosaponin B, metilprotodiostsin, terres-

*Address correspondence to this author at the University of Salento, DiSTeBA, campus Ecotekne, 73100 Lecce (LE), Italy;
E-mail: gp.disansebastiano@unisalento.it

#Present Address: Dipartimento di Bioscienze, Università degli Studi di Parma, Parco Area delle Scienze, 11/A, 43124 Parma, Italy

trozin H, prototribestin, gracillin [25]. Content, especially in terms of detectable saponins, varies with growth conditions and ecotype [20, 26-28] in addition to extraction methods. Since it has such a rich composition, it is not surprising that such diversified biological effects were observed for this plant extract.

Saponins are a diverse group of compounds widely distributed in the plant kingdom, which are characterized by their structure containing a triterpene or steroid aglycone and one or more sugar chains. Consumer demand for natural products coupled with their physicochemical (surfactant) properties and mounting evidence on their biological activity have led to the emergence of saponins as commercially significant compounds with expanding applications in food, cosmetics, and pharmaceutical sectors.

As a rich source of saponins, *T. terrestris* is a promising ingredient for many industries [29] but the research and development (R&D) activity willing to include this natural product in topic formulations for hygiene or cosmetic uses needs to be very carefully performed with the background knowledge.

Patent literature provides some examples on the different aspects of the preparation and characterization of *T. terrestris* extracts for topic uses. *T. terrestris* extracts comprising spirosteroid saponin have been characterized for the preparation of antifungal compositions and 17 distinct spironosaponins have been identified and associated by means of a common general chemical formula [30, 31]. Detailed methods for preparing cream using *T. terrestris* extracts with anti-bacterial, anti-inflammatory, anti-viral activities, and other activities for topical use on skin and mucosal tissues have been described [32, 33]. It has also been suggested to combine *T. terrestris* extracts with metals for preparing anti-viral pharmaceutical compositions [34, 35]. Several examples of plant extracts combinations including *T. terrestris* extracts are found in Asian patent literature. Some of such patent documents specifically refer to the usage involving topical administration such as pruritus and skin disorders [36], increasing the skin permeability and stimulating the generation of melanophore [37], improving skin tenderness or other cosmetic applications [38, 39].

In this work, we analyzed the application of *T. terrestris* extract to commercial uses through the analysis of three commercial extracts from different sources, all available on the Italian market, and compared their biological effect as biocide. Saponins measurement is difficult and reliable methods, mostly HPLC separation, should be referred to known standard molecules. Unfortunately the commercially available extracts have more approximate quantification standards (as the gravimetric method). For this reason we produced an extract from plants grown in Italy, in the area known as Salento, and used it as a reference. We tested the efficacy of the extract as ingredient in the formulation of a detergent for intimate hygiene to potentiate anti-*candida* effects. The selected extract appears as a very good ingredient but the need of accurate quality standards defined case by case, seems to be necessary to select the material on the market.

MATERIALS AND METHODS

Preparation of *Tribulus* extracts

T. terrestris L. full plants including roots and fruits, were harvested in Italy, in different sites of Salento peninsula, South of Apulia, in July 2010. Plant material was carefully identified by Prof. Zuccarello and Dr Di Sansebastiano with the support of Dr Accogli, Botanists and plant biologists at the Department of Biological and Environmental Sciences and Technologies (DiSTeBA) at University of Salento.

Fruits were separated from plants, washed, frozen in liquid nitrogen and lyophilized in a Christ Alpha 2-4 LSC freeze-dryer (Martin Christ Gefriertrocknungsanlagen GmbH, Osterode am Harz, Germany) for 24 h. The lyophilized material was ground to 500 μm in a laboratory mill (Retsch GmbH, Haan, Germany) to obtain a homogeneous powder. Saponins and other soluble molecules were initially extracted from this dry powder with a 70% ethanol solution for 24 hours. The solvent proportion was 200 ml each 120 gr of fruit powder to assure fluidity of the mixture during stirring extraction at 25°C. The resulting ethanol extract was cleared by centrifugation and filtered. Saponins were precipitated adding 2 volumes of cold acetone and centrifuging at 20000g for 30 min. The pellet, corresponding to about 2% of the starting material, was air dried for 30 min was resuspended in 70% ethanol at the concentration of 2 gr/ml. Three commercial extracts with a 40% declared content of saponins were also resuspended in 70% ethanol at the concentration of 2 gr/ml and compared with fruit extract extract.

HPLC Analysis

The analysis was carried out to compare chemical profile of the different extracts of *T. terrestris* using reverse phase HPLC with UV detector. The mobile phase that consisted of phosphoric acid buffer with pH-3 (A) and acetonitrile (B) was used for gradient elution. The flow rate was adjusted to 1.0 ml/min. The detection wavelength was at 203 nm. All separations were performed at ambient temperature. The plant material, (0,5g) was extracted two times with 5 ml of 50% aqueous acetonitrile by sonication for 15 min. The samples were centrifuged at 4900 rpm for 10 min. The supernatant was lyophilized for 15 min. The extract was dissolved in 50% aqueous acetonitrile [20]. Prior injection, all samples were filtered through a 0.45μm membrane. Each sample solution was injected in duplicate with injection volume of 20μl.

Antifungal Evaluation

Candida albicans strain MUCL 29800T [40]. The yeast was grown to exponential phase at 37°C for 18 h on a shaker in YPD liquid medium (1% yeast extract, 2% peptone, 2% glucose) or on a solid medium prepared by adding 4% agar. Extracts inhibitory activity was tested against the microorganism using a broth micro dilution method in 96 multiwell plates, in triplicate, as reported by Koneman [41] and recommended by the National Committee for Clinical Laboratory Standard [42]. Optical density measurements at 600nm were made in a TECAN Infinite.

Trolox Equivalent Antioxidant Capacity (TEAC) Assay

The antioxidant activity was measured using the ABTS discoloration method [43]. Samples B and E (Hydrophilic antioxidants) were centrifuged at 10,000 g for 7 min and the different supernatants were recovered and used for antioxidant activity measurements. The antioxidant activities were measured at 734 nm in a Cecil BioQuest CE 2501 spectrophotometer. The calibration curve was constructed, using freshly prepared Trolox solution for HAA determination. Values were obtained from three replicates as Trolox equivalent mg.

Toxicity

Human epithelial cells from A-253 line (ATCC, American Type Culture Collection Manassas, VA, USA) were maintained in a humidified atmosphere containing 5% CO_2 at 37 °C. Titration tests were carried out in 96 well plates: briefly, cells were exposed for 24 h to different concentrations of the extracts. Cell viability was assessed by neutral red test: cells were incubated for 2 h with complete medium with 0,05 mg/ml neutral red; this stain is actively accumulated in lysosomes of healthy cells. Following the incubation, cells were lysed with a ethanol/acetic acid solution and neutral red accumulation were measured by absorbance at 540 nm with a microplate reader. The cell vitality of cells incubated with the different products was expressed as percentage versus untreated cells (which absorbance values were considered as 100 % vitality).

A-253 cells retain the morphologic features typical of *epithelial cells.* Being derived from the submandibular region, they may well represent the most delicate mucosa epidermis.

Washing Simulation

Candida albicans cells in exponential growth phase. The yeast was grown to exponential phase at 37°C for 15 h on a shaker in YPD liquid medium. Aliquots of 1 ml of liquid culture were pelleted by rapid centrifugation (13000 rpm in a bench minifuge) in separated test tubes and resuspended in various detergent dilutions kindly provided by Ekuberg Pharma. After 5 minutes cells were pelleted by rapid centrifugation, resuspended in 200 microliter YPD and plated on solid YPD Petri dishes. After over-night culture the number of colonies was counted.

RESULTS

Extract Quality and Efficacy

Four *T. terrestris* extracts were used. Three commercial dried extracts with a 40% declared content in saponins were purchased from different Italian distributors. The plant origin was not always declared (Table **1**). We refer to these plant extracts as A, B and C. The fourth extract was obtained following a water/Ethanol extraction combined with a precipitation step in acetone. We refer to this as extract E. Biocide effect of extracts was tested on *Candida albicans* strain MUCL 29800T [40] liquid culture.

Commercial extracts declared Maltodextrin as excipient and colloidal anhydrous silica as auxiliary substance. All commercial extracts had an important insoluble residue; if added to *C. albicans* culture all induced an increase in fungus growth rate (not shown). Microscopy observation showed the presence of intact starch granules in commercial powder A. To eliminate the insoluble residue and make the extracts comparable, all of them were resuspended in a 70% ethanol solution (2g/mL) and filtered through a 0.2 micron filter.

HPLC analysis of the extracts revealed remarkable differences. The extract E shared with product C the highest similarity with only 58% of common peaks (Fig. **1**). The other extracts shared with E and among each other less than 40% of common peaks (not shown).

Solutions containing extracts A, B, C, E were diluted in YPD liquid culture medium where *Candida* was grown for 18 hours. OD absorbance at 600nm was simultaneously read in a multiwell plate for all samples and 3 to 5 independent experiments were performed.

Results shown in Fig. (**2**) give evidence that the minimal inhibitory concentration (MIC) has to be determined case by case, depending on the source of extract. The self-produced standard preparation, extract E, had a biological action stronger than that of 2 out of the 3 commercial sources but 1 of the commercial products, extract B, probably better titrated for the specific saponins responsible for its properties, had a very high activity. The extract B was then selected for further use.

Extract Antioxidant Activity and Toxicity

The selected extract B was analyzed to verify antioxidant activity and toxicity. Cytotoxicity and eventually chemo preventive role of saponins were discussed in a number of reviews and they depend on the specific molecular pattern [44]. In consideration of the high variability in the phytocomplex, assay case by case is necessary.

The antioxidant activity was measured using the ABTS discoloration method with the determination of trolox equivalent (TEAC). At the concentration of 1 mg/ml B produced the antioxidant activity of 1545.7 trolox equivalent

Table 1. General Information About the Products Used

	Extract			
	A	B	C	E
Saponin content	40%	40%	40%	n.d.
Excipients	maltodextrin	maltodextrin	maltodextrin	none
Auxiliary substance	colloidal anhydrous silica	maltodextrin	colloidal anhydrous silica	none
Plant organ	n.d.	fruit	fruit	fruit
Plant origin	n.d.	India	India	Italy (Salento)

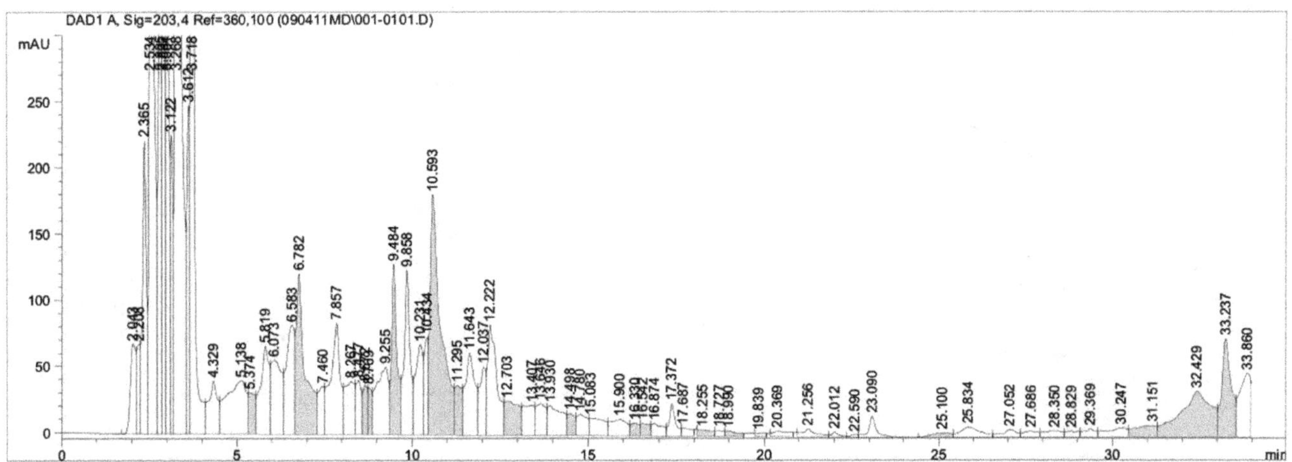

Fig. (1). HPLC-DAD chromatogram of the *T. terrestris* fruit extract E. Peaks representative were identified by their retention times. In grey the peaks shared chromatogram of commercial extract C.

(386.4 mg/ml Trolox), E produced the activity of 683.7 Trolox equivalent (170.9 mg/ml Trolox). A *Thymus vulgaris* extract treated in a similar way in terms of dry weight was used to evidence that *Tribulus* antioxidant activity was particularly high. In fact the same amount of dry extract from *Thymus* generated only a 29.1 Trolox equivalent activity (7.3 mg/ml).

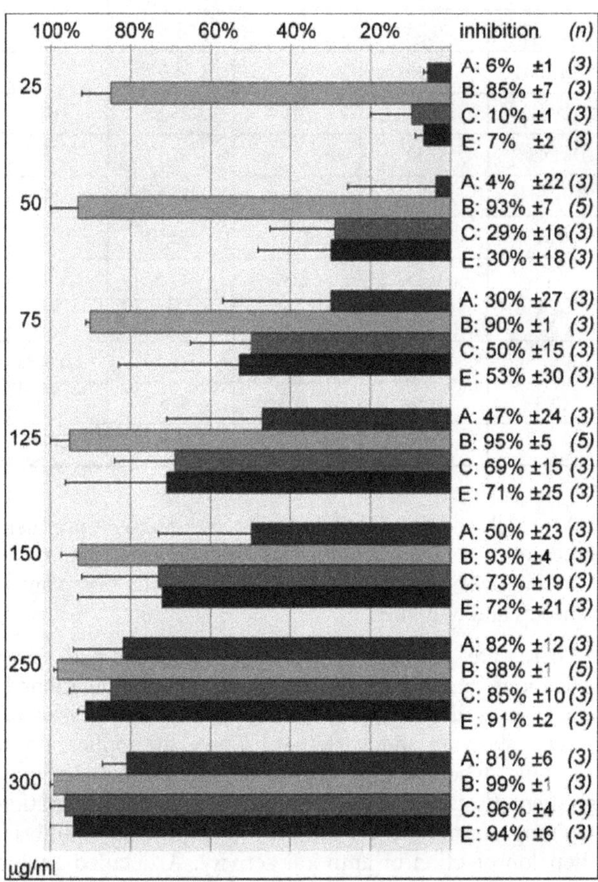

Fig. (2). Percentage of inhibition of *Tribulus* product dilutions on Candida growth. Error bars indicate SD. *(n)* indicates the number of experimental repeats.

Extract B cytotoxicity was measured using Neutral Red viability test on fibroblast cultures and compared with extract E and a raw fruit aqueous-extract (raw-E) was used as control (Fig. **3**). Extract B exerted high cytotoxic effect at 150-75 µg/ml, a 90% viability reduction resulted with respect to controls. At lower concentrations the toxicity significantly reduced, in fact at 25-10 µg/ml cells showed viability comparable with control. A similar trend was observed with product E, although it resulted in being toxic at lower concentrations. Extract E resulted to be much less toxic, in fact cell viability was comparable to control one already at 100 µg/ml. The raw aqueous-extract from fruit was obtained by extraction with a 70% ethanol solution and exhibited high toxicity, evidently for the action of other compounds additional to saponins.

Efficacy of *T. terrestris* Commercial Extract as a Control Agent

Commercial extract B (declared 40% saponins) was used in the formulation of a new product here designated as "DMX" at the final concentration of 0.1% w/v [45, 46] (DMX).DMX was compared with the same formulation without *Tribulus* extract (DMXnoT) and with one detergent already commercialized with 0.1% Triclosan instead of *Tribulus* extract (DMXtcs). In order to have an idea of general efficacy of similar products available on the market, three more detergents intimate feminine hygiene were selected from the same shelf in a shop and designated as C01, C02 and C03. Recovery of *Candida* cells after washing was evaluated as colonies growth on petri dish containing YPD medium (Fig. **4**). Data are reported in Table **2**. DMX showed a better performance (-87% of colonies growth) than DMXnoT (-65%). *Tribulus* appeared to be more effective than Triclosan in DMXtcs. Among competitors only C03 had better performances; C02, did not appear to affect fungi vitality. Such variability reminded the high variability in biological effects of extracts despite the generic quantification of ingredients.

DISCUSSION

Quality and efficacy of herbal medicines are directly linked to the quality of the medicinal herb raw materials. Three critical steps at the very beginning of the manufacturing process are: 1) cultivation/collection of authentic whole plants or plant parts, 2) sorting, drying and

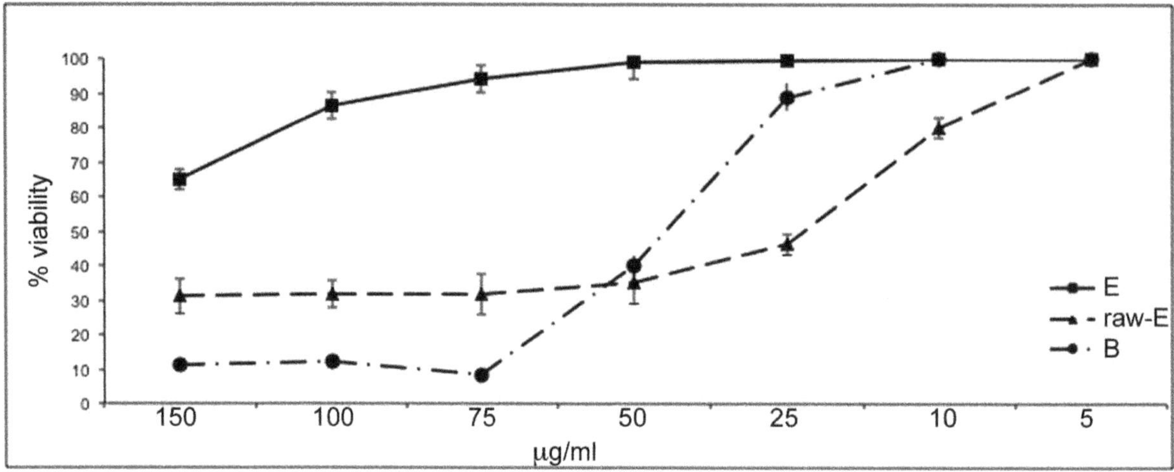

Fig. (3). Cytotoxic effect measured through cell viability exposed to different concentrations of 3 different extracts. Average data derived from 3 experimental repeats.

powdering of the herbal material, and, 3) non-targeted or targeted, solvent(s) based extractions of the herbal materials to enrich or to include 'active' or 'marker' compounds [47]. Any compromise in quality in each of these steps will permeate the sequential links in the manufacturing process.

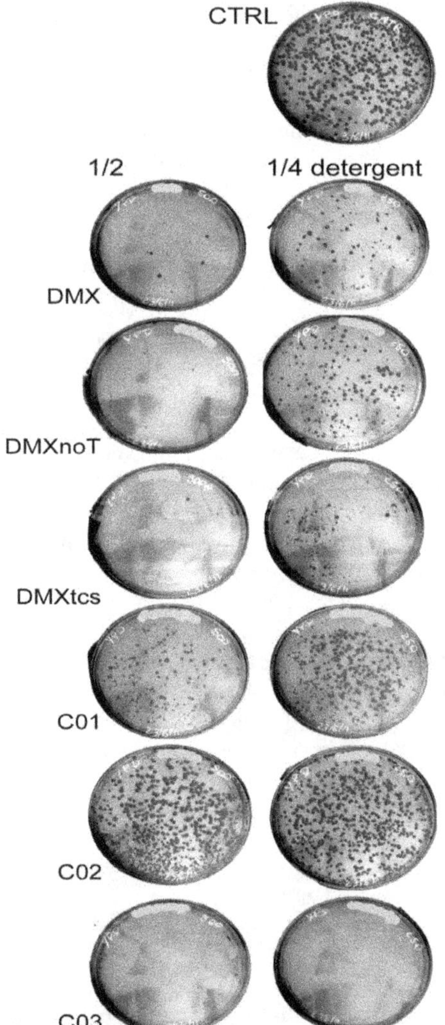

Fig. (4). Images of Candida's colonies grown on YPD medium after washing.

Table 2. Number of Colonies Grown from Candida's Cultures After Washing

Product	Dilution	Average	SD	Inhibition
CTRL	-	**576**	83,1	
DMX	0,50	**20**	3,6	
	0,25	**77**	3,6	-87%
DMXnoT	0,50	**22**	4,0	
	0,25	**201**	53,1	-65%
DMXtcs	0,50	**3**	0,6	
	0,25	**125**	71,1	-78%
C01	0,50	**236**	75,0	
	0,25	**428**	17,2	-26%
C02	0,50	**652**	113,3	
	0,25	**639**	33,0	0,00%
C03	0,50	**1**	0,6	
	0,25	**4**	2,0	-99%

As a rich source of saponins, *T. terrestris* is a promising ingredient for many industries and recent patents on dermatological applications support the use of this plant for cosmetics and hygiene.

There are a large number of patents and patent applications that describe technologies and compositions for medical uses that involve the preparation of *T. terrestris* extracts, showing the variety of fields of application for inventions wherein this plant is indicated as a major ingredient (Falciola and Di Sansebastiano, in preparation). They range from a beneficial effect on hormonal equilibrium to hepatoprotection or antiviral activity. A detailed analysis of patent information content is needed but, it is evident that many of them refer to applications in the field of sexual and fertility disorders correction. The physiological effects that justify the efficacy in general health and physiological performances appear strictly related to regulatory effects on hormonal balance [4, 25, 29].

Efficacy of *Tribulus* as an ingredient in dermatological application is also evident, being present in a minor but relevant and increasing number of patent applications. Nonetheless problems arise in the selection of the material to be used. The extracts of different origin may differ substantially [27]. Natural speciation processes normally influence 'variations' in wild-crafted medicinal plants. With the increasing demand for herbal medicines worldwide, there is a concomitant increase in cultivation of medicinal plants. Vegetative and clonal propagation and hybridization among cultivated sub-species/cultivars add to the variability in traits, making delineation of species difficult [48]. At present, most of the species are defined based on the 'typological species concept' on the premise that a group of plants of one 'type' share a number of diagnostic (fixed) traits. Taxonomic status of *T. terrestris* is complex because of its wide geographical distribution leading to highly variable morphology, ploidy and isozyme patterns. Moreover *Tribulus* can form panmictic populations, justifying variability [27, 49]. High levels of genetic polymorphism have been demonstrated in *T. terrestris* populations collected within the Indian sub-continent [50]. Fluctuating content of various saponins has been demonstrated within species, geographic distribution and spatiotemporal variation [47].

R&D activities willing to include this natural product in formulations for hygiene or cosmetic preparations face the preliminary problem represented by the qualitative evaluation of the material.

Tribulus extract contains a mixture of different compounds. Content, especially in terms of detectable saponins, varies with growth conditions and ecotype [20, 28] in addition to extraction methods. At least one commercial product of Bulgarian origin has indicated protodioscin and prototribestin as main components [1, 18], but the analysis of literature suggests that the characterization of the extract content does not take into account the intraspecific variability [50].

In this work, we collected three commercial extracts distributed in Italy and directly compared their biological effect as biocide since biochemical characterization could not be conclusive. Measurement by HPLC separation should be referred to standard molecules which is known to be related to the biological effect required by the product. Difficulties increase considering that steroidal saponins often lack chromophores for sensitive UV detection and accurate quantitation. Moreover the commercially available extracts have approximate quantification standards such as the gravimetric method.

We also included an extract performed from local plant material harvested, identified and directly processed. A preliminary HPLC analysis confirmed the evaluation problems since profiles appeared to be extremely diversified. We have no data to claim contamination from other materials or frauds; on the contrary we believe that differences may be due to plant material chemiotype, extraction method and conservation. Our goal was to select the material with the best biological activity. Once an effective extract was selected we tested its toxicity in comparison with a saponins enriched extract (E) and an aqueous raw-extract from fruits (raw-E). The reduced toxicity of E compared to raw-E showed how saponins do not have a strong toxicity when compared to other lipophilic compounds. The commercial product exhibited a higher cytotoxicity than extract E indicating a possible residual component of lipophilic compounds but such an effect disappeared far below the minimal concentration to produce an anti-Candida effect. The commercial extract B was then a good ingredient to be tested in the specific detergent formulation named DMX. The presence of *Tribulus* extract in DMX formulation led to an improvement in anti-*candida* performance compared to the "placebo" DMXnoT in which no specific biocides were used. The extract reduced the fungus recovery after washing as expected from a detergent aiming to control growth of potentially pathogenic flora.

The performance was superior to that of a DMX containing Triclosan (DMXtcs). Triclosan or TCS is a multi-purpose biocide widely used in personal care products. There are now growing concerns about its dispersal in the aquatic environment [51]. TCS safety for humans is also being questioned in the latest years and the use of such product will certainly be reduced in the next future. New and safer natural products are needed to potentiate products targeted to specific user categories. For example in the diabetic population, because of their poor glycemic control, the fungi are facilitated to colonize vagina and rectum [52] and require a stronger daily control.

Here we prove that natural products such as *Tribulus* fruit extracts, when properly selected from the market, can substitute triclosan and improve the performance in the control of potentially pathogenic skin flora.

CONFLICT OF INTEREST

The authors confirm that this article content has no conflict of interest.

ACKNOWLEDGEMENTS

This work was funded by the Italian program PO PUGLIA FSE 2007-2013 (to support DBM) and by Ekuberg pharma srl. We would like to thank L. Falciola (Promethera Biosciences, Belgium) for providing and reviewing information related to patent publications.

REFERENCES

[1] Evstatieva L, Tchorbanov B. Complex investigations of *Tribulus terrestris L.* for sustainable use by pharmaceutical industry. Biotechnol Biotechnol Equip 2011; 25: 2341-7.

[2] Tutin T. Flora Europaea. In: Tutin VNHTG, Burges DM, Morle DM, Valentine, Walters SM, Webb DA, Eds. Flora Europaea. vol. 2 Cambridge: Cambridge University Press 1968.

[3] Antonio J, Uelmen J, Rodriguez R, Earnest C. The effects of *Tribulus terrestris* on body composition and exercise performance in resistance-trained males. Int J Sport Nutr Exerc Metab 2000; 10: 208-15.

[4] Gauthaman K, Ganesan A. The hormonal effects of *Tribulus terrestris* and its role in the management of male erectile dysfunction - an evaluation using primates, rabbit and rat. Phytomedicine 2008; 15: 44-54.

[5] Huang J, Tan C, Jiang S. Terrestrinins A and B, two new steroid saponins from *Tribulus terrestris*. J Asian Nat Prod Res 2003; 5: 285-90.

[6] Iacono F, Prezioso D, Ruffo A, Di Lauro G, Romis L, Illiano E. Analyzing the efficacy of a new natural compound made of the alga *Ecklonia bicyclis*, *Tribulus terrestris* and BIOVIS (R) in order to improve male sexual function. J Womens Health 2011; 8: 282-7.

[7] Oh H, Park S, Moon H, Jun S, Choi Z, You Y. *Tribulus terrestris* inhibits caries-inducing properties of Streptococcus mutans. J Med Plants Res 2011; 5: 6061-6.

[8] Heidari M, Mehrani M, Pardakhty A. The analgesic effect of *Tribulus terrestris* extract and comparison of gastric ulcerogenicity of the extract with indomethacine in animal experiments. Ann N Y Acad Sci 2007; 1095: 418-27.

[9] Berkman Z, Tanriover G, Acar G, Sati L, Altug T, Demir R. Changes in the brain cortex of rabbits on a cholesterol-rich diet following supplementation with a herbal extract of *Tribulus terrestris*. Histol Histopathol 2009; 24: 683-92.

[10] Tuncer M, Yaymaci B, Satic L, *et al.* Influence of *Tribulus terrestris* extract on lipid profile and endothelial structure in developing atherosclerotic lesions in the aorta of rabbits on a high-cholesterol diet. Acta Histochem 2009; 111: 488-500.

[11] Kamboj P, Aggarwal M, Puri S, Singla SK. Effect of aqueous extract of Tribulus terrestris on oxalate-induced oxidative stress in rats. Indian J Nephrol 2011; 21: 154-9.

[12] Zang J, Zu Z, Jiang Y. Five furostanol saponins from fruits of *Tribulus terrestris* and their cytotoxic activities. Nat Prod Res 2009; 23: 1436-44.

[13] Xu Y, Xu T, Liu Y, *et al* D. Furostanol glycosides from leaves of the chinese plant *Tribulus terrestris*. Chem Nat Compd 2010; 46: 242-5.

[14] Tomova M, Gjulemetova R, Zarkova S, *et al*, Panov B. Method for the isolation of standardized mixtures os steroid saponins. Patent Application BG52085, 1986.

[15] Tomova M, Gjulemetova R, Zarkova S. Means for stimulating sexual activity. Patent Application BG27584, 1979.

[16] Gjulemetowa R, Tomowa M, Simowa M, Pangarowa T, Peewa S. Determination of furostanol saponins in the preparation Tribestan. Pharmazie 1982; 37: 296.

[17] Nalwaya N, Jarald E, Asghar S, Ahmad S. Diuretic activity of a herbal product UNEX. Int J Green Pharm 2009; 3: 224-6.

[18] Kostova I, Dinchev D. Saponins in *Tribulus terrestris* - chemistry and bioactivity. Phytochem Rev 2005; 4: 111-37.

[19] Gauthaman K, Ganesan A, Prasad R. Sexual effects of puncturevine (*Tribulus terrestris*) extract (protodioscin): an evaluation using a rat model. J Altern Complement Med 2003; 9: 257-65.

[20] Ivanova A, Lazarova I, Mechkarova P, Semerdjieva I, Evstatieva L. Intraspecific variability of biologically active compounds of different populations of *Tribulus terrestris* in Thracian floristic region. Biotechnol Biotechnol Equip 2011; 25: 2357-61.

[21] De Combarieu E, Fuzzati N, Lovati M, Mercalli E. Furostanol saponins from *Tribulus terrestris*. Fitoterapia 2003; 74: 583-91.

[22] Conrad J, Dinchev D, Klaiber I, Mika S, Kostova I, Kraus W. A novel furostanol saponin from *Tribulus terrestris* of Bulgarian origin. Fitoterapia 2004; 75: 117-22.

[23] Akram M, Asif H, Akhtar N, *et al.* Tribulus terrestris Linn.: A review article. J Med Plants Res 2011; 5: 3601-5.

[24] Li T, Zhang Z, Zhang L, Huang X, Lin J, Chen G. An improved facile method for extraction and determination of steroidal saponins in *Tribulus terrestris* by focused microwave-assisted extraction coupled with GC-MS. J Sep Sci 2009; 32: 4167-75.

[25] Kozlova O, Perederiaev O, Ramenskaia G. Determination by high performance chromatography, steroid saponins in a biologically active food supplements containing the extract of *Tribulus terrestris*. Vopr Pitan 2011; 80: 67-71.

[26] Dincheva D, Jandab B, Evstatievac L, Oleszekb W, Aslanid M, Kostova I. Distribution of steroidal saponins in *Tribulus terrestris* from different geographical regions. Phytochemistry 2007; 69: 176-86.

[27] Nikolova M, Ivanova A, Lazarova I, Peev D, Valyovska N. Variability of some biologically active compounds of *Tribulus terrestris L.3* Agric Sci Technol 2011; 3: 150-4.

[28] Szakiel A, Paczkowski C, Henry M. Influence of environmental abiotic factors on the content of saponins in plants. Phytochem Rev 2011; 10: 471-91.

[29] Francis G, Kerem Z, Makkar H, Becker K. The biological action of saponins in animal systems: a review. Br J Nutr 2002; 88: 587-605.

[30] Chen H, Xu Y, Jian Y. Application of *Tribulus* spirosteroid saponin compound in preparation of antifungal medicine. Patent Application CN1428349, 2004.

[31] Zhang JD, Xu Z, Cao YB, *et al.* Antifungal activities and action mechanisms of compounds from *Tribulus terrestris L.* J Ethnopharmacol 2006; 103: 76-84.

[32] Alexis B. Natural, Anti-Bacterial, Anti-Inflammation, Anti-Virus, Anti-Herpes Cream. Patent Application WO2001/011971, 2001.

[33] Alexis B. Treatment of vulvovaginitis with spirostanol enriched extract from *Tribulus terrestris*. Patent Application US2005/0112218, 2005.

[34] Alexiev B. Pharmacological composition based on biologically active substances obtained from *Tribulus terrestris*. Patent Application WO2003/070262, 2003a.

[35] Alexiev B. Pharmacological substance from *Tribulus terrestris*. Patent Application WO2003/070261, 2003b.

[36] Li A. Chinese herb medicine for treating pruritus skin diseases. Patent Application TW201014611, 2010.

[37] Zhang Y. Formulas of internal medicine and external medicine for treating leucoderma. Patent Application CN102240337, 2011.

[38] Ke X. Formula of Chinese medicine capable of allowing skin to be white and tender. Patent Application CN102188631, 2010.

[39] Jing H. Pawpaw coix seed facial mask. Patent Application CN102100658, 2009.

[40] Bleve G, Rizzotti L, Dellaglio F, Torriani S. Development of reverse transcription (RT)-PCR and real-time RT-PCR assays for rapid detection and quantification of viable yeasts and molds contaminating yogurts and pasteurized food products. Appl Environ Microbiol 2003; 69: 4116-22.

[41] Koneman EW. Color atlas and textbook of diagnostic microbiology. 2nd ed. Roma A. Delfino, Philadephia: Lippincott: Williams & Wilkins 1995; pp. 550-605.

[42] NCCLS, N. C. f. C. L. S. Performance standards for antimicrobial susceptibility testing; eleventh informational supplement In *M100-S11*, vol. 22 (N. C. f. C. L. Standards). Wayne, Pa: NCCLS 2001.

[43] Tlili I, Hdider C, Lenucci M, Riadh I, Jebari H, Dalessandro G. Bioactive compounds and antioxidant activities of different watermelon (Citrullus lanatus (Thunb.) Mansfeld) cultivars as affected by fruit sampling area. J Food Compost Anal 2011; 24: 307-14.

[44] Podolak I, Galanty A, Sobolewska D. Saponins as cytotoxic agents: a review. Phytochem Rev 2010; 9: 425-74.

[45] Coleman J, Okoli I, Tegos G, *et al.* E. Characterization of plant-derived saponin natural products against *Candida albicans*. ACS Chem Biol 2010; 5: 321-32.

[46] Kim K, Kim YS, Han I, Kim MH, Jung M, Park HK. Quantitative and qualitative analyses of the cell death process in *Candida albicans* treated by antifungal agents. PLoS ONE 2011; 6: e28176.

[47] Govindaraghavana S, Hennellb JR, Sucher NJ. From classical taxonomy to genome and metabolome: Towards comprehensive quality standards for medicinal herb raw materials and extracts. Fitoterapia 2012; 83(6): 979-88.

[48] Dugo G, Di Giacomo A. Citrus : the genus citrus. New York, London: Taylor & Francis 2002.

[49] Varghese M, Yadav S, Thomas J. Taxonomic status of some of the *Tribulus* species in the Indian sub-continent. Saudi J Biol Sci 2006; 13: 7-12.

[50] Srivastava P, Sarwat M, Das S. Analysis of genetic diversity through AFLP, SAMPL, ISSR and RAPD markers in *Tribulus terrestris*, a medicinal herb. Plant Cell Rep 2008; 27: 519-28.

[51] Von der Ohe P, Schmitt-Jansen M, Slobodnik J, Brack W. Triclosan-the forgotten priority substance? Environ Sci Pollut Res Int 2012; 19: 585-91.

[52] Nowakowska D, Kurnatowska A, Stray-Pedersen B, Wilczyński J. Species distribution and influence of glycemic control on fungal infections in pregnant women with diabetes. J Infect 2004; 48: 339-46.

Immune Alterations in IgE and Non IgE-Associated Atopic Dermatitis

Giampaolo Ricci*, Elisabetta Calamelli and Francesca Cipriani

Pediatric Unit, Department of Medical and Surgical Sciences, S. Orsola - Malpighi Hospital, University of Bologna, Bologna, Italy

Abstract: Atopic dermatitis is a complex disease in which a strong interaction between alterations of skin barrier and the adaptive immune system coexists. In the recent years, new findings have underlined the importance of skin proteins, especially filaggrin, which participate to the outmost layers of the skin. To strengthen this physical barrier, many factors are available, such as antimicrobial peptides, chemokines and cytokines produced by keratinocytes. Skin disruption can easily allow the allergen penetration and the local keratinocytes can promote the adaptive immune response toward a Th2 phenotype. On the other side, allergic Th2 cytokines may downregulate the production of skin barrier proteins, facilitating the penetration of allergens. Moreover, data on murine models show the absolute relevance of the systemic immune system to develop clinical skin reaction. Since the clinical aspect of patients with AD does not show different patterns whatever is the prevalent underlying mechanism, in clinical practice it is difficult to translate the different endotypes beside the IgE and non IgE associated forms. The aim of this review is to point out to the most recent knowledge in this field, which makes AD more difficult to frame in a unique clinical entity.

Keywords: Atopic dermatitis, endotype, filaggrin, IgE, immune system, skin barrier, Th2.

INTRODUCTION

In 1970, few years after the discovery of IgE (1966), Johansson *et al.* published a paper where, describing the spectrum of diseases with high IgE levels, indicated among these atopic eczema and classified it into two subgroups: atopicum eczema (frequently with high IgE) and non-atopicum eczema (a skin disease with the same features - skin lesions and their distribution pattern- but without evidence of IgE sensitization to aero- or food allergens) [1]. This was the first observation in which a difference in atopic eczema was underlined after the discovery of IgE. Indeed, in 1933, Wise and Sulzberger had already proposed the definition of "atopic dermatitis" (AD) to emphasize its close association with other atopic diseases, especially allergic rhino-conjunctivitis and asthma [2]. The possible link with the immune system and allergic diseases stimulated numerous studies to investigate the underlying pathogenic mechanisms.

THE FIRST IMMUNOLOGICAL STUDIES

In the course of the years, the immunological studies on AD followed the progressive update knowledge: among the earlier ones is paradigmatic the work published in 1975 by the group guided by Rebecca Buckley, that described an alteration of cell-mediated immunity in inverse relationship with the level of total IgE, detected analyzing peripheral white cells of subjects with atopic eczema [3]. Thus far, in these initial studies lymphocytes were differentiated into two main sub-groups through the formation of rosettes E. However, these researches strongly reflected on the clinical level: in 1978 the Lancet published a double-blind trial conducted by the Institute of Child Health in London [4]. In this study, authors highlighted the advantages of an exclusion diet in children suffering from AD with more severe clinical features; these data have been later confirmed by further observations. These studies lead to profound changes in clinical practice: from this time the elimination diet had a stronger impact on the therapeutic strategies of paediatricians.

In order to better define the disease, clinician tried to separate the two distinct forms of AD: one characterized by the presence of high IgE and associated allergic manifestations (also named "extrinsic AD") and the other one with normal IgE without allergic symptoms (or "intrinsic AD"), with a high prevalence of the former type but different percentage in relation to age and severity of the disease (Table **1**) [5-16].

In the meantime, the immunological network incredibly complicated: with the advent of monoclonal antibodies an important step in the knowledge of the immune system had been made. It was possible to distinguish different subtypes of lymphocytes with different functions; this allowed much more accurate results to be obtained, and moved the target organ from the blood to the skin.

In 1981 the first data on T cell subsets using monoclonal antibodies in AD patients appeared: Leung *et al.* reported data about *in vitro* cellular reactivity from 22 patients with AD by using monoclonal antibodies to recognize different peripheral lymphocytes [17]. Patients with AD showed a lower rate of T3+ cells (now named CD3+) and T8+ cells (now named CD8+) but not of T4+ (now named CD4+)

*Address correspondence to this author at the Pediatric Unit, Department of Medical and Surgical Sciences, S. Orsola- Malpighi Hospital - University of Bologna, Via Massarenti, 9, 40138 Bologna, Italy;
E-mail : giampaolo.ricci@unibo.it

Table 1. Prevalence of non IgE-associated type atopic dermatitis (AD) in different studies.

Reference	No. of Patients	Pts with Non IgE-Associated AD, n (%)	Age (Years)
Wüthrich *et al.* 1990 [5]	37	9 (24%)	14-60
Hochreutener 1991 [6]	40	15 (30%)	1-7
Walker *et al.* 1993 [7]	25	5 (20%)	17-56
Kägi *et al.* 1994 [8]	33	14 (42%)	19-55
Cabon *et al.* 1996 [9]	59	27 (45%)	0-12
Wüthrich 1999 [10]	93	17 (18%)	37
Schäfer *et al.* 1999 [11]	2201	726 (25%)	5-14
Fabrizi *et al.* 1999 [12]	72	8 (11%)	36
Akdis *et al.* 1999 [13]	1151	117 (10%)	11-51
Laske & Niggemann 2004 [14]	345	93 (27%)	1-24
de Benedictis *et al.* [15]	2184	764 (35%)	1-2
Ricci *et al.* 2014 [16]	184	15 (8%)	8-18

compared to controls. An interesting finding was the higher T4+/T8+ ratio observed in 17 of 22 patients with atopic dermatitis but not in the control subjects.

The main characteristics that suggested an immune pathogenesis in AD were summarized by Donald Leung in 1995 as listed below: increased IgE levels, skin test sensitization to multiple allergens, higher spontaneous histamine release by basophils, lower number of CD8 suppressor/cytotoxic lymphocytes with less effective function, higher expression on mononuclear cells surface of the low-affinity receptor for IgE CD23, increased rate of Th2-like cells secreting IL-4 and IL-5, and decreased rate of numbers of those ones secreting IFN-γ with a significant inverse correlation between *in vitro* IFN-γ production and *in vivo* IgE serum concentrations in AD patients [18]. Furthermore, other studies confirmed the increased number of T cells producing Th2-like cytokines such as IL-4, IL-5 and IL-13 in response to specific allergens, but decreased number of T cells producing IFN-γ in peripheral blood samples of patients with AD [19, 20].

At the same time the immunological studies were also directed to the comprehension of skin function; it was found that the skin cells were able to recognize antigens and to elicit a systemic immune response. Spergel *et al.* [21] described the mechanism of epicutaneous sensitization in a murine model: the induction of allergic sensitization by ovalbumin, a well known allergenic protein, leads to an increase in levels of total and ovalbumin-specific serum IgE and to the development of the atopic dermatitis skin lesions, with a local appreciable infiltrate of CD3+ T cells, eosinophils and neutrophils, and expression of IL-4, IL-5 and INF-γ mRNA. These cutaneous immunohistological features corresponded to the Th2 response (increased IL-4, IL-5, and IL-13 levels) of the acute phase of AD, while chronic lesions showed meanly a prevalence of Th1-cytokines (IL-12 and IFN-γ). The two types of AD did not show dramatic differences in the expression of inflammatory cytokines: IL-5 and IFN-γ were detectable in similar amounts, while IL-4 and IL-13 showed a lower expression in non IgE AD, especially in the lesional skin.

THE ADVENT OF GENETIC STUDIES

The new advance on basic science is promptly reflected on clinical research: with the advent of the new technologies of gene analysis, the skin barrier became the protagonist. In 2002, Coxson and Moffatt [22] understood that a gene or a cluster of genes, coding for proteins involved in the formation of the deep layers of the skin, may play a key role in the pathogenetic mechanisms of atopic dermatitis, including allergic sensitization. But only in 2006 data from a cohort of Irish patients with AD were published in Nature Genetics [23]: authors found alterations in the nucleotidic sequence of the gene encoding for filaggrin. This protein is the most important among those of the so called "epidermal differentiation complex" and is fundamental to preserve the skin barrier integrity. Moreover, filaggrin is able to promote the aggregation of the keratin filaments and its functional defects have described as a risk factor for the onset of AD. Furthermore, in subjects with AD two variants of this gene (R510X and 2282del4) were associated with the occurrence of allergic asthma. Otherwise, these alterations of the gene of filaggrin were observed in not more than 30% of patients, so that was insufficient to explain the pathogenesis of AD. Later, further studies on additional proteins that might contribute to the integrity of the skin barrier had been performed, and other skin proteins (e.g. loricrin, claudine 1) have been associated to the development of AD [24, 25].

THE IMMUNE RESPONSE: WHAT WE KNOW NOW

The contribution of multiple cell types, and the existence of multiple cytokine patterns at different evolution stages give an idea of the high complexity of the mechanisms involved in the immune response in patients with AD.

The Skin Immune Response

A model to study the immune response is to analyze the cellular skin infiltrate after atopy patch test (APT) to house dust mites (HDM). Epicutaneous application of HDM frequently induces eczema in the nonlesional skin of 40-50% of patients with AD. By using immunohistochemistry and molecular analysis, it has been shown that also cytotoxic T cells are implicated in the pathogenesis of these lesions; the analyses from a murin model showed that very few CD8+ T cells infiltrating the skin (about 5% among the CD45+ cells) are sufficient to trigger the HDM-induced AD lesions and their presence is even indispensable, because mice depletion with anti-CD8 monoclonal Abs completely suppressed the inflammatory process [26]. In a recent study, patients with mild to moderate AD were enrolled on the basis of the positivity of APT to HDM; in nine patients the skin biopsy showed that CD8+ T cells are involved in the early phase of the response to allergen exposure. A hypothesis is that the apoptosis of keratinocytes and the epidermal spongiosis, which are both pathological hallmarks of AD, are due to the cytotoxic activity of CD8+ cells [26].

Recently, *in vivo* studies evidenced new relevant details in the skin immune response. In certain allergic tissue reactions potent agents with vasodilator and permeability functions were recognized to be expressed by the inflammatory cells in the lesional skin, such as the calcitonin gene-related peptide (CGRP) and the vascular endothelial growth factor (VEGF). Skin biopsy specimens from atopic dermatitis lesions were collected after various times from the cutaneous allergen exposure and analysed by using single and double immunohistochemistry and *in situ* hybridization: neutrophils and $CD3^+$ T lymphocytes were the main $CGRP^+$ cells detected at the late-phase of the reaction (i.e., 6 hours) [27]. In the setting of allergic inflammation, the wide CGRP production by neutrophils may clarify the characteristic vasodilation that can be observed in the late-phase of the skin reaction: thus it could be at least in part a neutrophil-dependent phenomenon [27]. Otherwise, in patients with chronic AD and in those with psoriasis, the lesional skin biopsy specimens show that dendritic cells (DC) did not increase a preferential T-cell subsets in a disease-specific manner. The capacity of each DC subset to increase Th1, Th2, Th17 and Th22 subsets was the same in the two diseases, but an upregulation of specific chemokine expression such as CCL17, CCL18, and CCL22 was observed only in patients with AD [28]. Moreover, in patients with AD, cutaneous biopsy showed an impaired IFN-γ-mediated signaling pathway and a decreased IFN-γ production both in DCs and in their precursor cells; this condition might contribute to the Th2 bias [29]. On the other side, the increased IFN-γ responses suggest the role of multiple new factors involved in the mechanisms of apoptosis and inflammation in the development of AD [30]. Also other mediators, such as TNF-α and the TNF-like weak inducer of apoptosis (TWEAK), cooperate in the induction of keratinocyte apoptosis and in the lesional production in AD patients [31]. Indeed, during disseminated viral infections such as eczema herpeticum, which is caused by herpes simplex virus, patients suffering from AD showed a mixture of defects both in the skin barrier function and in the innate and adaptive immune responses. In particular, an impaired IFN-γ response was observed in human AD complicated by eczema herpeticum: indeed genetic variants as single nucleotide polymorphisms were found in IFN-γ and IFNGR1 genes and they were significantly related with eczema herpeticum and abnormal IFN-γ production [32].

Also mutations of STAT6 (signal transducer and activator of transcription 6) gene increase make patients with AD more prone towards disseminated viral skin infections [33]. Also the cellular transcription factor Specificity protein (Sp)-1 is involved in diverse cellular functions and represents a critical player during the antiviral responses of skin keratinocytes. Sp1 deficiency in AD patients with viral infection may contribute to increase the risk to develop a disseminated infection of the skin [34].

Recently, the molecular and cellular pathogenetic mechanisms of lesional and nonlesional AD (intrinsic and extrinsic) have been studied in 51 patients with severe AD by using the gene expression assay (real-time PCR). While a prominent infiltrate of T cells and DCs was observed in lesional skin of both types of AD, patients with the intrinsic form (n=9) showed a Th17 immune response more increased than those with extrinsic AD (n=42) [35]. Moreover, higher activation of all inflammatory axes, with a particular involvement of Th17 and Th22 cytokines, including the Th2 products, was detected in patients with intrinsic AD. A positive association between Th17-related molecules and severity of AD, assessed by SCORAD index, was found only in patients with intrinsic AD, whereas patients with extrinsic AD showed a characteristic positive association between the SCORAD index and Th2 cytokine levels (IL-4 and IL-5) and inverse association with proteins involved in the skin differentiation (e.g. loricrin and periplakin) [35].

AGAINST THE BIPHASIC MODEL

The current model to describe the skin inflammation in AD largely descends from experimental studies performed by using APTs with environmental allergens to induce acute lesions and simulate the acute phase of the disease [36, 37].

As previously described, AD pathogenesis is characterized as a biphasic T cell-mediated disease: an early Th2 pattern which predominates in the acute phase and a late Th1 pattern which prevails in the chronic phase [36, 37]. On the basis of an experimental model comparing spontaneous acute AD lesions with chronic lesions from the same patient should permit the develop of a new viewpoint [38]. This new perspective to explore this mechanism was recently performed: biopsy specimens from acute lesion, chronic lesion (>72 hours duration), and nonlesional skin and blood samples from the same patient were collected from 17 patients with moderate-to-severe AD. A significant increases in gene expression levels of Th2 (i.e. IL-4, IL-13, and IL-31) and Th22 (i.e. IL-22) cytokines was associated with the onset of acute lesions; the quantitative gene expression showed also a raise of some other inflammation products as IL-31, IL-22, S100A7, S100A8, and S100A9 with a positive correlation between the SCORAD index and IL-22 mRNA expression [38]. Th1 products induced by interferon, in particular IFN-γ, was also decreased in acute skin lesions. A small increase of Th17-cytokines were observed in acute disease associated with a higher increase in IL17-regulated products (CCL20, peptidase inhibitor 3 elafin, and lipocalin 2). Instead IL-22 mRNA and its associated products (S100A7, S100A8, S100A9, and IL-32) showed a progressive increase and were detected both in acute and in chronic lesions [39]. The chronic phase is also characterized by an intensified release of Th2-related cytokines with the exception of IL-4; indeed a decrease of IL-4 levels has been observed from acute to chronic lesions [38]. The result of skin inflammation is a marked activation of the gene cluster codifying for proteins of the Epidermal differentiation complex and located on chromosome 1q, with an increased expression of S100A7, S100A8 and S100A9 genes. The hyperexpression of these genes induces a rapid increase in the synthesis of S100 proteins by epidermal keratinocytes both in acute and in chronic AD skin lesions. The S100A7, S100A8, and S100A9 proteins play important roles in the inflammation process, such as stimulation of T cells, monocytes, and neutrophils chemotaxis, as well as an action as a proinflammatory mediators in patients with multiple inflammatory diseases [40-43].

Innate Immune System

In the skin innate immunity is expressed through different cells and functional proteins. The first observation demonstrated a higher and massive recruitment of eosinophils into the skin in AD than in healthy individuals with a long-lasting eosinophil survival [44, 45]. Eosinophils' function is mainly as effector cells, but they may also play a role in immunoregulation mechanism, by promoting the cytokine switch from a Th2- pattern in acute lesions to a prevalent Th1-like pattern in the chronic stage of the disease [46, 47]. The number of eosinophils in peripheral blood is elevated in both IgE and non IgE associated forms [8, 48].

Recent observations demonstrated the relevance of the local defences, in which antimicrobial peptides (AMPs) are essential in the clearance of microbial pathogens and in maintaining epidermal barrier efficiency [49]. AMPs include different proteins: in addition to the β-defensin family (HBD1, 2 and 3) and LL-37 (cathelicidin), other proteins show antimicrobial activity such as S100 family proteins and ribonuclease. AMPs are mainly synthesized in the stratum granulosum, incorporated into lamellar bodies, and then discharged into the stratum corneum.

Furthermore, it has been shown a reduction of LL-37, HBD2 and HBD3 levels in the epidermis of lesional skin of patients with AD if compared to those affected by psoriasis [50, 51], but an increase of these levels when comparing with nonatopic healthy controls [51].

The deficiency of cathelicidin confers to patients with AD a higher susceptibility towards viral infections. Although evidences from murine model of cathelicidin-deficient mice showed an increased viral replication in the site of inoculation, they did not develop disseminated skin viral infection [52]. This observation suggests that the mechanism underlying cathelicidin deficiency is insufficient alone to explain the etiopathology of disseminated viral infections and other immunological alterations should be involved in patients with eczema herpeticum. The action of cathelicidin seems to be different but complementary to the mechanism of action of IFN: indeed while cathelicidin acts extracellularly by damaging the viral envelope, IFN inhibits the intracellular viral transcription and translation [53]. Therefore in patients with AD both intracellular and extracellular defects in the antiviral response of the host are involved in increasing the susceptibility to viral infections.

Keratinocytes can modulate the release of inflammatory mediators (e.g., cytokines, chemokines, and AMPs) through the expression of specific receptors for the effectors of the innate immune response overall defined pattern recognition receptors (PRRs). The relation between AD and the innate immune receptors system has been clearly reviewed by Kuo *et al.*, who remarked their synergic action in the production of pro-Th2 cytokines, as the Thymic Stromal Lymphopoietin (TSLP), IL-25 and IL-33, which drive the immune response towards a Th2 pattern [54].

TSLP is preferentially produced by epithelial cells such as keratinocytes and mucosal cells of the airway; the TSLP expression level is increased in the epidermal layers of AD patients if compared with healthy subjects and it shows a correlation with SCORAD index, in particular with the dry skin score [55].

In 10 adult patients with mild to moderate AD, it was observed that the epicutaneous application of HDM using the APTs promotes the induction of TSLP and of CCL17/ Thymus and activation-regulated chemokine (TARC), as a potential indicators of TSLP bioactivity [56, 57].

ADAPTIVE IMMUNE SYSTEM

After the review article by Leung *et al.* issued in 1995 [18], an intriguing paper by Akdis *et al.* was published in 1999 [13]. The authors investigated the immunologic mechanisms among 1151 chronic AD patients (10% of them with non- IgE associated AD) and they found that skin T cells were always implicated in both the subtypes of AD, responding to staphylococcal enterotoxin B, superantigens and cytokines (IL-2, IL-5, IL-13 and INFγ). Interestingly, skin T cells from non-IgE associated form expressed lower IL-13 and IL-5, while IL-4 was not found in any of the two types. Moreover, authors found a relevant expression of CD23 in the activated B cells of patients with IgE associated AD, while the non-IgE associated form was mainly characterized by the absence IL-13-induced-B cells and subsequent IgE secretion.

Recently, new lymphocytes' phenotypes and cytokines have been identified. Th22 cells, originally identified as circulating T-cell clones with skin-homing properties, express receptors for chemokines (CLA, CCR4, CCR6 and CCR10.7) and do not coproduce IL-17, IL-4, or IFN γ. In thirteen patients with severe chronic AD a raised rate of T cells characterized by skin-homing capability and expressing both IL-13 and IL-22 was found. Indeed, this peculiar subtype of T-cells named "IL-13/IL-22-coproducing T cells" might act a potential key role in the pathogenesis of the disease [58].

Furthermore, not only Th2 cells have been identified as producers of IL-31, since also DCs, monocytes and mast cells are implicated in IL-31 synthesis: these cells have been isolated in the skin of subjects affected by AD and the expression of IL-31 was found to be raised also in the sera of these patients with a strong correlation with the grade of severity of the disease [59]. In addition, IL-31 plays a relevant role also in the process of skin differentiation: in a human 3-dimensional skin model filaggrin was observed to be downstream regulated by IL-31 [59].

Also the role of IL-10 is crucial in modulating the adaptive immune system: IL-10 owns suppressive properties both on DCs' maturation and subsequent cytokines expression, and on Th1 cell differentiation. Simultaneously, it contains properties of effector T-cells and enhances the function of Tregs, suggesting that the interaction between the different cell subsets (DCs, Tregs and effector T cells) is crucial in down-regulating an unbalanced activation of the immune system [60]. Studies on IL-10-deficient (IL-$10^{-/-}$) mice have shown that DC-specific IL-$10R^{-/-}$ rodents have an intensified hypersensitivity reactions towards contact haptens, arguing that the pathway of IL-10 signalling is crucial in limiting the contact hypersensitivity reaction, while it is not essential in T-cell priming [61]. In the end, IL-10, suppressing the expression of proinflammatory cytokines from monocytes and macrophages, plays also a critical role in modulating the responses of both the adaptive and innate immune systems [60, 61].

Also the interactions between the endocrine and the immune systems play an influent role in AD [62]: levels of corticotropin-releasing hormone (CRH) receptor expressed by T cells were significantly lower in subjects with AD compared to controls. In contrast, in the healthy population, CRH induces the upregulation of IL-4 by Th2 cells and the inhibition of Th1 cells-induced IFN-γ secretion. In subjects with AD, T cells were not shown to secrete IL-4 and IFN-γ after CRH treatment, while CRH significantly inhibits the synthesis of IL-10 from Tregs, giving an explanation to the stress-induced recurrences of AD skin lesions [62].

The relation between immune system and the development of AD skin lesions has been distinctly observed in a murine model showing the importance of the adaptive immunity in the spontaneous appearance of skin lesions. Filaggrin-deficient flaky tail (ft) mice (*Flgft/ft*) show spontaneous skin inflammation that imitates human AD. The breeding of *Flgft/ft* with Balb/c Rag2-deficient (*Rag2−/−*) generated mice with a lack of function of filaggrin as well as of T and B lymphocytes (*Rag2−/−/Flgft/ft*) [63]: these *Rag2−/−/Flgft/ft* mice didn't develop skin lesions during the observation period of 32 weeks, confirming that T cells and the adaptive immune system give an essential contribution to the development of skin inflammation [63].

A link between cytokines and AD has been shown by recent results from genome-wide association studies [64]. Data were obtained from a public repository about independent populations from two birth cohorts from the United Kingdom (ALSPAC, 12 set 7) and Germany (Multicenter Allergy Study [MAS]): a significant association was detected for 318 genetic markers related to the expression of pro-inflammatory genes, identifying novel genetic risk factors for AD. A mutation in the amino acidic sequence of the IL-6 receptor (IL-6R Asp358Ala; rs2228145) resulting in a functional change of the protein, has been significantly associated with AD, in particular with the persistent forms [64].

THE INTERACTIONS AMONG SKIN IMMUNE RESPONSE AND THE INNATE AND ADAPTIVE IMMUNE SYSTEM

The interplay among skin barrier and the innate and adaptive immune system in AD has been clearly summarized in recent review articles [65, 66]. When the barrier function is compromised, haptens and protein antigens easily penetrate in the skin, promoting the switch toward a Th2-cytokine pattern. Th2 (IL-4, IL-13, and IL-31) and Th22 (IL-22) cytokines act as suppressors of the major final differentiation of skin proteins in keratinocytes (i.e., filaggrin and loricrin), enhancing thê barrier disruption [35, 38, 63]. Moreover, IL-4 and IL-13 have inhibitors capacity on the production of AMPs, directly inhibiting the expression of HBD-2 and HBD-3 and, indirectly, of hBD-3 and LL-37 (*via* inhibition of STAT6 activation) and subsequently suppression of TNF-α/NF-κB and IFN-γ production. On the other hand, IL-17 and IL-22 cytokines, derived from the recently identified T-cell subsets, have many effects on epidermal keratinocytes, enhancing the production of proinflammatory mediators such as S100A7, S100A8, and S100A9 proteins. In addition, keratinocytes by themselves release cytokines, chemokines and AMPs, which enhance the production of pro-Th2 cytokines, including TSLP, IL-25, and IL-33, and drive the immune response to surface antigens toward a Th2 profile. Finally TSLP stimulate DCs and induces the expression of cell-surface activation markers to promote Th2-skewed inflammatory responses (Table **2**).

Table 2. Major interactions between skin barrier/innate immunity and adaptive immunity in AD patients.

Main Links Between Innate and Adaptive Immunity in AD
1. **Eosinophils** act as immunoregulatory cells, playing a role in the switch from a Th2-cytokine pattern in acute lesions of AD to a more Th1-like pattern in the chronic stage
2. **TSLP** (secreted by keratinocytes) stimulate DCs and induces the expression of cell-surface activation markers to promote Th2-skewed inflammatory responses
3. **Keratinocytes** release cytokines, chemokines and AMPs, which acts producing pro-Th2 cytokines, including TSLP, IL-25, and IL-33, and drive the immune response to surface antigens toward a Th2 profile.

Main Links Between Adaptive Immunity and Skin Barrier/Innate Immunity in AD
1. **IL-4**, **IL-13** cytokines have inhibitors capacity on epidermal differentiation and production of antimicrobial peptides; they could inhibit the expression of **hBD-2** and **hBD-3** and might indirectly inhibit **hBD-3** and **LL-37** *via* inhibition of **STAT6** activation and subsequently inhibit **TNF-α/NF-κB and IFN-γ production**
2. **IL-17** and **IL-22** cytokines derived from the recently identified T-cell subsets have many effects on **epidermal keratinocytes**, **S100A7**, **S100A8**, and **S100A9 mRNAs** (human keratinocytes).
3. **T$_H$2 (IL-4**, **IL-13**, and **IL-31**) and **T$_H$22** (**IL-22**) cytokines were shown to suppress the major final differentiation proteins (i.e., filaggrin and loricrin)

DCs: dendritic cells; TSLP: thymic stromal lymphopoietin.

FROM THE OLD NOMENCLATURE TO THE "UNIFYING HYPOTHESIS"

In the last years the nomenclature and classification of AD has been revised: initially AD was classified in two subtypes named "extrinsic" (associated with atopic sensitization) and "intrinsic". The intrinsic type was not associated with specific IgE sensitization and with any of the clinical manifestation of other atopic diseases and was characterized by normal levels of total serum IgE. Later, the nomenclature changed and the current classification called the extrinsic form as "IgE-associated" and the intrinsic one as "non-IgE-associated AD" [67, 68]. However, a recently proposed model unified these two subtypes, considering them as different stages of the same pathogenetic process: indeed, while in the early infancy the non-IgE associated form is predominant, at a later stage the allergic sensitization occurs in most of the patients determining the switch to the IgE-associated phase [69-71].

CONCLUSION

AD is a complex disease in which many actors contribute to develop the clinical phenotypes. Nevertheless, many of these are not directly bound to the pathogenetic mechanism implicated: the two main actors are the primitive skin barrier defects (in particular the alterations of the filaggrin gene) and the immune system Th2-directed (i.e. cells, cytokines and chemokines allergic-oriented). The primitive barrier defect facilitates the passage of allergens and antigens; this contact actives innate immunity to develop a Th2 oriented response. On the other hand, allergic Th2 cytokines may downregulate the production of barrier proteins facilitating the income of allergens. These two main alterations may interact with different proportion each other (Fig. **1**) determining many potential distinct endotypes, even if the phenotypic appearance of the skin shows similar characteristics in both pathways.

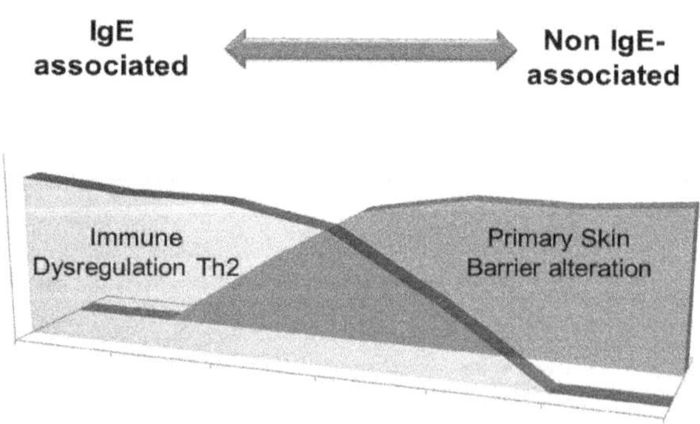

Fig. (1). Schematic representation of the two main alterations implicated in the development of the IgE and non IgE associated forms of atopic dermatitis. Both the primitive skin barrier defects and the immune dysregulation of Th2 system may interact the one with the other in different proportions, determining many potential distinct endotypes. On the one hand, the primitive barrier defect facilitates the passage of allergens and antigens and stimulate the innate immunity to develop a Th2-oriented response. On the other hand, allergic Th2 cytokines down-regulate the production of barrier proteins and facilitate the income of allergens.

It is difficult to translate in clinical practice such complex pathogenesis: the majority of patients (about 80%) have an "IgE-associated AD", as recently suggested to be defined by Thomas Bieber [71]. Some patients, with the "non-IgE associated" form, seem to show an immune alteration profile only at the skin level, where together with the increase of IL5 and IL13, a wider production of IL17 appears to be stimulated, supporting the hypothesis of a link with an autoimmune course. Since skin disruption can easily allow allergen penetration and the local keratinocytes can promote an allergic immune response, the clinical intervention should be addressed to the strict control of the skin inflammation by the application of emollients with antinflammatory and proactive properties in order to interrupt this mechanism. On the other hand, a wider effort should be addressed to evaluate which is the allergic sensitization pattern of the patient, in particular during the paediatric age, since at this stage preventive strategies are still possible and effective. Meanwhile, how much the sensitization directly influences the course of AD should be determined by the physician on the basis of the clinical severity of the diseases and on the results of the allergic response.

ABBREVIATIONS

AD	=	Atopic dermatitis
AMPs	=	Antimicrobial peptides
APT	=	Atopy patch test
CGRP	=	Calcitonin gene-related peptide
CRH	=	Corticotropin-releasing hormone
DC	=	Dendritic cell
HBD	=	β-defensin
HDM	=	House dust mites
PRRs	=	Pattern recognition receptors
Sp-1	=	Specificity protein-1
STAT6	=	Signal transducer and activator of transcription 6 gene
TSLP	=	Thymic stromal lymphopoietin
TWEAK	=	TNF-like weak inducer of apoptosis
VEGF	=	Vascular endothelial growth factor

CONFLICT OF INTEREST

The authors confirm that they have no conflict of interest.

ACKNOWLEDGEMENTS

Declared none.

REFERENCES

[1] Johansson SG, Bennich H, Berg T, Högman C. Some factors influencing the serum IgE levels in atopic diseases. Clin Exp Immunol 1970; 6: 43-7.

[2] Wise F, Sulzberger MB. Footnote on the problem of eczema. Neurodermatitis and lichenification. In: Wise F, Sulzberger MB, Eds. The 1933 year book of dermatology and syphilology: Chicago, Year Book Publishers 1933; 38-9.

[3] McGeady SJ, Buckley RH. Depression of cell-mediated immunity in atopic eczema. J Allergy Clin Immunol 1975; 56: 393-406.

[4] Atherton DJ, Sewell M, Soothill JF, Wells RS, Chilvers CE. A double-blind controlled crossover trial of an antigen-avoidance diet in atopic eczema. Lancet 1978; 25: 401-3.

[5] Wutrich B, Joller-Jemelka H, Helfenstein U, Grop PJ. Levels of soluble interleukin-2 receptors correlate with the severity of atopic dermatitis. Dermatologica 1990; 181: 92-7.

[6] Hochreutener H. Clinical aspects and allergy-immunologic parameters in 40 children 0-7 years of age with atopic dermatitis [Klinische Aspekte und allergologisch-immunologische parameter bei 40 Kindern von 0-7 Jahren mit atopischer Dermatitis]. Monatsschr Kinderheilkd 1991; 139: 618-25.

[7] Walker C, Kagi MK, Ingold P, *et al.* Atopic dermatitis: correlation of peripheral blood T cell activation, eosinophilia and serum factors with clinical severity. Clin Exp Allergy 1993; 23: 145-53.

[8] Kagi MK, Wutrich B, Montano E, *et al.* Differential cytokine profiles in peripheral blood lymphocyte supernatants and skin biopsies from patients with different forms of atopic dermatitis, psoriasis and normal individuals. Int Arch Allergy Immunol 1994; 103: 332-40.

[9] Cabon N, Ducombs G, Mortureux P, Perromat M, Taieb A. Contact allergy to aeroallergens in children with atopic dermatitis: comparison with allergic contact dermatitis. Contact Dermatitis 1996; 35: 27-32.

[10] Wutrich B. Clinical aspects, epidemiology and prognosis of atopic dermatitis. Ann Allergy Asthma Immunol 1999; 83: 464-70.

[11] Schafert T, Heinrich J, Wjst M, *et al.* Association between severity of atopic eczema and degree of sensitization to aeroallergens in schoolchildren. J Allergy Clin Immunol 1999; 104: 1280-4.

[12] Fabrizi G, Romano A, Vultaggio P, *et al.* Heterogeneity of atopic dermatitis defined by the immune response to inhalant and food allergens. Eur J Dermatol 1999; 9:380-4.

[13] Akdis CA, Akdis M, Simon D, *et al.* T cells and T cell-derived cytokines as pathogenic factors in the nonallergic form of atopic dermatitis. J Invest Dermatol 1999; 113: 628-34.

[14] Laske N, Niggemann B. Does the severity of atopic dermatitis correlate with serum IgE levels? Pediatr Allergy Immunol 2004; 15: 86-8.

[15] de Benedictis FM, Franceschini F, Hill D, *et al.* The allergic sensitization in infants with atopic eczema from different countries. Allergy 2009; 64: 295-303.

[16] Ricci G, Dondi A, Neri I, Ricci L, Patrizi A, Pession A. Atopic dermatitis phenotypes in childhood. Ital J Pediatr. 2014; 12; 40: 46.

[17] Leung DY, Rhodes AR, Geha RS. Enumeration of T cell subsets in atopic dermatitis using monoclonal antibodies. J Allergy Clin Immunol 1981; 67: 450-5.

[18] Leung DY. Atopic dermatitis: the skin as a window into the pathogenesis of chronic allergic diseases. J Allergy Clin Immunol 1995; 96: 302-18.

[19] Kimura M, Tsuruta S, Yoshida T. Unique profile of IL-4 and IFN gamma production by peripheral blood mononuclear cells in infants with atopic dermatitis. J Allergy Clin Immunol 1998; 102: 238-44.

[20] Kimura M, Tsuruta S, Yoshida T. Correlation of house dust mite-specific lymphocyte proliferation with IL-5 production, eosinophilia, and the severity of symptoms in infants with atopic dermatitis. J Allergy Clin Immunol 1998; 101: 84-9.

[21] Spergel JM, Mizoguchi E, Brewer JP, Martin TR, Bhan AK, Geha RS. Epicutaneous sensitization with protein antigen induces localized allergic dermatitis and hyperresponsiveness to methacholine after single exposure to aerosolized antigen in mice. J Clin Invest 1998; 101: 1614-22.

[22] Cookson WO, Moffatt MF. The genetics of atopic dermatitis. Curr Opin Allergy Clin Immunol 2002; 2: 383-7.

[23] Palmer CN, Irvine AD, Terron-Kwiatkowski A, *et al.* Common loss-of-function variants of the epidermal barrier protein filaggrin are a major predisposing factor for atopic dermatitis. Nat Genet 2006; 38: 441-6.

[24] Sugawara T, Iwamoto N, Akashi M, *et al.* Tight junction dysfunction in the stratum granulosum leads to aberrant stratum corneum barrier function in claudin-1-deficient mice. J Dermatol Sci 2013; 70: 12-8.

[25] Gschwandtner M, Mildner M, Mlitz V, *et al.* Histamine suppresses epidermal keratinocyte differentiation and impairs skin barrier function in a human skin model. Allergy 2013; 68: 37-47.

[26] Hennino A, Jean-Decoster C, Giordano-Labadie F, *et al.* CD8+ T cells are recruited early to allergen exposure sites in atopy patch test reactions in human atopic dermatitis J Allergy Clin Immunol 2011; 127: 1064-7.

[27] Kay B. Calcitonin gene-related peptide- and vascular endothelial growth factor-positive inflammatory cells in late-phase allergic skin reactions in atopic subjects. J Allergy Clin Immunol 2011; 127: 232-7.

[28] Fujita H, Shemer A, Suarez-Farinas M, *et al.* Lesional dendritic cells in patients with chronic atopic dermatitis and psoriasis exhibit parallel ability to activate T-cell subsets. J Allergy Clin Immunol 2011; 128: 574-82.

[29] Gros E, Petzold S, Maintz L, Bieber T, Novak N. Reduced IFN-γ receptor expression and attenuated IFN-γ response by dendritic cells in patients with atopic dermatitis. J Allergy Clin Immunol 2011; 128: 1015-21.

[30] Rebane A, Zimmermann M, Aab A, *et al.* Mechanisms of IFN-γ-induced apoptosis of human skin keratinocytes in patients with atopic dermatitis. J Allergy Clin Immunol 2012; 129: 1297-306.

[31] Zimmermann M, Koreck A, Meyer N, *et al.* TNF-like weak inducer of apoptosis (TWEAK) and TNF-a cooperate in the induction of keratinocyte apoptosis. J Allergy Clin Immunol 2011; 127: 200-7.

[32] Leung DY, Gao PS, Grigoryev DN, *et al.* Human atopic dermatitis complicated by eczema herpeticum is associated with abnormalities in IFN-γ response. J Allergy Clin Immunol 2011; 127: 965-73.

[33] Howell MD, Gao P, Kim BE, *et al.* The signal transducer and activator of transcription 6 gene (STAT6) increases the propensity of patients with atopic dermatitis toward disseminated viral skin infections J Allergy Clin Immunol 2011; 128: 1006-14.

[34] De Benedetto A, Slifka MK, Rafaels NM, *et al.* Specificity protein 1 is pivotal in the skin's antiviral response. J Allergy ClinImmunol 2011; 127: 430-38.

[35] Suárez-Fariñas M, Dhingra N, Gittler J, *et al.* Intrinsic atopic dermatitis shows similar TH2 and higher TH17 immune activation compared with extrinsic atopic dermatitis. J Allergy Clin Immunol 2013; 132:361-70.

[36] Grewe M, Walther S, Gyufko K, Czech W, Schopf E, Krutmann J. Analysis of the cytokine pattern expressed *in situ* in inhalant allergen patch test reactions of atopic dermatitis patients. J Invest Dermatol 1995; 105: 407-10.

[37] Thepen T, Langeveld-Wildschut EG, Bihari IC, *et al.* Biphasic response against aeroallergen in atopic dermatitis showing a switch from an initial TH2 response to a TH1 response *in situ*: an immunocytochemical study. J Allergy Clin Immunol 1996; 97: 828-37.

[38] Gittler JK, Shemer A, Suarez-Fari~nas M, *et al.* Progressive activation of TH2/TH22 cytokines and selective epidermal proteins characterizes acute and chronic atopic dermatitis. J Allergy Clin Immunol 2012; 130: 1344-54.

[39] Eyerich S, Eyerich K, Pennino D, *et al.* Th22 cells represent a distinct human T cell subset involved in epidermal immunity and remodeling. J Clin Invest 2009; 119: 3573-85.

[40] Boniface K, Bernard FX, Garcia M, Gurney AL, Lecron JC, Morel F. IL-22 inhibits epidermal differentiation and induces proinflammatory gene expression and migration of human keratinocytes. J Immunol 2005; 174: 3695-702.

[41] Roth J, Vogl T, Sorg C, Sunderkotter C. Phagocyte-specific S100 proteins: a novel group of proinflammatory molecules. Trends Immunol 2003; 24: 155-8.

[42] Goyette J, Geczy CL. Inflammation-associated S100 proteins: new mechanisms that regulate function. Amino Acids 2011; 41: 821-42.

[43] Eckert RL, Broome AM, Ruse M, Robinson N, Ryan D, Lee K. S100 proteins in the epidermis. J Invest Dermatol 2004; 123: 23-33.

[44] Bruijnzeel P, Storz E, Van Der Donk E, Bruijnzeel-Koomen C. Skin eosinophilia in patients with allergic asthma, patients with nonallergic asthma, and healthy controls. II. 20-Hydroxy-leukotriene B_4 is a potent *in vivo* and *in vitro* eosinophil chemotactic factor in nonallergic asthma. J Allergy Clin Immunol 1993; 91: 634-42.

[45] Wedi B, Raap U, Lewrick H, Kapp A. Delayed eosinophil programmed cell death *in vitro*: a common feature of inhalant allergy and extrinsic and intrinsic atopic dermatitis. J Allergy Clin Immunol 1997; 100: 536-43.

[46] Gleich GJ. Mechanisms of eosinophil-associated inflammation. J Allergy ClinImmunol 2000; 105: 651-63.

[47] Sampson AP. The role of eosinophils and neutrophils in inflammation. Clin Exp Allergy 2000; 30(s1): 22-7.

[48] Kapp A, Werfel T. Allergic inflammation: skin. Allergy 1999; 55: 23-4.

[49] Schittek B. The antimicrobial skin barrier in patients with atopic dermatitis. Curr Probl Dermatol 2011; 41: 54-67.

[50] Nomura I, Goleva E, Howell MD, *et al.* Cytokine milieu of atopic dermatitis, as compared to psoriasis, skin prevents induction of innate immune response genes. J Immunol 2003; 171: 3262-9.

[51] Ong PY, Ohtake T, Brandt C, *et al.* Endogenous antimicrobial peptides and skin infections in atopic dermatitis. N Engl J Med 2002; 347: 1151-60.

[52] Howell MD, Jones JF, Kisich KO, Streib JE, Gallo RL, Leung DY. Selective killing of vaccinia virus by LL-37: implications for eczema vaccinatum. J Immunol 2004; 172: 1763-7.

[53] Leung DY, Gao PS, Grigoryev DN, *et al.* Human atopic dermatitis complicated by eczema herpeticum is associated with abnormalities in IFN-g response. J Allergy Clin Immunol 2011; 127: 965-73.

[54] Kuo IH, Yoshida T, De Benedetto A, Beck LA. The cutaneous innate immune response in patients with atopic dermatitis. J Allergy Clin Immunol 2013; 131: 266-78.

[55] Sano Y, Masuda K, Tamagawa-Mineoka R, *et al.* Thymic stromal lymphopoietin expression is increased in the horny layer of patients with atopic dermatitis. Clin Exp Immunol 2012; 171: 330-7.

[56] Landheer J, Giovannone B, Mattson JD, *et al.* Epicutaneous application of house dust mite induces thymic stromal lymphopoietin in nonlesional skin of patients with atopic dermatitis. J Allergy Clin Immunol 2013; 132: 1252-4.

[57] Morita E, Takahashi H, Niihara H *et al.* Stratum corneum TARC level is a new indicator of lesional skin inflammation in atopic dermatitis. Allergy 2010; 65: 1166-72.

[58] Teraki Y, Sakurai, Izaki AS. IL-13/IL-22-coproducing T cells, a novel subset, are increased in atopic dermatitis J Allergy Clin Immunol 2013; 132: 971-4.

[59] Cornelissen C, Marquardt Y, Czaja K, J. *et al.* IL-31 regulates differentiation and filaggrin expression in human organotypic skin models. J Allergy Clin Immunol 2012; 129: 426-33.

[60] Sabat R, Grütz G, Warszawska K *et al.* Biology of interleukin-10. Cytokine Growth Factor Rev 2010; 21: 331-44.

[61] Boyman O, Werfel T, Cezmi A. Akdis. The suppressive role of IL-10 in contact and atopic dermatitis. J Allergy Clin Immunol 2012; 129: 160-1.

[62] Oh SH, Park CO, Wu WH, *et al.* Corticotropin releasing hormone downregulates IL10 production by adaptive forkhead box protein 3 negative regulatory T cells in patients with atopic dermatitis. J Allergy Clin Immunol. 2012; 129: 151-9.

[63] Leisten S, Oyoshi MK, Galand C, Hornick JL, Gurish MF, Geha RS. Development of skin lesions in filaggrin-deficient mice is dependent on adaptive immunity. J Allergy Clin Immunol 2013; 131: 1247-50.

[64] Esparza-Gordillo J, Schaarschmidt H, Liang L, *et al.* A functional IL-6 receptor (IL6R) variant is a risk factor for persistent atopic dermatitis. J Allergy Clin Immunol 2013; 132: 371-7.

[65] Kabashima K. New concept of the pathogenesis of atopic dermatitis: Interplay among barrier, allergy, and pruritus as a trinity. J Dermatol Sci 2013; 70: 3-11.

[66] Levin J, Fallon Friedlander S, Del Rosso JQ. Atopic dermatitis and the stratum corneum: part 3: the immune system. Allergy 2001; 56: 841-9.

[67] Schmid-Grendelmeier P, Simon D, Simon HU, Akdis CA, Wüthrich B. Epidemiology, clinical features, and immunology of the "intrinsic" (non-IgE-mediated) type of atopic dermatitis (constitutional dermatitis). in atopic dermatitis. J Clin Aesthet Dermatol 2013; 6: 37-44.

[68] Johansson SG, Bieber T, Dahl R, *et al.* Revised nomenclature for allergy for global use: report of the Nomenclature Review Committee of the World Allergy Organization, October 2003. J Allergy Clin Immunol 2004; 113: 832-6.

[69] Bieber T. Atopic dermatitis. N Engl J Med 2008; 358 :1483-94.

[70] Dondi A, Ricci L, Neri I, Ricci G, Patrizi A. The switch from non-IgE-associated to IgE-associated atopic dermatitis occurs early in life. Allergy 2013; 68: 259-60.

[71] Bieber T. Atopic dermatitis 2.0: from the clinical phenotype to the molecular taxonomy and stratified medicine. Allergy 2012; 67: 1475-82.

Permissions

All chapters in this book were first published in TODJ, by Bentham Open; hereby published with permission under the Creative Commons Attribution License or equivalent. Every chapter published in this book has been scrutinized by our experts. Their significance has been extensively debated. The topics covered herein carry significant findings which will fuel the growth of the discipline. They may even be implemented as practical applications or may be referred to as a beginning point for another development.

The contributors of this book come from diverse backgrounds, making this book a truly international effort. This book will bring forth new frontiers with its revolutionizing research information and detailed analysis of the nascent developments around the world.

We would like to thank all the contributing authors for lending their expertise to make the book truly unique. They have played a crucial role in the development of this book. Without their invaluable contributions this book wouldn't have been possible. They have made vital efforts to compile up to date information on the varied aspects of this subject to make this book a valuable addition to the collection of many professionals and students.

This book was conceptualized with the vision of imparting up-to-date information and advanced data in this field. To ensure the same, a matchless editorial board was set up. Every individual on the board went through rigorous rounds of assessment to prove their worth. After which they invested a large part of their time researching and compiling the most relevant data for our readers.

The editorial board has been involved in producing this book since its inception. They have spent rigorous hours researching and exploring the diverse topics which have resulted in the successful publishing of this book. They have passed on their knowledge of decades through this book. To expedite this challenging task, the publisher supported the team at every step. A small team of assistant editors was also appointed to further simplify the editing procedure and attain best results for the readers.

Apart from the editorial board, the designing team has also invested a significant amount of their time in understanding the subject and creating the most relevant covers. They scrutinized every image to scout for the most suitable representation of the subject and create an appropriate cover for the book.

The publishing team has been an ardent support to the editorial, designing and production team. Their endless efforts to recruit the best for this project, has resulted in the accomplishment of this book. They are a veteran in the field of academics and their pool of knowledge is as vast as their experience in printing. Their expertise and guidance has proved useful at every step. Their uncompromising quality standards have made this book an exceptional effort. Their encouragement from time to time has been an inspiration for everyone.

The publisher and the editorial board hope that this book will prove to be a valuable piece of knowledge for researchers, students, practitioners and scholars across the globe.

List of Contributors

N.G. Ilina and M. Yu. Denisov
Novosibirsk State University (NSU) 630090 Pirogova Street 2, Novosibirsk, Russia

Yu M. Krinitsyna
Novosibirsk State University (NSU) 630090 Pirogova Street 2, Novosibirsk, Russia
Institute of Regional Pathology and Pathomorphology 630117 Ak.Timakova street 2, Novosibirsk, Russia

I. G. Sergeeva
Novosibirsk State University (NSU) 630090 Pirogova Street 2, Novosibirsk, Russia
Institute International Tomography Center of the Russian Academy of Sciences, laboratory of translational brain research 630090 Institutskaia Street 3, Novosibirsk, Russia

Hiroshi Amano
Graduate School of Engineering, Akasaki Research Center, Nagoya University, Furo-cho, Chikusa-ku, Nagoya 464-8603, Japan

Kan Torii, Takuya Furuhashi and Akimichi Morita
Department of Geriatric and Environmental Dermatology, Nagoya City University Graduate School of Medical Sciences, Nagoya 467-8601, Japan

Lara El Hayderi, Marie Caucanas and Arjen F. Nikkels
Department of Dermatology, University Hospital of Liège, Liège, Belgium

Nikolay P. Serdev
Medical Centre "Aesthetic Surgery, Aesthetic Medicine", Sofia, Bulgaria

Hideki Nagase, Yoshinori Nakachi, Keiji Ishida and Mamoru Kiniwa
Tokushima Research Center, Taiho Pharmaceutical Co., Ltd., Tokushima, Japan

Satoshi Takeuchi
Department of Dermatology, Graduate School of Medical Sciences, Kyushu University, Fukuoka, Japan

Ichiro Katayama
Department of Dermatology, Osaka University Graduate School of Medicine, Osaka, Japan

Yoshinari Matsumoto
Department of Dermatology, Aichi Medical University School of Medicine, Aichi, Japan

Fukumi Furukawa
Department of Dermatology, Wakayama Medical University, Wakayama, Japan

Shin Morizane
Department of Dermatology, Okayama University Graduate School of Medicine, Dentistry and Pharmaceutical Sciences, Okayama, Japan

Sakae Kaneko
Department of Dermatology, Shimane University Faculty of Medicine, Shimane, Japan

Yoshiki Tokura
Department of Dermatology, University of Occupational and Environmental Health, Kitakyushu, Japan (Department of Dermatology, Hamamatsu University School of Medicine, Hamamatsu, Japan)

Motoi Takenaka
Department of Dermatology and Allergology, Nagasaki University Hospital, Nagasaki, Japan

Yutaka Hatano
Department of Dermatology, Faculty of Medicine, Oita University, Oita, Japan

Yoshiki Miyachi
Department of Dermatology, Kyoto University Graduate School of Medicine, Kyoto, Japan

Mahsa Amir, Jeffrey H. Dunn, Melanie R. Bui, Laura Huff and Sofia Mani
University of Colorado School of Medicine, Aurora, CO, USA

Jodi Duke
University of Colorado Skaggs School of Pharmacy and Pharmaceutical Sciences, Aurora, CO, USA

Robert Dellavalle
University of Colorado School of Medicine, Aurora, CO, USA
Dermatology Service, Department of Veterans Affairs Medical Center, Denver, CO, USA

P. Alex McNally
University of Colorado School of Medicine, Department of Surgery, CO, USA

Ashley Hamstra
Loma Linda University Medical Center, Department of Dermatology, CA, USA

Gian-Pietro Di Sansebastiano, Maria De Benedictis, Dario Lofrumento, Anna Montefusco, Vincenzo Zuccarello, Giuseppe Dalessandro and Gabriella Piro
University of Salento, DiSTeBA, Campus Ecotekne, 73100 Lecce (LE), Italy

Davide Carati
EKUBERG Pharma s.r.l, Via Pozzelle n.36 73025 Martano (LE), Italy

Miriana Durante
CNR, Istituto di Scienze delle Produzioni Alimentari (ISPA), Campus Ecotekne, 73100 Lecce (LE), Italy

S. Cao and A. F. Nikkels
Department of Dermatology, University Hospital of Liège, Sart Tilman, Liège, Belgium

Tim Kiesewetter
School of Medicine, University of Cologne, Cologne, Germany

Liana Ariza
Department of Community Health, School of Medicine, Federal University of Ceará, Fortaleza, Brazil

Maria M. Martins
Faculty of Veterinary Medicine, Federal Universidade of Uberlândia, Uberlândia, Brazil

Júlio Mendes
Institute of Biomedical Sciences, Federal Universidade of Uberlândia, Uberlândia, Brazil

Jean E. Limongi
Institute of Biomedical Sciences, Federal Universidade of Uberlândia, Uberlândia, Brazil
Centre of Control of Zoonotic Diseases, Municipal Health Secretariat of Uberlândia, Minas Gerais, Brazil

Juliana Junqueira da Silva
Centre of Control of Zoonotic Diseases, Municipal Health Secretariat of Uberlândia, Minas Gerais, Brazil

Cláudia M. Lins Calheiros
Institute of Biological Sciences and Health, Federal University of Alagoas, Maceió, Brazil

Heiko Becher
Institute of Public Health, University of Heidelberg, Heidelberg, Germany

Jorg Heukelbach
Department of Community Health, School of Medicine, Federal University of Ceará, Fortaleza, Brazil
Anton Breinl Centre for Public Health and Tropical Medicine, School of Public Health, Tropical Medicine and Rehabilitation Sciences, James Cook University, Townsville, Australia

Toshiko Harada
Takarazuka University School of Nursing, Japan

Arianna Giannetti, Giampaolo Ricci, Valentina Piccinno, Federica Bellini, Roberto Rondelli and Andrea Pession
Pediatric Unit, Department of Gynecologic, Obstetric and Pediatric Sciences University of Bologna, Bologna, Italy

Arianna Dondi
Pediatric Unit, Department of Gynecologic, Obstetric and Pediatric Sciences University of Bologna, Bologna, Italy
Dermatology Unit, Department of Specialist, Diagnostic and Experimental Medicine, University of Bologna, Bologna, Italy

Annalisa Patrizi
Dermatology Unit, Department of Specialist, Diagnostic and Experimental Medicine, University of Bologna, Bologna, Italy

Mikiko Uede and Fukumi Furukawa
Department of Dermatology, Wakayama Medical University, Japan

Chikako Kaminaka and Yuki Yamamoto
Department of Dermatology, Wakayama Medical University, Japan
Department of Cosmetic Dermatology and Photomedicine, Wakayama Medical University, Japan

Nozomi Yonei
Department of Dermatology, Public Naga Hospital, Japan

Akihiko Fujisawa, Masatoshi Jinnin and Hironobu Ihn
Department of Dermatology and Plastic Surgery, Faculty of Life Sciences, Kumamoto University, Japan

Kiyofumi Egawa
Department of Dermatology, The Jikei University School of Medicine, Tokyo, Japan
Department of Microbiology, Kitasato University School of Allied Health Science, Sagamihara, Japan

Yumi Honda
Department of Surgical Pathology, Kumamoto University Hospital, Kumamoto, Japan

Masahide Kuroki
Department of Biochemistry, Faculty of Medicine, Fukuoka University, Fukuoka, Japan

N. Boufflette
Departments of Dermatology

J. E. Arrese
Departments of Dermatopathology

P. Leonard
Departments of Infections Diseases, University Hospital of Liège, Liège, Belgium

Annie Crissinger
Department of Pharmacy, Cleveland Clinic Foundation, Cleveland, OH, USA

Nicholas V. Nguyen
Department of Dermatology, University of Colorado, Aurora, CO, USA

Deon V. Canyon, Chauncey Canyon, Sami Milani and Rick Speare
Office of Public Health Studies, University of Hawaii at Manoa, 1960 East-West Rd, Biomed Building #T103, Honolulu, HI 96822, USA

C. Rodríguez-Cerdeira
Department of Dermatology, CHUVI/ University of Vigo, Vigo, Spain

E. Sánchez-Blanco, A. Gutierrez and A. Rodriguez-Rodriguez
University of Vigo, Vigo, Spain

B. Sánchez-Blanco
Department of Emergency, CHUVI, Vigo, Spain

Christine Schopper, Eva Maria Valesky, Roland Kaufmann and Markus Meissner
Department of Dermatology, Venereology und Allergology, Johann Wolfgang Goethe-University, Frankfurt am Main, Germany

Katsuhiro Hitomi, Seiichi Izaki, Yuichi Teraki, Yuko Aso, Megumi Yokoyama, Saori Takamura, Yumiko Inoue and Yoshiki Sato
Department of Dermatology, Saitama Medical Center, Saitama Medical University, Kawagoe, Saitama, Japan

Neena Philips
School of Natural Sciences, University College, Fairleigh Dickinson University, Teaneck, NJ, USA

Mio Nakamura
Wayne State University School of Medicine, Detroit, MI, USA

Amir M. Ghaznavi, Vigen Darian and Aamir Siddiqui
Division of Plastic and Reconstructive Surgery, Department of Surgery, Henry Ford Health System Detroit, MI, USA

Anne Mundstock, Rawad Abdayem, Fabrice Pirot and Marek Haftek
Université Lyon 1, EA4169 "Fundamental, clinical and therapeutic aspects of the skin barrier function"; 8 avenue Rockefeller, 69373 Lyon, France

Anna Bulgheroni, Linda Frisenda, Alessandro Subissi and Federico Mailland
Scientific Department, Polichem S.A., Lugano CH, Switzerland

Ebtisam Elghblawi
Dermatology OPD, STJTL, Tripoli, Libya

Zamir Calamita, Ana Cristina Rizzo Alonso, Lorena Carla Oliveira da Costa and Andrea Bronhara Pelá Calamita
Marília Medical School (FAMEMA), São Paulo, Brazil

L. Raty, V. Failla and A. F. Nikkels
Departments of Dermatology

R. Andrianne, M. Fillet and D. Waltregny
Departments of Urology, CHU du Sart Tilman, University of Liège, Belgium

Satoshi Kamiyama and Isamu Akasaki
Department of Materials Science and Engineering, Faculty of Science and Technology, Meijo University, 1-501 Shiogamaguchi Tempaku-ku, Nagoya 468-8502, Japan

Shunko A. Inada
Department of Materials Science and Engineering, Faculty of Science and Technology, Meijo University, 1-501 Shiogamaguchi Tempaku-ku, Nagoya 468-8502, Japan
Department of Geriatric and Environmental Dermatology, Nagoya City University Graduate School of Medical Sciences, Nagoya 467-8601, Japan

Kimiko Maruyama, Takaharu Ikeda, Katsunori Tanaka and Fukumi Furukawa
Department of Dermatology, Faculty of Medicine, Wakayama Medical University, Japan

V. Failla, N. Nikkels-Tassoudji, M. Sabatiello, V. de Schaetzen and A. F. Nikkels
Department of Dermatology, University Hospital of Liège, Liège, Belgium

Carmen Rodríguez-Cerdeira
Dermatology Department, CHUVI and University of Vigo, Vigo, Spain

José Telmo Pera-Grasa
University of Vigo, Vigo. Spain

A, Molares
FIDI Xeral-Calde, Hospital Lucus Augusti, Lugo, Spain

Rafael Isa-Isa
Institute of Dermatology and Skin Surgery, Santo Domingo, Dominican Republic

Roberto Arenas-Guzmán
Dermatology Department, Hospital Dr, Manuel Gea González, D.F., México

Anne Cécile Zoung-Kanyi Bissek, Earnest N. Tabah, Emmanuel Kouotou, Julius Y. Fonsah, Alfred K. Njamnshi, Paul Koueke and Walinjom F. T. Muna
Department of Internal Medicine and Specialties (Dermatology & Neurology Units), Faculty of Medicine & Biomedical Sciences, University of Yaoundé I, Yaoundé, Cameroon

Guillaume Chaby and Catherine Lok
Centre Hospitalier Universitaire, Amiens Sud, France

Salvador Gonzalez
Dermatology Service, Memorial Sloan-Kettering Cancer Center, New York, USA
Dermatology Service, Ramon y Cajal Hospital, Madrid, Spain

Yolanda Gilaberte
Dermatology Service, Hospital San Jorge, Huesca, Spain

Angeles Juarranz
Biology Department, Sciences School, Universidad Autónoma de Madrid, Madrid, Spain

Giampaolo Ricci, Elisabetta Calamelli and Francesca Cipriani
Pediatric Unit, Department of Medical and Surgical Sciences, S. Orsola - Malpighi Hospital, University of Bologna, Bologna, Italy

Index

www.ingramcontent.com/pod-product-compliance
Lightning Source LLC
Chambersburg PA
CBHW080657200326
41458CB00013B/4895

* 9 7 8 1 6 3 9 2 7 0 6 3 7 *